Pediatric Sleep Medicine

STEPHEN H. SHELDON, DO

Associate Director, Sleep Disorders Center
University of Chicago Hospitals
Clinical Associate, Department of Pediatrics
Wyler Children's Hospital
Chicago, Illinois

JEAN-PAUL SPIRE, MD

Professor of Neurology and Neurosurgery
Director, Neurophysiology Laboratories and Sleep Disorders Center
University of Chicago
Chicago, Illinois

HOWARD B. LEVY, MD

Director, Pediatric Ecology Programs
Pediatric Center of Chicago
Chicago, Illinois

W. B. SAUNDERS COMPANY

Harcourt Brace Jovanovich, Inc.

Philadelphia / London / Toronto / Montreal / Sydney / Tokyo

W. B. SAUNDERS COMPANY
Harcourt Brace Jovanovich Inc.

The Curtis Center
Independence Square West
Philadelphia, Pennsylvania 19106

Library of Congress Cataloging-in-Publication Data

Sheldon, Stephen H.
Pediatric sleep medicine/Stephen H. Sheldon, Jean-Paul Spire, Howard B. Levy.
p. cm.
ISBN 0-7216-3374-9
1. Sleep disorders in children. I. Spire, Jean-Paul. II. Levy, Howard B. III. Title.
[DNLM: 1. Diagnosis, Differential. 2. Sleep Disorders—in infancy & childhood. 3. Sleep Disorders—therapy. WM 188 S544p]
RJ506.S55S54 1992
618.92'8498—dc20
DNLM/DLC
for Library of Congress 91-46869
CIP

Editor: Judith Fletcher

Designer: Joan Sinclair

Production Manager: Frank Polizzano

PEDIATRIC SLEEP MEDICINE ISBN 0-7216-3374-9

Printed in Mexico

Last digit is the print number: 9 8 7 6 5 4 3 2 1

This book is dedicated to our wives:

Jeannie Sheldon
Ikuko Mizuno
and
Urmila Chaudhry-Levy

Contributors

ERIC BELL, MA, RPsgT

Laboratory Director, Sleep Disorders Center, The Methodist Hospitals, Inc.; Psychology Intern, Parter-Starke Services, Merrillville, Indiana

Appendix 1 Introduction to Polysomnography

ALEXANDER Z. GOLBIN, MD, PhD

Assistant Professor, Psychiatry Department, University of Illinois; Chairman, Child Psychiatry and Sleep Disorders Service, Cook County Hospital, Chicago, Illinois

Parasomnias

Preface

Sleep Disorders Medicine has become a unique specialty. It has been distinguished from other fields of specialization by its focus on the human organism during the sleep rather than the waking state. Dr. William Dement eloquently described the need for this differentiation in his welcome address to the 1985 Anniversary Meeting of the Association of Professional Sleep Societies:*

> ***The Sleep Research Society was born 25 years ago when a small group of sleep researchers met at the University of Chicago to discuss sleep state scoring; and for some reason, they kept meeting. . . .***
>
> ***As we drew back the curtain of the night, we began to realize that all was not well in the land of sleep. This fascinating, working, sleeping brain was failing in millions of human beings. For example, we learned that it fails to accomplish its task of restoration, so that the many victims of the narcolepsy syndrome cannot stay awake during the day; it fails to maintain proper breathing during sleep in millions of our citizens; and, it fails to maintain sleep through the night in additional millions. Its functions deteriorate with age, and its delicate and exquisite organization is buffeted by drugs and alcohol, jet lag, and schedule change.***
>
> ***Finally, we learned enough to offer assistance to those millions of disenfranchised human beings with sleep disorders. And to make this help the best possible, the Association of Sleep Disorders Centers was organized. And, that was amazingly just ten short years ago.***

It has become clear that the human organism functions differently when asleep. The extrapolation from many basic physiological principles identified in wakefulness must be cautious, and thus to fully understand human medicine, one must investigate it *awake and also asleep*.

Sleep of children holds special significance: 50% of an infant's life is spent sleeping; newborns, infants, and young children all sleep differently from adults. The ontogenetic development of sleep follows an orderly, reproducible pattern governed by the development of the central nervous system as closely and methodically as all other neurodevelopmental landmarks. Consideration of normal and abnormal human development, therefore, must include an adequate assessment of sleep and sleep-wake cycles and must assume equal importance to all other neurodevelopmental milestones.

While the structure of sleep has been well defined, however, the function of sleep remains obscure, beyond the pedestrian observation that we have to sleep in order to remain awake the next day. Human subjects cannot be totally sleep deprived indefinitely, as they will reveal electroencephalographic (EEG) evidence of sleep while appearing behaviorally awake, or will uncontrollably fall asleep during normal waking hours.

Since sleep constitutes such a large portion of the newborn's and young infant's day, it must hold special significance in development, but the cause or effect has yet to be determined. Both animal and human studies suggest that sleep is an important variable

*Association of Sleep Disorders Centers—Clinical Sleep Society—Sleep Research Society Meeting, Seattle, WA, July 9, 1985.

in acquiring and retaining new knowledge obtained during wakefulness. Does disordered sleep have an effect on learning disabilities, reading disorders, developmental delays, or behavior disorders? Does keeping term or premature infants in a well-lit nursery 24 hours a day for our own convenience disrupt their normal ultradian rhythmicity? Does continual taking of vital signs, drawing blood, and administering medications without paying attention to normal biological rhythms affect outcome? Sleep and chronobiology have rarely, if ever, been controlled for in neonatal outcome studies, despite the fact that the premature infant's normal developmental environment is dark for 24 hours. Sleep-activity cycles can be identified as early as 28 weeks of gestation, and approximately 90% of sleep is active sleep (REM sleep correlate) during this period of life. The chronobiology of the sleep of these very fragile individuals must be investigated.

Reference to disordered sleep is found throughout literature, extending beyond biblical times. Well-known examples include the Charles Dickens character of the fat boy, Joe, from the classic *The Posthumous Papers of the Pickwick Club,* who possessed features of hypersomnolence, obesity, and obstructive sleep apnea. Dickens' description of the symptoms was precise. "Pickwickian syndrome" now describes the clinical constellation of obstructive sleep apnea with obesity, carbon dioxide retention, decreased ventilatory drive to increased PCO_2, and excessive daytime sleepiness. Sleep paralysis is to be found in Edgar Allen Poe's tale of the "Premature Burial" and a character in Herman Melville's *Moby Dick* suffered from narcolepsy. James Thurber wrote of insomnia, Bellini's *La Sonnambula* centered on sleepwalking, and Washington Irving's Rip Van Winkle suffered from alcoholism and hypersomnia.

Sleep research can be traced back to the latter part of the 19th century when spontaneous neuroelectrical discharges in the brains of sleeping animals were described. Classic observations, such as eye movements during sleep and the fact that dreaming occurred during eye movement activity, were suggested in 1868 by Griesinger. Freud described muscle relaxation associated with dreaming in 1895, and MacWilliams observed increases of blood pressure, pulse rate, and changes in respiratory patterns associated with this sleep state.

The first recording of human neuroelectrical activity was performed by Hans Berger in 1929. From 1929 to 1938 he conducted a series of extraordinary observations that confirmed earlier animal studies. He also demonstrated that electrical activity originating in neuronal tissue was modulated by sensory input and that clinical epileptic seizures were associated with abnormal discharges.

Differentiation of sleep into spontaneously occurring, discontinuous states was first described by Loomis, Harvey, and Hobart in 1937. Changes between sleep states were described as originating from "internal stimuli." This discovery provided the groundwork for the current research of neural mechanisms responsible for sleep.

Although suggested more than 75 years earlier, it was not until 1953 that human REM sleep was first described by Aserinsky and Kleitman at the University of Chicago. They described an active EEG pattern during this state, rapid eye movements, increased heart rate, and increased respirations. The majority of subjects (75%) reported dreams involving visual imagery when awakened from this state (compared with 9% describing dreams when awakened from other sleep states). In 1957, Dement and Kleitman reported that REM and non-REM (NREM) sleep cycled throughout the night. They proposed a classification system that differentiated REM from NREM sleep and divided NREM sleep into four distinct stages.

Based on these studies, the need for standardization of a system to score sleep was apparent. In 1960, the Association for the Psychophysiological Study of Sleep (APSS) was formed originally to adopt a standard scoring system. At the inaugural meeting, the opportunity to discuss research diverted these efforts. Because of serious unreliability of scoring certain sleep stages, an *ad hoc* committee of the APSS, co-chaired by Drs. Allen Rechtschaffen and Anthony Kales, was formed under the auspices of the UCLA Brain Information Service. The committee's charge was to standardize terminology and a scoring system to be used universally by sleep researchers. The result was the publication of *A Manual of Standardized Terminology, Techniques, and Scoring System for Sleep Stages of Human Subjects* in 1968. This work remains the standard today. These standards, however, were appropriate for adult subjects, and interest in characteristics of sleep in infants and children required similar standardization. A second *ad hoc* committee co-chaired by Drs. Thomas Anders, Robert Emde, and Arthur Parmelee met in 1969 and 1970, and *A Manual for Standardized Terminology, Techniques, and Criteria for Scoring of States of Sleep and Wakefulness in Newborn Infants* was published in 1971. In 1979, a nosology of sleep disorders was published through a combined effort of the APSS and the Association of Sleep Disorders Centers (ASDC). The American Sleep Disorders Association, in association with the European Sleep Research Society, Japanese Society of Sleep Research, and the Latin American Sleep Society, has recently refined this work and published *The International Classification of Sleep Disorders: Diagnostic and Coding Manual* (1990).

The following is a textbook on sleep disorders in children. It is the opinion of the authors that the fundamental differences of childhood sleep and its disturbances should be discussed separately from those of adolescents and adults. This volume is intended to shed some light into the night for primary care practitioners of children as well as for those sleep disorders professionals who are involved in the evaluation and treatment of children with disordered sleep.

SHS

JPS

HBL

Contents

1

Introduction to Sleep and Its Disorders

FUNCTION OF SLEEP

The first question asked about a biological function is an explanation of its purpose, yet the exact function of sleep remains elusive. Historically, physicians have, seemingly wisely, recommended sleep for the treatment of many ailments. This inexpensive prescription has been based on the assumption that sleep must have a unique restorative purpose. However, no study has documented that sleep cures anything.[1] Circadian rhythms of various biological processes, for example, the immune system, appear to be modulated by sleep; lymphocyte functions are dramatically altered at sleep onset and during sleep.[2] Specific pokeweed mitogen response and natural killer cell activity are altered with sleep in healthy young men. Interleukin-1-like activities are followed by interleukin-2-like activities during sleep, and the activity of interleukin-1 and interleukin-2 is disrupted with sleep deprivation.[3] Narcoleptic patients present disordered diurnal patterns of immune function.[4] However, what clinical effect these changes produce or how they may be therapeutically modified is unknown. The relationship between the immune system and sleep is obviously important and possesses many clinical implications.

Theories of sleep function fall into several major and overlapping categories. An understanding of these hypotheses provides a basis for comprehension of the varied effects disordered sleep may have on health and disease.

Restoration Theory

Sherington suggested in 1946 that sleep was a state required for enhanced tissue growth and repair.[5] This theory holds that certain somatic and cerebral deficits occur as a result of wakefulness and that sleep either allows or induces physiological processes to repair or restore these deficits. This restoration, in turn, allows normal daytime functioning.[6-8] Special focus has been placed on restoration of both somatic function and central nervous system (CNS) function. Non–rapid eye movement (NREM) sleep is thought to function in reparation of body tissue, and REM sleep in restoration of brain tissue. Supporting evidence, however, is empirical and indirect. The theoretical role of NREM sleep in repair of somatic tissue comes from investigations that have shown the following:

1. Slow-wave sleep (SWS) increases following sleep deprivation.[9]
2. The percentage of SWS is increased during developmental years.[10]
3. Total sleep duration increases with body mass.[11]
4. Release of growth hormone occurs at sleep onset, and peak levels occur during SWS in prepubertal children.[12]

5. The release of many endogenous anabolic steroids (prolactin, testosterone, and luteinizing hormone) occurs in a sleep-dependent cycle.[13,14]
6. The nadir of the release of catabolic steroids, such as corticosteroids, occurs during the first hours of sleep, coincident with the largest percentage of SWS.[15]
7. Increased mitosis of lymphocytes and increased rate of bone growth occur during sleep.[16]
8. The SWS percentage of total sleep time gradually increases in response to a graded increase of physical exercise.[17]

Contrary and conflicting observations exist: For example, although peak rates of cell division occur during sleep, this appears not to be due to sleep itself. Increased mitosis is demonstrable after a night without sleep, is positively influenced by oral glucose load, and is negatively influenced by cortisol secretion.[18] Similarly, in adolescents and adults somatomedin levels are highest during waking, not during sleep as they are in prepubertal children.[19]

REM sleep has been thought to function in the restoration of CNS function. This state is characterized by intense CNS activation. REM sleep may have evolved to "reprogram" innate behaviors and to incorporate learned behaviors and knowledge acquired during wakefulness.[20] Synthesis of CNS proteins is increased during REM sleep.[21] REM sleep also appears in significantly higher proportions in the fetus and newborn, gradually decreasing over the first few years of life. Increased protein synthesis during this sleep state may be critical in the development of the CNS.

Evolutionary and Adaptive Theories

Development of many physiological functions follows an orderly progression that mirrors phylogenetic development. It has been suggested that the development of sleep in the human organism follows this same phylogenetic pattern. Evidence for this theory is scant. Animals sleep in many different ways, which are more often influenced by the environment and life-style than by evolution of the species.[22] SWS and REM sleep rebound are characteristically seen after sleep deprivation in dogs, cats, rabbits, and humans.[23] Definitive REM sleep, however, has never been documented in dolphins. Dolphins do not have a pulmonary reflex to hypoxemia and therefore have completely voluntary control of breathing. Presumably sleep would be associated with impaired respiratory neural control. Actually, dolphins appear to exhibit hemispheric sleep; that is, when dolphins appear to sleep, slow-wave electroencephalographic (EEG) patterns are seen over one hemisphere while the other hemisphere shows waking rhythm.[24,99] If the evolutionary theory is true, animals with highly complex CNS function, such as dolphins, should follow this pattern. It stands to reason that if the dolphin slept in the same manner as the dog, cat, and human, survival in its aquatic environment would be impossible. Skeletal muscle atonia during REM sleep (as currently understood) would result in drowning. Therefore the life-style and environment of the dolphin play a much more significant role than phylogeny in the pattern of sleep development in this species.

In some species sleep may function to enhance survival. Animals that graze for food tend to sleep in short bursts, a behavior that may provide time for sufficient food seeking and for vigilance against predators.[25] Carnivorous animals that do not require large amounts of time for foraging and that are relatively safe from predation tend to sleep for long periods.

Sleep may also be an instinctive behavior, a patterned response to stimuli that conserves energy, prevents maladaptive behaviors, and promotes survival.[26] According to the evolutionary theory of sleep, REM sleep cortical activation may perform additional survival functions.[27]

Energy Conservation Theory

Sleep may function to conserve energy. Mammal species exhibit a high correlation between metabolic rate and total sleep time.[28] According to this view, energy reduction is greater during sleep than during periods of quiet wakefulness and sleep provides periods of enforced rest, barring the animal from activity for extended periods. Endothermic animals exhibit SWS. During NREM sleep, endogenous thermoregulation continues, although functioning at levels below wakefulness. Poikilothermic species, on the other hand, do not exhibit clear SWS patterns.

It is doubtful that the energy conservation theory explains the function of sleep in humans. The reduction in metabolism that occurs during sleep in humans is minimal. Although the hypothesis is intriguing, energy conservation theory has been disputed and evidence exists that increase in sleep time does not correlate with increased metabolic rate.[29,30] Only approximately an 8% to 10% reduction in metabolic rate occurs during sleep when compared with relaxed wakefulness. This is insignificant considering an adult human's basal metabolic expenditure.

Learning Theory

A particularly interesting theory centers on the role of sleep in the process of learning and memory. A significant body of knowledge suggests that retention of new information depends on activation of some brain function, which occurs at a critical period after the registration of this information.[31,32] Two pivotal phases appear to exist. The first is consolidation. Medication that causes stimulation of the reticular activating system and cortical excitation during the first 90 seconds after acquisition of new information appears to enhance memory and increase retention. Although the consolidation phase of learning is important, it cannot be considered definitive for fixation of information because processing continues for a long time.[31]

The second critical phase of information processing seems to occur during REM sleep. Two theories have been proposed: the *passive* hypothesis (unlearning theory) and the *active* hypothesis, which suggests that there are active consolidation mechanisms. Several facts support an active process. Considerable brain activity occurs during REM sleep: brain oxygen consumption increases, cerebral blood flow increases, and cortical and reticular neurons are intensely active, indicating an active, functional process.

Over the past 50 years beneficial effects of sleep on the retention of memories acquired during wakefulness have been documented.[33,34] REM sleep appears to hold special significance. Despite evidence from animal and human studies the exact function of REM sleep in childhood development and learning remains unknown. Diverse reasons have been proposed for children's learning difficulties, but no single factor appears to be consistent for all individuals. Most diagnostic and treatment protocols have focused empirically on the child's daytime capabilities.

Minor neurological and EEG abnormalities have been described in children with hyperactivity syndrome.[35] These abnormalities have been associated with specific or global learning difficulties. The syndrome was previously described as "minimal cerebral dysfunction." Neurological and EEG abnormalities associated with this "hyperactivity" syndrome, however, have been shown to be nonspecific and variable,[36] resulting in a change in the syndrome's name to "attention deficit hyperactivity disorder."

It is noteworthy that of 115 reading-disabled (dyslexic) children studied by Levinson, 97% revealed evidence of cerebellar-vestibular dysfunction. Ninety-six percent of 22 blinded neurological examinations and 90% of 70 completed electronystagmograms indicated similar cerebellar-vestibular dysfunction.[37] Ottenbacher and associates explored the relationship between vestibular function as measured by duration of postrotatory nystagmus and human figure drawing ability in 40 children labeled as learning disabled.[38] Chronological age and postrotatory nystagmus durations both varied significantly from human figure drawing skills. The variables of intelligence quotient and sex were nonsignificant. DeQuiros and Schrager have also identified vestibular dysfunction in some learning-disabled children and described another related syndrome they termed "vestibular-oculomotor split," which results in impaired ocular fixation, impaired scanning ability, and poor eye-head coordination.[39]

Despite the evidence that some children with learning disabilities display soft or nonfocal neurological signs[40] and have low scores on tests of visual-motor integration, reading achievement, and ocular scanning,[41] contrary evidence of normal vestibular responses to rotation in dyslexic children has been published. Brown and associates measured eye movements provoked by sinusoidal rotation of the subjects at low frequencies.[42] Gain, phase, and asymmetry of the responses were calculated from the eye velocity and stimulus velocity waveforms. There were no differences between the dyslexic and control groups in any of the measurements. These results led Brown and associates to conclude that there were "no clinically measurable differences in this aspect of vestibular function" in their carefully selected population of dyslexic and control children. Their conclusions, however, were based on evidence obtained during the waking state. Vestibular nuclei play a major role in the control of eye movements when awake and asleep. If these nuclei are destroyed, eye movements during REM sleep are absent. In a pilot study of four reading-disabled children a significant difference was found in the mean angular velocity of eye movements during REM sleep when compared with three normally reading control subjects.[43]

The phasic events of rapid eye movements are correlated with cerebellar-vestibular control.

Pompeiano and associates have shown that lesions of the medial and descending vestibular nuclei in the cat eliminated all phasic inhibition of sensory input, spinal reflexes, and all motor output associated with phasic REM bursts, including eye movements themselves.[44,45] They have also demonstrated that intense spontaneous discharges from neurons of the vestibular nuclei occur synchronously with the ocular activity of REM sleep. Nystagmus evoked by rotation can be most readily induced during sleep at the time of phasic events of REM sleep.[46] In Wernicke-Korsakoff syndrome, in which the vestibular nuclei are often damaged, eye movements are absent during REM sleep.[47] These observations partially confirm the influences of vestibular mechanisms on the phasic activity of REM sleep.

Normal subjects have shown an age-related development of phasic inhibition of auditory evoked potentials during the ocular activity of REM sleep, as well as an age-related increase in the duration of the REM bursts.[48] It seems that central vestibular influences underlie these events and that vestibular control of phasic activity follows a developmental maturation schedule.

Considering the preceding evidence, a relationship may exist between the cerebellar-vestibular control of REM phasic events and phasic REM sleep's importance in learning and memory. As yet, however, this relationship remains a mystery.

Significant literature nonetheless supports a relationship between REM sleep, phasic REM activity, and learning. Sleep patterns in hyperkinetic children and normal children were studied by Busby, Firestone, and Pivik.[49] Analysis of sleep pattern variables revealed a significantly longer REM onset latency and a greater absolute and relative amount of movement time for the hyperkinetic group than for control subjects. No other sleep parameter differentiated the groups.

Clinical observations have suggested that disturbances of motility and perception are fundamental symptoms of childhood autism. The nature of these disturbances indicates a maturational delay in the development of complex motor patterns and the modulation of sensory input.[48] Sleep studies have provided some evidence for a maturational delay in the differentiation of REM sleep patterns and the development of phasic excitatory and inhibitory mechanisms during REM sleep in autistic children. These findings implicate a failure of central vestibular control over sensory transmission and motor output during REM sleep. The hypothesis that a dysfunction of central vestibular mechanisms underlies the delayed organization and differentiation of the REM sleep state is supported by observations of altered vestibular nystagmus in the waking state in autistic children.[48]

Studies in animals and humans support the importance of REM sleep in learning. Lucero conducted experiments showing that animals subjected to consecutive learning experiences, when compared with control animals, had a significant increase in REM sleep duration, a nonsignificant increase in total sleep time, and no changes in SWS duration.[50] Increase in REM sleep time observed after incremented learning suggests that REM sleep might be involved in the processing of information acquired during wakefulness. Such processing might consist of the transformation of a "labile program" acquired in the learning session into a more "stable program" devoid of superfluous information.

Major evidence of the importance of REM sleep in facilitating recall of complex associative information has been documented by Scrima.[51] The beneficial effect of isolated REM and isolated NREM sleep on recall was tested in 10 narcoleptic subjects. The results for complex associative tasks indicated significant differences between three conditions for free recall. Recall was significantly better after isolated REM than after isolated NREM sleep or wakefulness and was significantly better after NREM sleep than after wakefulness. The results were consistent with the proposed neuronal activity correlates theory of Emmons and Simon[52] that REM sleep actively consolidates or integrates complex associative information and that NREM sleep passively prevents retroactive interference of recently acquired complex associative information.

Newborn animals and human infants show a greater proportion of REM sleep with respect to total sleep time than adults,[53,54] and a progressive decrease in that proportion as growing continues is paralleled by a decrease in learning ability.[24] Fishbein has shown that REM sleep deprivation, both before and after learning, disrupts primarily long-term memory processes.[55] Evidence has been provided that learning induces a protracted augmentation of paradoxical sleep time, lasting for at least 24 hours.[56] This work, together with previous works, suggests that REM sleep augmentation may be a neurobiological expression of the long-term process of memory consolidation. Fishbein was able to augment REM sleep using behavioral techniques of learning. Therefore one psychobiological function of

REM sleep may be to process and maintain information during wakefulness.

Results obtained from nondeprivation studies of animals provide consistent support for the hypothesis that REM sleep is functionally related to learning. Studies employing multiple training sessions suggest either that prior REM sleep prepares the organism for subsequent learning or that REM sleep facilitates consolidation and retrieval of prior learning. Given the equivocal nature of prior REM deprivation literature, the second interpretation seems more reasonable.[57]

Impaired cognitive functioning has been documented in studies conducted on sleep-deprived physicians. In one investigation, cognitive functioning in acutely and chronically sleep-deprived house officers was evaluated.[58] Analysis of data revealed significant deficits in primary mental tasks involving basic rote memory, language and numerical skills, and tasks requiring high-order cognitive functioning and intellectual abilities.

Acquisition of many simple learning tasks in animals is followed by augmentation of REM sleep without any modification of NREM sleep.[31] Augmentation of REM sleep after learning has also been described in human infants.[59] Sleep may be particularly important for RNA and DNA synthesis linked to memory processes. Evidence indicates that during sleep RNA is more actively synthesized, less rapidly degraded, or more slowly transported into the cytoplasm.[60]

Like infants, older children and adults may have increased REM sleep following learning. Hartman has demonstrated an increase of REM sleep time occurring after days of increased learning, mental stress, and especially demanding events.[61] If learning does cause an increase in REM sleep, brain-damaged patients who are improving should have a higher proportion of REM sleep than patients who show no improvement. Following up nine patients with severe traumatic brain damage, Ron and associates found a correlation between cognition and REM sleep improvement in seven of these individuals.[62] Greenberg and Dewan compared the percentage of REM sleep in improving and nonimproving aphasic patients and found that the latter patients did in fact have lower levels.[63] In 32 patients with Down's syndrome, phenylketonuria, and other forms of brain damage, Feinberg found a positive relationship between the amount of eye movement during REM sleep and estimates of intellectual function,[10] and in a comparison of 38 individuals with normal brain function and 15 with brain damage, he showed that mentally retarded patients had less REM sleep.[64] REM sleep was linked with development of the visual system in a recent study by Oksenberg and co-workers.[65] They reported significant changes in the microscopic anatomy of the visual cortex in REM sleep–deprived cats.

In spite of evidence from human and animal studies, the exact function of sleep in the process of learning, memory, and child development is still speculative.

Unlearning Theory

An antithetical hypothesis for the function of REM sleep in learning and memory involves a process of *unlearning*. No single memory center appears to exist in the brain.[66] Many parts of the CNS participate in the representation of a single event. However, localization of memory of a single event generally involves a limited number of neural pathways, and each collection of neurons within which a memory is equivalently represented probably contains a "set" of no more than a thousand neurons. These interconnected assemblies of cells could store associations.[67,68] If the cells involved in the "memory" of an event form mutual synapses, when part of that event is encountered again, regeneration of the activity of the entire neuronal set would occur. Therefore Crick and Mitchison proposed that the function of REM sleep is to remove certain undesirable modes of interaction in cell networks in the cerebral cortex.[69] This would be accomplished during REM sleep by a "reverse learning" mechanism, so that the activity of dreaming weakens, rather than strengthens, the trace of the unconscious dream in the brain. A mathematical and computer model of a network of 30 to 1,000 neurons has been developed by Hopfield, Feinstein, and Palmer.[70] Their model network has a content-addressable memory or "associative memory," which allows it to learn and store many memories. A particular memory can be evoked in its entirety when the network is stimulated by a large enough subpart of the information of that memory. When memories are learned, spurious information is created and can also be evoked. Applying an "unlearning" process, similar to the learning process but with a reversed sign and starting from a noise input, enhanced the performance of the network in accessing real memories and minimizing spurious ones.

Thus sleep (in particular REM sleep) may reduce or prevent unwanted, unnoticed, or spurious material acquired during wakefulness. Isolation of the cortex from environmental stimuli may be necessary for the removal of inhibiting or competitive stimuli, inappropriate behavior patterns, and overloading of neuronal networks, permitting reprogramming and consolidation of more vital material.

Other Hypotheses

Presence of circulating hypnotoxin(s) has received some attention in the literature. This theory holds that during wakefulness there is accumulation of sleep-producing "toxin(s)," the presence of which stimulates or results in sleep. Once the toxin(s) has been modified by sleep, awakening occurs. Investigation of many substances claimed to be released after sleep deprivation and thalamic stimulation has failed to produce convincing evidence for this theory.[71] Craniophagus and thoracophagus twins have independent sleep-wake cycles, despite sharing circulatory or nervous systems or both.[72]

Sleep may be required for the normal functioning of the motor system and skeletal musculature. Muscle aching and change in skeletal muscle enzyme activity have been reported following NREM sleep deprivation.[73] Although sleep deprivation does not drastically affect the ability to work, physical performance follows a definite circadian rhythm.[74] Sleep also has a profound effect on certain diseases that affect the motor system, including Parkinson's disease[75] and hereditary progressive dystonia.[76]

Although all theories of the function of sleep have had significant support, evidence against each theory exists. The function of sleep may have a simple explanation or may be one of the more complex biological mechanisms. A unitary explanation of the function of sleep is probably unrealistic. The exact function and purpose of sleep may prove to be a combination or a series of integrations of all proposed hypotheses.

SLEEP DEPRIVATION

Experiments conducted to unravel the meaning and function of various physiological processes have involved abolition of the process followed by observations of the consequences of its absence. For many years researchers have attempted to identify the repercussions of total sleep deprivation, partial deprivation, and deprivation of various sleep stages. Unfortunately, these studies have been less fruitful in determining the function of sleep than investigations obliterating other physiological mechanisms.

Total sleep deprivation studies in animals have shown significant deleterious effects. In early experiments constant activity was necessary to keep animals awake for prolonged periods, confounding the results. In 1983 Rechtschaffen and co-workers described an ingenious experimental method that controlled for the stimuli used to keep the animals awake.[77] Experimental and control rats were placed on a platform that rotated and awakened an experimental animal whenever it fell asleep. Activity of the experimental and control animals was kept constant. Experimental animals suffered severe pathological changes from the sleep deprivation. Changes ranged from severely debilitated appearance (ungroomed and yellowed fur) to intense neurological abnormalities (ataxia and motor weakness) and death. Interestingly, EEG amplitude fell to less than half of normal waking values before the experimental animals died. Necropsy findings included pulmonary edema, atelectasis, gastric ulcerations, gastrointestinal hemorrhage, edema of the limbs, testicular atrophy, scrotal damage, bladder enlargement, hypoplasia of the liver and spleen, and hyperplasia of the adrenal glands (indicating a significant stress response). Body weight decreased in both experimental and control animals, but the loss was significantly greater in the experimental, sleep-deprived animals. Interestingly, the animals that ate the most lost the most weight. In addition there was a surprisingly high correlation between the amount of paradoxical (REM) sleep in the experimental animals and the survival time.

In comparison, effects of total sleep deprivation on human subjects have been remarkably few. Although brief psychotic episodes have been reported in some subjects, long-term psychological effects do not appear to result.[78] The only certain and reproducible effect of total sleep deprivation has been *sleepiness*.

Fatigue, decline in perceptual, cognitive, and psychomotor capabilities, and increasing transient ego disruptive episodes have been reported by Kales and co-workers during sleep deprivation.[79] As the experiment continued, reality testing became impaired and regressive behavior was noted. Tests for thought disorders showed shifts in thought processes to a more childlike level of cognition; however, no obvious evidence of schizophrenic thinking was seen.

Performance may also be hampered by sleep deprivation. Vigilance and performance on reaction time tests have been shown to be significantly impaired by the loss of as little as one night's sleep.[80] In a study of 44 men participating in a strenuous combat course in Norway, vigilance, reaction time, code testing, and profile of mood state were significantly impaired after 24 hours of sleep deprivation. Complaints of symptoms occurred first, followed by disturbances of senses and behavior. Horne and associates have reported that after 60 hours of continuous wakefulness, inherent capacity for signal detection exhibited a stepwise decline during deprivation, falling sharply during the usual sleep period time and leveling out during the daytime.[81] A clear circadian rhythm overlays the decline caused by deprivation. It was concluded that changes in inherent capacity seem to be consistent with a brain "restitutive" role for sleep function.

Significant physiological changes after total sleep deprivation have been reported. Rebound of Stage 4 sleep on the first recovery day and REM rebound on the second and third recovery days were documented by Berger and Oswald in 1962 and Williams and associates in 1964.[9,82] Kales and co-workers reported that after 205 hours of sleep deprivation, subjects had significant increases in Stage 4 sleep and REM sleep and significant decreases in Stage 2 sleep.[79] On the first two recovery nights alterations in REM sleep were noted. Subjects showed an increase in REM percentage, the appearance of sleep-onset REM periods (SOREMPs), a decrease in REM latency, and a decrease in inter-REM intervals. These occurred most dramatically in subjects who had the greatest psychological disturbances during the deprivation period.

Significant changes in performance and sleep physiology have been documented in subjects only partially deprived of sleep. In 1974 Webb and Agnew reported the results of an experiment conducted on 15 subjects restricted to 5½ hours of sleep a night for 60 days.[83] The initial effect was an increase in the absolute volume of Stage 4 sleep. By the fifth week of the experiment the volume of Stage 4 sleep returned to the baseline level. The initial effect on REM sleep was a sharp reduction from the baseline. During the course of the experiment, REM sleep was reduced by 25%. Latency to the onset of Stage 4 sleep and latency to the onset of REM sleep were also reduced. The only behavioral change associated with continued sleep restriction was a decline in performance on the Wilkinson Vigilance Task. Initially the subjects experienced difficulty in arousing in the morning and felt drowsy during the day, but this did not continue throughout the experiment. Mood scales showed no significant changes. The authors concluded that the chronic loss of as much as 2½ hours of sleep per night is unlikely to have major behavioral consequences. However, with partial sleep restriction significant physiological effects were documented (especially in REM sleep) by polysomnography. Restricting sleep by early morning waking generally deprives the subject of REM and Stage 2 sleep but leaves NREM Stage 4 intact. Recovery nights, however, show a substantial increase in NREM Stage 4 volume, suggesting that high-voltage, slow-wave sleep is to some extent a function of total sleep time.[84]

Children's response to acute restriction in sleep is similar to that in adults but shows some major differences. When sleep has been restricted by 4 hours or more, children show decreases in all stages of sleep except SWS; reduction in sleep onset latency, Stage 4 latency, and REM latency; and reduction in wakefulness during the sleep period. Carskadon, Harvey, and Dement studied the effect of acute, partial restriction of sleep in nine children between the ages of 11 and 13.2 years.[85] Children were permitted to sleep 10 hours on baseline and recovery nights and 4 hours on a single restricted night. No significant differences were found on any performance test. Unfortunately, the tests were brief, which may have had a significant impact on the outcome. Kleitman[71] and Wilkinson[85a] have emphasized that duration of performance of a task is a major factor determining a test's sensitivity to sleep loss. On the other hand, significant changes did occur on objective sleep testing. The Multiple Sleep Latency Test (MSLT) showed a significant increase in daytime sleepiness during the morning following sleep restriction. This suggests that children are more severely affected by sleep restriction than adults. Polysomnography findings were comparable to those in adults, *but children did not show recover rebound of SWS and REM sleep as reported for adults*. Although children appear to tolerate a single night of restricted sleep without a decrement in performance on brief tasks, perhaps more prolonged restriction and prolonged tasks similar to those required in school would show decrements. Children seem to require more time to recuperate fully from nocturnal sleep restriction than adults. The extent of daytime sleepiness that occurs is not trivial. With additional nights of partial sleep deprivation, cumulative sleepiness might rapidly become a significant problem. The effects of sleep restriction on daytime sleepiness, school performance, and behavior of children may be greater than previously realized.

In 1972 Dement powerfully described possible outcomes of restricted sleep on wakefulness[86]:

> After an excessively long period of wakefulness, the state of sleep becomes preemptive. When we enforce wakefulness, we are probably preventing or minimizing activity in the neural systems that subserve sleep induction and maintenance. As the potency of these systems increase during the period of their induced inactivity, they may begin to intrude upon wakefulness in an ever more aggressive manner.
>
> The notion of total sleep deprivation could be somewhat illusory, and could result merely in a redistribution of activity in sleep and arousal systems in which NREM sleep would occur in the form of hundreds of microsleeps.

Microsleeps have been well documented in both human and animal studies.[87-89] Kales and associates described disorientation and misperceptions during sleep deprivation that seemed to be associated with "lapses" that became more frequent as deprivation continued.[79] Armington and Mitnick found that sleep deprivation eventually produced brain wave patterns that were more or less continuously at the NREM Stage 1 level, although the subjects appeared to be awake.[87] The most consistent result of modest amounts of sleep loss in humans is the occurrence of these microsleep periods.[88] Microsleeps increase in frequency throughout periods of sleep deprivation. Since gross waking behavior is not affected, these lapses may have significant consequences on performance and its assessment, especially for the school-age child whose consistent attentiveness is required for success in school. Since the perceptual shutdown can occur before EEG changes are apparent at the outset of sleep, sleep-deprived subjects may have many more such episodes than EEG patterns alone would suggest.[86]

PHYLOGENETIC CONSIDERATIONS

Understanding sleep in humans requires reflection on sleep in other species. Although periods of sluggish activity can be documented in reptiles, they do not appear to have physiological sleep.[90] Although only a relatively small number of mammalian species have been studied, it appears that most, if not all, birds and mammals sleep. Quiescent periods, intervals of reduced responsiveness to environmental stimuli, rapid reversibility of state, specific postures, and characteristic EEG changes have been observed.[91] All these criteria, however, need not be present concomitantly, and quiescence is not always equivalent to inactivity. Ritualistic activity and behaviors precede sleep in many species, including humans. Timing of sleep varies among species; some consolidate sleep into a single period and others distribute sleep throughout a 24-hour continuum.

Sleep in birds is remarkably similar to sleep in mammals. Two distinct types of sleep with comparable electrophysiological activity have been documented. Major differences appear to be in the pattern of sleep and the greater number of sleep states observed in avian species.[92]

Zeplin and Rechtschaffen studied available sleep data on more than 50 mammalian species.[93] Sleeping patterns were correlated with metabolic rates, gestational periods, and brain weights. Animals with lower metabolic rates tend to sleep less than those with higher metabolic rates. Species that have longer sleep periods tend to be smaller and to have shorter life spans. Meddis replicated this study on a sample of 65 species and obtained similar results.[94]

NREM-REM cycling appears to be the basic organization of sleep in most species studied. Although the quality and quantity of NREM and REM sleep vary considerably, a regularly patterned series of state changes occurs with demonstrable slowing of the EEG and the presence of spindling activity.[91] Paradoxical sleep has been recorded in almost all mammalian species studied. Characteristics of this sleep state include desynchronization (activation) of CNS electrical activity, skeletal muscle atonia, periodic twitching, and physiological instability (especially of the cardiovascular and respiratory systems). Changes in thermoregulation and high arousal thresholds are present. Rhythmical theta activity and pontogeniculate-occipital (PGO) spikes are typically seen on EEG during mammalian paradoxical sleep.

Phylogenetic development of REM sleep has been studied by Allison and Van Twyver.[95] REM sleep appears to have developed approximately 130 million years ago. Allison and Cicchetti concluded that the volume of REM sleep correlated with life-style, risk of predation, and degree of exposure of the sleep environment.[25]

REM sleep is the preponderant state early in life in most mammals (including humans). Although considered to be ontogenetically primitive, REM sleep may play a significant role in the development of the CNS. Premature newborn humans spend approximately 90% of their total sleep time in active sleep. This falls rapidly to about 50% by term. A gradual decrease continues throughout the first few years of life to about 20% to 25%. This level remains remarkably constant throughout the remainder of the life cycle.[54]

Jouvet-Mounier, Astic, and Lacote have studied the ontogenetic development of sleep of infant cats, rats, and guinea pigs.[96] More than 70 animals underwent electrocortical, electroocular, electromyographic, and behavioral monitoring from birth to 50 days of age. REM sleep was the preponderant form of sleep in these species. The species varied significantly in the degree of development at birth, with rat pups the most immature, kittens intermediate, and guinea pigs the most mature. Degree of immaturity at birth correlated highly with the volume of paradoxical sleep recorded during the perinatal period. At birth rat pups exhibited 70% paradoxical sleep, which decreased rapidly to near adult levels by 30 days of life. Decrease of paradoxical sleep in kittens was considerably slower. Infant guinea pigs showed the lowest volume of paradoxical sleep (7%), but this was still approximately double the volume seen in the adult animal. Maturation of SWS is late in comparison with paradoxical sleep, and the time spent in paradoxical sleep and SWS varies during the first postnatal month. These variations are different among species. Newborn kittens have a more highly developed cortex than rat pups.[97] Cortical neurons in kittens mature rapidly and show the histological characteristics of adult cortical neurons by the twelfth postnatal day, concomitant with the appearance of SWS. In contrast, the cortex of the newborn guinea pig appears histologically the same as that of the adult.[98]

Sleeping dolphins and porpoises are fascinating and of particular ontogenetic interest because of the complexity of the cetacean CNS. Mukhametov has studied the neurophysiology of sleep in the bottle-nose dolphin *(Tursiops truncatus)* and the porpoise *(Phocoena phocoena)*.[99] He showed that the main characteristics of sleep in these marine mammals are unihemispheric SWS and the apparent absence of paradoxical sleep. EEG characteristics are typical for the mammalian brain and show three distinct stages: desynchronization; intermediate synchronization with sleep spindles, theta activity, and delta waves; and maximal synchronization with slow waves comprising more than 50% of each recording period. In all dolphins studied, unihemispheric SWS was the main type of sleep recorded. Interestingly, this type of sleep is not found in other mammals. Synchronization of the EEG occurs in one hemisphere, while the opposite hemisphere reveals desynchronization. These cycles of synchrony and desynchrony appear to be independent. Each hemisphere exhibits different volumes of SWS, and deprivation of SWS in one hemisphere does not result in contralateral rebound. Ipsilateral rebound is noted in the SWS-deprived hemisphere only. Mukhametov attempted to identify neurophysiological and behavioral correlates of paradoxical sleep in 30 animals of two species and did not find evidence of paradoxical sleep in dolphins or porpoises. Proving the complete absence of paradoxical sleep is difficult, however, since testing of dolphin fetuses and calves has not yet been possible. Whether these characteristics represent a phylogenetic, developmental, or adaptive phenomenon is unknown. Unraveling the mystery has fascinating teleological implications.

BEHAVIORAL AND PHYSIOLOGICAL CONSIDERATIONS

At first glance sleep appears to be a simple process, a required part of our 24-hour life cycle. Little attention is paid to the sleeping state because human life-style focuses primarily on interactions with the environment and daily fragments of disengagement seem of secondary importance. Time spent in activities not related to goal attainment, pursuit of sustenance, fulfillment, happiness, or success appears to be an intrusive, unwelcome gap. The importance of such gaps, however, in permitting the individual to function and interact appropriately with the environment during the waking state has only recently been discovered.

Any definition of sleep is complex from both a behavioral and a physiological perspective. In simplest terms sleep has been defined as a reversible disengagement from and unresponsiveness to the external environment, regularly alternating with engagement and responsiveness in a circadian manner. This definition is now known to be significantly incomplete and simplistic, since sleep is a highly active and complex state.

It seems easy to determine when an individual is sleeping. Behavioral correlates include a recumbent position, closed eyelids, quiescence, and diminished responsiveness to external stimuli. These behaviors are fairly consistent between individuals. Sleep onset, however, requires complex interactions of learned behaviors and physiological processes. Absence of sudden external stimuli; a suitable, safe, comfortable environment; relaxation of postural muscles; and learned stereotypical behaviors associated with bedtime are required.[100] Evidence suggests that rhythmical, monotonous sensory stimulation promotes sleep.[101] Whether this effect is behavioral, physiological, or a combination is speculative.

Sleep onset and maintenance are not passive physiological processes. Isolation of the cerebrum from the brainstem and spinal cord (cerveau isolé) produces a state indistinguishable from physiological sleep.[102] A series of exquisite experiments identified neurons of the reticular formation that received collateral input from somatic, visceral, and special sensory pathways and sent ascending projections dorsally and ventrally to the basal forebrain.[103-105] These collections of neurons were termed the reticular activating system. Complex projections of neurons from the reticular formation to the posterior hypothalamus-subthalamus, the basal forebrain, and then the cortex are responsible for the maintenance of wakefulness.[106]

Although sleep was initially thought to result from a decrease in the activity of the reticular activating system, brainstem transection experiments resulting in diminished sleep suggested that sleep-inducing structures must also be present in the central nervous system.[107] These sleep-inducing structures appear to be located in the lower brainstem, specifically the dorsal medullary reticular formation and nucleus of the solitary tract. Lesions in this area produced EEG activation in a sleeping animal.[108-109] A sleep facilitation center appears to be present in the rostral hypothalamus,[110] and cortical synchrony can be elicited by stimulation of the midline thalamus.[111] Sleep-inducing neurons are also found in the preoptic area and basal forebrain. Gamma-aminobutyric acid (GABA) neurons located in the cortex, as well as neurons in the hypothalamus and basal forebrain, are vital for production of SWS.[106]

Sleep onset therefore results from a complex series of events involving changes in levels of somatic, visceral, and special sensory input; active inhibition of neuron networks that produce cortical desynchronization; and active stimulation of neuronal systems and pathways responsible for cortical synchrony. The rhythmical organization of these activities is extremely complex and appears to be controlled by neurons in the suprachiasmatic nucleus.[112] Jouvet described a separate system of neurons in the upper pons that controlled the induction and manifestations of REM sleep.[113] This system was under the influence of an "oscillator," which was separate from (although linked to) the oscillator which controlled the rhythmicity of the sleep-wake cycle. According to Hobson and McCarley a cholinergic, "REM-on" system of neurons is located primarily in the mesencephalic, medullary, and pontine gigantocellular tegmental fields but may be widespread.[114] Discharges from these neurons are responsible for REM sleep epiphenomena of cortical desynchronization, conjugate eye movements, decrease in muscle tone by active inhibition of alpha motor neurons, muscular twitching, and cardiorespiratory irregularities. It has also been shown that a self-inhibitory, aminergic, "REM-off" system of neurons, located in the dorsal raphe nuclei, locus ceruleus, and nucleus peribrachialis lateralis, interacts with the opposing system, resulting in alternations between NREM and REM sleep.

The behavioral, neurochemical, and neurophysiological mechanisms of the sleep-wake cycle and electrophysiological cycles during sleep itself are complex and intensely integrated. Many characteristics have yet to be elucidated. Sleep may prove to be one of the most complex physiological processes known. Its implications in fetal and childhood development may be more significant than our wildest dreams.

REFERENCES

1. Rechtschaffen A: The function of sleep: methodological issues. In Drucker-Colin R, Shkurovich M, and Sterman MB (eds): The functions of sleep. New York, Academic Press, 1979, p 1.
2. Moldofsky H: Immunology and sleep. Presented at the First Annual Meeting of the Association of Professional Sleep Societies, Columbus, Ohio, June 15-20, 1986.
3. Moldofsky H et al: The effect of 40 hours of wakefulness on immune functions in humans. II. Interleukins-1- and -2-like activities. Sleep Res 1988; 17:34.
4. Moldofsky H et al: Disordered diurnal patterns of immune functions in three patients with narcolepsy-cataplexy. Sleep Res 1988;17:223.
5. Sherington CS: Man on his nature. Cambridge, Eng, Cambridge University Press, 1946, p 413.
6. Oswald I: Sleep. Harmondsworth, Middlesex, Eng, Penguin Books, 1974.
7. Hartmann E, Orzack MH, and Branconnier R: Deficits produced by sleep deprivation: Reversal by D- and L-amphetamine. Sleep Res 1974;3:151.
8. Adam K and Oswald I: Sleep is for tissue restoration. J Coll Phys 1977;11:376.
9. Berger R and Oswald I: Effects of sleep deprivation

on behavior, subsequent sleep and dreaming. J Ment Sci 1962;108:457.
10. Feinberg I: The ontogenesis of human sleep and the relationship of sleep variables to intellectual function in the aged. Comp Psychiatry 1968;9:138.
11. Adam K: Body weight correlates with REM sleep. Br Med J 1977;1:813.
12. Sassin JF et al: Human growth hormone release relation to slow-wave sleep and sleep-waking cycles. Science 1969;165:513.
13. Sassin JF et al: The nocturnal rise of human prolactin is dependent on sleep. J Clin Endocrinol Metab 1973;37:436.
14. Boyar RM et al: Human puberty: simultaneous augmented secretion of luteinizing hormone and testosterone during sleep. J Clin Invest 1974;54:609.
15. Weitzman ED and Hellman L: Temporal organization of the 24-hour pattern of the hypothalamic-pituitary axis. In Ferin M et al (eds): Biorhythms and human reproduction. New York, Wiley, 1974, p 371.
16. Valk IM and van der Bosch JSG: Intra-daily variation of the human ulnar length and short term growth—a longitudinal study in eleven boys. Growth 1974;42:107.
17. Griffin SJ and Trinder J: Physical fitness, exercise and human sleep. Psychophysiology 1978;15:447.
18. Fisher LB: The diurnal mitotic rhythm in the human epidermis. Br J Dermatol 1968;80:75.
19. Finkelstein JW et al: Age-related change in the twenty-four hour spontaneous secretion of growth hormone. J Clin Endocrinol Metab 1972;35:665.
20. Jouvet M: The function of dreaming: a neurophysiologist's point of view. In Gazzaniga MS and Blakemore C (eds): Handbook of Psychobiology. New York, Academic Press, 1975, p 499.
21. Giuditta A et al: Synthesis of brain RNA and DNA during sleep. In Borbely A and Valtax JL (eds): Sleep mechanisms. Berlin, Springer-Verlag, 1984, p 146.
22. Bert J: Sleep in primates under natural conditions and in the laboratory. In Koella WP and Levin P (eds): Sleep 1976: Third European Congress of Sleep Research. Basel, S Karger, 1977, p 152.
23. Webb WB: Sleep stage responses of older and younger subjects after sleep deprivation. Electroencephalogr Clin Neurophysiol 1981;52:368.
24. Kovalzon VM: Brain temperature variations in ECoG in free-swimming bottle-nose dolphins. In Koella WP and Levin P (eds): Sleep 1976: Third European Congress of Sleep Research. Basel, S Karger, 1977, p 239.
25. Allison T and Cicchetti DV: Sleep in mammals: ecological and constitutional correlates. Science 1976;194:732.
26. McGinty DJ, Harper TM, and Fairbanks MK: Neuronal unit activity and the control of sleep states. In Weitzman E (ed): Advances in sleep research. New York, Spectrum, 1974, p 173.
27. Snyder F: Toward an evolutionary theory of dreaming. Am J Psychiatry 1966;123:121.
28. Zepelin H and Rechtschaffen A: Mammalian sleep, longevity, and energy conservation. Brain Behav Evolution 1974;10:425.
29. Carpenter AC and Timiras PS: Sleep organization in hypo- and hyperthyroid rats. Neuroendocrinology 1982;34:438.
30. Eastman C and Rechtschaffen A: Effects of thyroxin on sleep in the rat. Sleep 1979;2:215.
31. Block V, Hennevin E, and Leconte P: The phenomenon of paradoxical sleep augmentation after learning: experimental studies of its characteristics and significance. In Fishbein W (ed): Sleep, dreams and memory. Jamaica, NY, Spectrum, 1981, pp 1-18.
32. Smith C and Butler S: Paradoxical sleep at selective times following training is necessary for learning. Physiol Behav 1982;29:469.
33. Jenkins J and Kallenbach K: Oblivescence during sleep and waking. Am J Psychol 1924;35:605.
34. VanOrmer EG: Retention after intervals of sleep and waking. Arch Psychol 1932;137:5
35. Carter S and Gold A: The syndrome of minimal cerebral dysfunction. In Barnett MH and Einhorn A (eds): Pediatrics. New York, Appleton-Century-Crofts, 1972.
36. Dykman RA et al: Specific learning disabilities: an attentional deficit syndrome. In Myklebust HR (ed): Progress in learning disabilities. New York, Grune & Stratton, 1971.
37. Levinson HN: Dyslexia: a solution to the riddle. New York, Springer-Verlag, 1980, p 73.
38. Ottenbacher K et al: Human figure drawing ability and vestibular processing in learning disabled children. J Clin Psychol 1984;40:1084.
39. DeQuiros JB and Schrager OL: Neuropsychological fundamentals in learning disabilities. San Rafael, Calif, Academic Therapy Press, 1978.
40. Steinberg M and Rendle-Short J: Vestibular dysfunction in young children with minor neurologic impairment. Dev Med Child Neurol 1977;19:639.
41. Ottenbacher K et al: Nystagmus and ocular fixation difficulties in learning-disabled children. Am J Occup Ther 1979;33:717.
42. Brown B et al: Dyslexic children have normal vestibular response to rotation. Arch Neurol 1983;40:370.
43. Sheldon SH, Spire JP, and Levy HB: REM sleep eye movements in reading disabled children. Sleep Res 1990;19:128.
44. Pompeiano O: The neurophysiological mechanisms of the postural and motor events during desynchronized sleep. In Kety SS, Evarts EV, and Williams HL (eds): Sleep and altered states of consciousness. Baltimore, Williams & Wilkins, 1967, p 351.
45. Pompeiano O: Mechanisms of sensorimotor integration during sleep. Prog Physiol Psychol 1970;3:1.
46. Reding GR and Fernandez C: Effects of vestibular stimulation during sleep. Electroencephalogr Clin Neurophysiol 1968;24:75.
47. Appenzeller C and Fisher AP: Disturbances of rapid eye movements during sleep in patients with lesions of the nervous system. Electroencephalogr Clin Neurophysiol 1968;25:29.
48. Ornitz EM: Development of sleep patterns in autistic children. In Clemente C, Purpura DP, and Mayer FE (eds): Sleep and the maturing nervous system. New York, Academic Press, 1972, p 363.
49. Busby K, Firestone P, and Pivik RT: Sleep patterns in hyperkinetic and normal children. Sleep 1981;4:366.
50. Lucero MA: Lengthening of REM sleep duration consecutive to learning in the rat. Brain Res 1979;20:319.
51. Scrima L: Isolated REM sleep facilitates recall of complex associative information. Psychophysiology 1982;19:252.
52. Emmons W and Simon C: Response to material presented during various levels of sleep. J Exp Psychol 1956;51:89.

53. Parmelee HA, Schulz HR, and Disbrow MA: Sleep patterns of the newborn. J Pediatr 1961;58:241.
54. Roffwarg HP, Dement WC, and Fisher C: Preliminary observations on the sleep patterns in neonates, infants, children, and adults. In Harms E (ed): Problems of sleep and dreams in children. London, Pergamon Press, 1963.
55. Fishbein W: Disruptive effects of rapid-eye-movement sleep deprivation on long-term memory. Physiol Behav 1971;6:279.
56. Fishbein W, Kastaniotis C, and Chattman D: Paradoxical sleep: prolonged augmentation following learning. Brain Res 1974;71:61.
57. McGrath MJ and Cohen DB: REM sleep facilitation of adaptive waking behavior: a review of the literature. Psychol Bull 1978;85:24.
58. Hawkins MR et al: Sleep and nutritional deprivation and performance of house officers. J Med Educ 1985;60:530.
59. Paul K and Dittrichova J: Sleep patterns following learning in infants. In Levin P and Koella U (eds): Sleep: 1974. Basel, S Karger, 1975, p 388.
60. Parkes JD: Sleep and its disorders. Major problems in neurology, vol 14. London, WB Saunders, 1985, p 44.
61. Hartman E: The functions of sleep. New Haven, Conn, Yale University Press, 1976.
62. Ron S et al: Time-related changes in the distribution of sleep stages in brain injured patients. Electroencephalogr Clin Neurophysiol 1980;48:432.
63. Greenberg R and Dewan EM: Aphasia and rapid-eye-movement sleep. Nature 1969;223:183.
64. Feinberg I: Eye movement activity during sleep and intellectual function in mental retardation. Science 1968;159:1256.
65. Oksenberg et al: Effect of REM sleep deprivation during the critical period of neuroanatomical development of the cat visual system. Sleep Res 1986;15:53.
66. Squire LR: Memory and the brain. New York, Oxford University Press, 1987, p 123.
67. Kohonen T: Associative memory. New York, Springer-Verlag, 1977.
68. Palm G: Neural assemblies: an alternative approach to artificial intelligence. New York, Springer-Verlag, 1982.
69. Crick F and Mitchison G: The function of dream sleep. Nature 1983;304:111.
70. Hopfield JJ, Feinstein DI, and Palmer RG: "Unlearning" has a stabilizing effect in collective memories. Nature 1983;304:158.
71. Kleitman N: Sleep and wakefulness. Chicago, University of Chicago Press, 1963, p 552.
72. Webb WB: The sleep of conjoined twins. Sleep 1978;1:205.
73. Moldofsky H and Scarisbrick P: Induction of neurasthenic musculoskeletal pain syndrome by selective sleep stage deprivation. Psychosom Med 1976; 38:35.
74. Nicholson AN and Marks J: Insomnia. Lancaster, Eng, MTP, 1983, p 22.
75. Marsden CD: "On-off" phenomenon in Parkinson's disease. In Rinne UK, Klinger M, and Stamm G (eds): Parkinson's disease—current progress, problems and management. Amsterdam, Elsevier/North Holland, 1980, p 241.
76. Segawa M et al: Hereditary progressive dystonia with marked diurnal fluctuation. Adv Neurol 1976; 14:215.
77. Rechtschaffen A et al: Physiological correlates of prolonged sleep deprivation in rats. Science 1983;221:182.
78. Passouant P et al: Etude polygraphique des narcolepsies au cours du nychemore. Rev Neurol (Paris) 1968;118:431.
79. Kales A et al: Sleep patterns following 205 hours of sleep deprivation. Psychosom Med 1979;32:189.
80. Glenville M et al: Effects of sleep deprivation on short duration performance measures compared to the Wilkinson Auditory Vigilance Task. Sleep 1978;1:169.
81. Horne JA, Anderson NR, and Wilkinson RT: Effects of sleep deprivation on signal detection measures of vigilance: implications for sleep function. Sleep 1983;6:347.
82. Williams HL et al: Response to auditory stimulation, sleep loss, and EEG stages of sleep. Electroencephalogr Clin Neurophysiol 1964;16:269.
83. Webb WB and Agnew HW: The effect of a chronic limitation of sleep length. Psychophysiology 1974;11:265.
84. Dement W and Greenberg S: Changes in total amount of stage 4 sleep as a function of partial sleep deprivation. Electroencephalogr Clin Neurophysiol 1966;20:523.
85. Carskadon MA, Harvey K, and Dement WC: Acute restriction of nocturnal sleep in children. Perceptual Motor Skills 1981;53:103.
85a. Wilkinson RT: Sleep deprivation: performance tests for partial and selective sleep deprivation. In Abt LE and Riess BF (eds): Progress in clinical psychology, vol 8. New York, Grune & Stratton, 1968, pp 28-43.
86. Dement WC: Sleep deprivation and organization of the behavioral states. In Clemente C, Purpura D, and Mayer F (eds): Sleep and the maturing nervous system. New York, Academic Press, 1972, p 319.
87. Armington J and Mitnick L: Electroencephalogram and sleep deprivation. J Appl Physiol 1959;14:247.
88. Williams H, Lubin A, and Goodnow J: Impaired performance with acute sleep loss. Psychol Monogr 1959;73:1.
89. Friedman L, Bergmann BM, and Rechtschaffen A: Effects of sleep deprivation on sleepiness, sleep intensity, and subsequent sleep in rats. Sleep 1979;1:369.
90. Cartwright RD: A primer on sleep and dreaming. Reading, Mass, Addison-Wesley, 1978, p 19.
91. Zepelin H: Mammalian sleep. In Kryger MH, Roth T, and Dement WC (eds): Principles and practice of sleep medicine. Philadelphia, WB Saunders, 1989, p 30.
92. Amlaner CJ and Ball NJ: Avian sleep. In Kryger MH, Roth T, and Dement WC (eds): Principles and practice of sleep medicine. Philadelphia, WB Saunders, 1989, p 50.
93. Zeplin H and Rechtschaffen A: Mammalian sleep, longevity, and energy conservation. Brain Behav Environ 1974;10:425.
94. Meddis R: The evolution of sleep. In Mayes A (ed): Sleep mechanisms and function in humans and animals: an evolutionary perspective. Berkshire, Eng, Van Nostrand Reinhold (UK), 1983.
95. Allison T and Van Twyver H: The evolution of sleep. Natural History 1970;79:56.
96. Jouvet-Mounier D, Astic L, and Lacote D: Ontogenesis of the states of sleep in rat, cat, and guinea

pig during the first postnatal month. Dev Psychobiol 1970;2:216.

97. Nobak CR and Purpura DP: Postnatal ontogenesis of neurons in cat neocortex. J Comp Neurol 1961;117:291.
98. Peters HG and Bademan H: The form and growth of stellate cells in the cortex of the guinea pig. J Anat 1963;97:111.
99. Mukhametov LM: Sleep in marine mammals. Exp Brain Res 1984;8:227.
100. Konorski J: Integrative action of the brain. Chicago, University of Chicago Press, 1967, p 531.
101. Gastaut H and Bert B: Electroencephalographic detection of sleep induced by repetitive sensory stimuli. In Wolstenholme GEW and O'Connor M (eds): On the nature of sleep. London, Churchill, 1961, p 260.
102. Bremer F: Quelques propriétés de l'activité electrique du cortex cerebral "isole." CR Soc Biol (Paris) 1935;118:1241.
103. French JD and Magoun HW: Effects of chronic lesions in central cephalic brain stem of monkeys. Arch Neurol Psychiatry 1952;69:591.
104. Lindsley DB, Bowden JW, and Magoun HW: Effect upon the EEG of acute injury to the brain stem activating system. Electroencephalogr Clin Neurophysiol 1949;1:475.
105. Moruzzi G: The sleep-waking cycle. Ergeb Physiol 1972;64:1.
106. Jones BE: Basic mechanisms of sleep-wake states. In Kryger MH, Roth T, and Dement WC: Principles and practice of sleep medicine. Philadelphia, WB Saunders, 1989, p 121.
107. Barini C et al: Effects of complete pontine transections of the sleep-wakefulness rhythm: the midpontine pretrigeminal preparation. Arch Ital Biol 1959;97:1.
108. Freemon FR, Salinas-Garcia RF, and Ward JW: Sleep patterns in a patient with a brain stem infarction involving the raphe nucleus. Electroencephalogr Clin Neurophysiol 1974;36:657.
109. Westmoreland BF et al: Alpha-coma. Arch Neurol 1975;32:713.
110. Nauta WJH: Hypothalamic regulation of sleep in rats: an experimental study. J Neurophysiol 1946;9:285.
111. Morison RS and Dempsey EW: A study of thalamocortical relations. J Physiol 1942;135:281.
112. Hanada Y and Kawamura H: Sleep-waking electrocorticographic rhythms in chronic cerveau isolé rats. Physiol Behav 1981;26:725.
113. Jouvet M: Paradoxical sleep: a study of its nature and mechanisms. In Himwich WA and Schade JP (eds): Sleep mechanisms: progress in brain research. Amsterdam, Elsevier, 1965.
114. Hobson JA: The cellular basis of sleep cycle control. Adv Sleep Res 1974;1:217.

2

Normal Sleep in Children and Young Adults

SLEEP ONSET

Sleep onset is not a unitary event. Identification of a specific time of transition from wakefulness to sleep is difficult from both a behavioral and a physiological perspective. For practical purposes sleep onset can be correlated with certain behavioral and physiological changes that occur over a period of time. In addition to behaviors typically associated with sleep (e.g., eyelids closed, recumbency, quiescence), behavioral changes consist of modulation in responsiveness to auditory and visual stimuli, decrease in the ability to perform even simple tasks, and alterations in memory of events occurring several moments before sleep onset. Changes in electroencephalographic (EEG) activity commonly associated with the sleeping state are not always perceived by the individual as sleep, and conversely, individuals may believe they have slept without obvious documentable EEG changes from the normal waking state.[1]

It is generally (although not unequivocally) believed that sleep is heralded by two major electrophysiological events: (1) disappearance of alpha activity on EEG and its replacement by a relatively low-voltage, mixed-frequency (RLVMF) pattern and (2) appearance of slow, rolling, sometimes disconjugate eye movements on electrooculogram. At sleep onset the electromyogram (EMG) may reveal a gradual fall in muscle tone, but this does not always occur and a discrete fall in tone below that of waking may not be appreciated. Environmental perceptions during this period vary considerably. Thoughts become fragmented, although most individuals will report that they are not sleeping during periods of Stage 1 sleep.[2]

Ability to perform simple behavioral tasks ceases during the transition to sleep, and continued performance of activity for a few seconds after EEG changes to an RLVMF pattern is considered an example of simple *automatic behavior*.[3] *Perceptual disengagement* from the environment at sleep onset can be demonstrated by a lack of response to visual and auditory stimuli[4] and return of the response to the stimuli only after the EEG reverts to a waking pattern. Central nervous system integration of stimuli, however, appears to persist after sleep onset, since the arousal threshold for meaningful stimuli is significantly less than for nonmeaningful stimuli.[5]

Vague and fragmentary visual imagery is often reported during the transition from wakefulness to sleep. Generalized or localized involuntary muscle contractions may occur during this period and are termed *hypnic myoclonia*.[2] These hypnic jerks, which are often associated with altered perceptions or imagery of falling, are a normal occurrence and may appear more frequently during times of stress and altered or irregular sleep-wake schedules.

Guilleminault and Dement have described amnesic properties associated with the transition from wakefulness to sleep.[6] Subjects who were awakened 30 seconds after sleep onset could recall words heard over headphones presented at 1-minute intervals, beginning 10 minutes before sleep onset. In contrast, when the subjects were permitted to sleep for 10 minutes after sleep onset, words presented 6 to 10 minutes before falling to sleep could be repeated, but those presented within the 5 minutes before sleep onset could not be recalled. Guilleminault and Dement concluded that if sleep persists for approximately 10 minutes, memory of events occurring during the few minutes before sleep onset is lost.

NORMAL COURSE OF EVENTS

Healthy Young Adults

In normal, healthy young adults, sleep is entered through non–rapid eye movement (NREM) sleep (whereas infants normally enter sleep through REM sleep). At sleep onset the EEG converts to an RLVMF pattern, theta activity appears, and eye movements become slow, rolling, pendulous, and disconjugate. The EMG reveals that muscle tone changes little from waking levels (Fig. 2–1). Variable perceptual disengagement from the environment occurs. Arousal thresholds are low but vary when meaning is assigned to the stimulus (e.g., an individual may respond to his or her name but not to another name). Stage 1 sleep lasts for a brief time and is followed by transition to Stage 2 sleep. Stage 2 is identified by the appearance of *sleep spindles* and *K-complexes* on EEG (Fig. 2–2). Sleep spindles are 9 to 13 cycles per second (cps) waveforms, of waxing and waning amplitude, lasting greater than 0.5 second. K-complexes are large vertex prominent, slow waves, having an amplitude of at least 75 μV with an initial negative deflection, followed by a positive deflection and then return to the baseline of the recording pen. These two EEG waveforms are characteristic of sleep and do not occur in any other state. Arousal thresholds are higher in Stage 2 than in Stage 1 (i.e., a greater stimulus amplitude is required for arousal), and the same stimulus that may cause arousal from Stage 1 may cause a K-complex to appear in Stage 2, but not arousal. After approximately 5 to 25 minutes of Stage 2 sleep the EEG shows a gradual increase in high-voltage (at least 75 μV) waves with a frequency of no more than 2 cps. When these slow waves comprise greater than 20% but less than 50% of each recording epoch, Stage 3 sleep begins. Stage 4 is identified by slow waves comprising greater than 50% of the recording epoch (Fig. 2–3). The distinction between Stage 3 and Stage

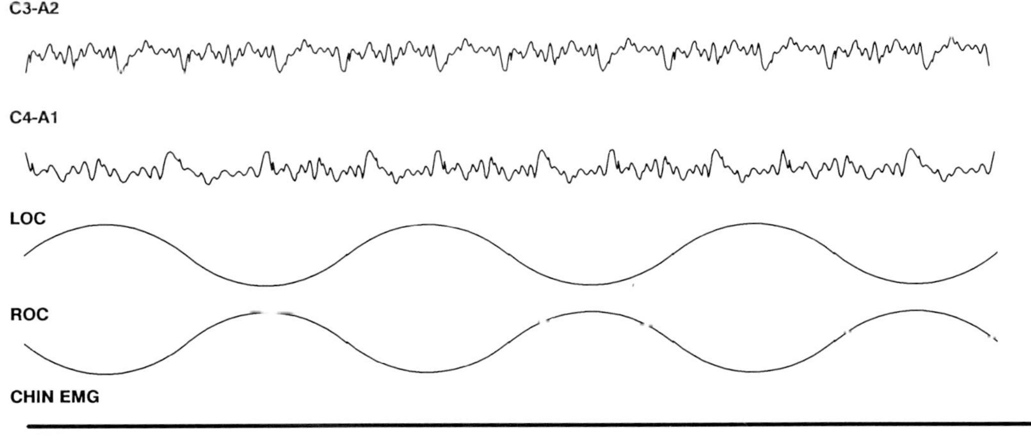

FIGURE 2–1. Stage 1 sleep. Stage 1 is characterized by relatively low-voltage, mixed-frequency EEG; slow, rolling eye movements; and tonic EMG activity.

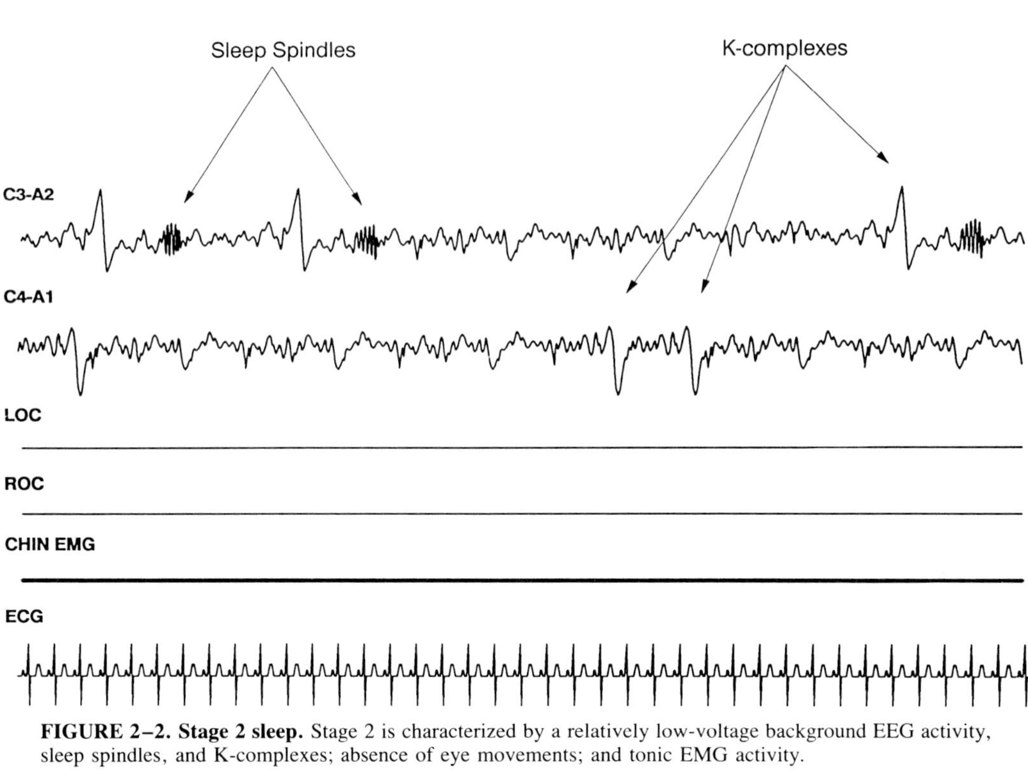

FIGURE 2–2. Stage 2 sleep. Stage 2 is characterized by a relatively low-voltage background EEG activity, sleep spindles, and K-complexes; absence of eye movements; and tonic EMG activity.

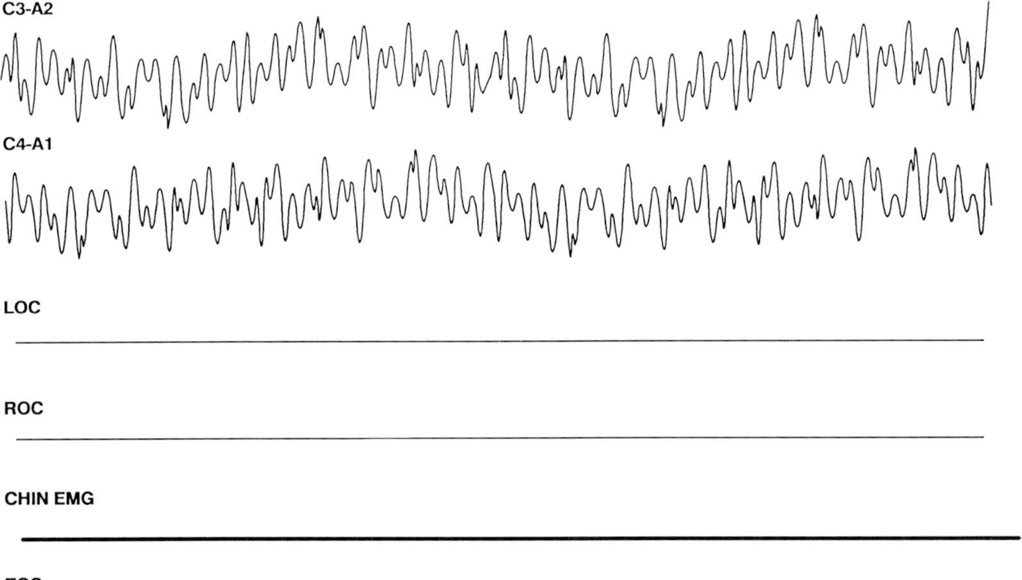

FIGURE 2–3. Stage 4 sleep. Stage 4 is characterized by high-voltage, slow-wave EEG activity; absence of eye movements; and tonic EMG activity.

4 is somewhat arbitrary, since physiological characteristics of Stage 3 and Stage 4 are almost identical. Stage 3 is relatively short, lasting only a few minutes during the first sleep cycle, and may be considered a transition stage to Stage 4. Stages 3 and 4 are often combined and termed *slow-wave sleep* (SWS). Arousal thresholds are considerably higher in SWS than in other sleep stages. During the first cycle of the sleep period, SWS lasts about 20 to 40 minutes and ends with a series of body movements followed by an arousal (ascent to a lighter or higher NREM stage).

The first REM period of the night typically occurs 70 to 100 minutes after sleep onset (Fig. 2–4). It is brief, lasting usually less than 10 minutes, and is often missed during the first night of recording in the laboratory. Arousal threshold is variable during REM sleep and is generally considered to be similar to that in Stage 2. Interestingly, if the stimulus for arousal during REM sleep is incorporated into dream content, it is less likely to result in arousal.

NREM sleep and REM sleep then cycle throughout the remainder of the sleep period at intervals of approximately 90 to 120 minutes (Fig. 2–5). SWS is most prominent early in the sleep period (first third to first half of the night) and decreases as the night progresses. REM periods, on the other hand, become longer and more intense throughout the sleep period, with the longest and most intense REM episode occurring in the early morning hours.

Although internal and external variability exists, volume of sleep stages across sleep periods is relatively constant. As shown in Figure 2–6, Stage 1 comprises 2% to 5%; Stage 2, 45% to 55%; SWS, 13% to 23%; and REM, approximately 20% to 25%. Wake after sleep onset accounts for less than 5%. Normally four to six cycles of sleep stages occur per night. Table 2–1 shows a comparison of sleep stages.

Newborns, Infants, and Children

Observation of newborns, infants, and children reveals that sleep occupies a major portion of their lives. A newborn infant spends approximately 70% of every 24 hours in this state. In contrast, adults spend 25% to 30% of their time sleeping. The major "work" of the waking child has been said to be play. Because sleep occupies such a large portion of a child's life, the major "work" of childhood is more likely sleep.

Characteristics of sleep in normal infants vary significantly from normal sleep in adults. Pre-

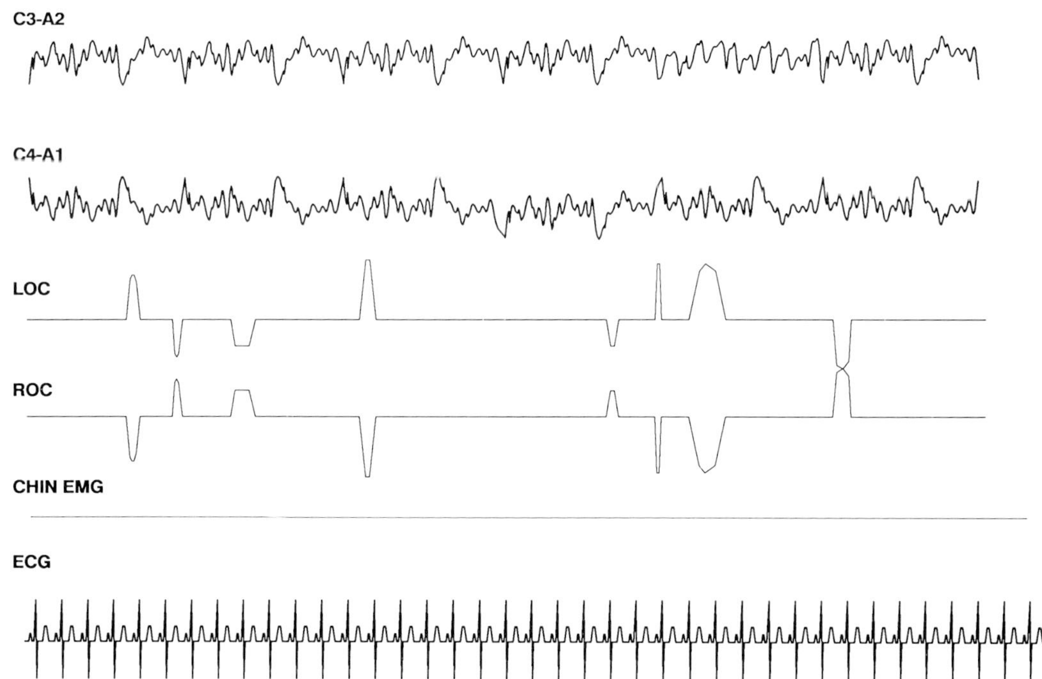

FIGURE 2–4. Stage REM sleep. REM sleep is characterized by a relatively low-voltage, mixed-frequency background EEG activity, with bursts of notched theta (sawtooth) waves; rapid, saccadic, conjugate eye movements; and chin muscle tone significantly decreased from waking and NREM levels.

TYPICAL SLEEP ARCHITECTURE
Across a Single Night's Sleep

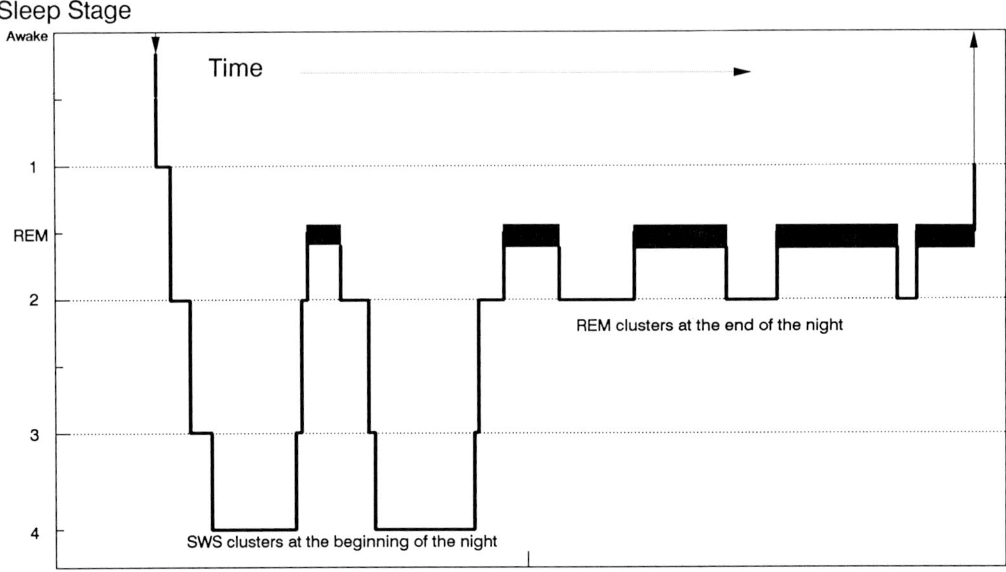

FIGURE 2–5. Typical progression of sleep stages across a single night's sleep in a healthy young adult. SWS tends to cluster during the early hours of the sleep period and decreases as the night progresses. REM sleep increases in volume throughout the night and clusters during the latter hours of the sleep period.

Normal Healthy Young Adult

Stage 2
Stage 1
Awake
REM
SWS

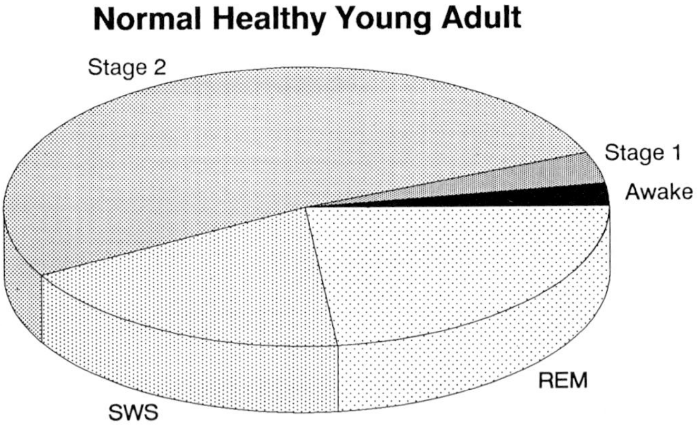

Stage	Percent of Total Recording Time
Wake after sleep onset	Less than 5%
Stage-1	2% to 5%
Stage-2	45% to 55%
Slow-wave Sleep	13% to 23%
REM	20% to 25%

FIGURE 2–6. Sleep stage volumes in normal healthy young adults.

TABLE 2–1. Comparison of Polysomnographic Characteristics of Stages of Sleep and Wake

	EEG	EOG	EMG	AROUSAL THRESHOLD
Awake	Alpha rhythm predominates, especially in occipital region	Clear saccadic eye movements present	Tonic	
Stage 1	RLVMF pattern; vertex sharp waves may appear	Slow, rolling eye movements present	Tonic	Altered perceptions of environment; arousal threshold weak; perception of not sleeping
Stage 2	RLVMF background; sleep spindles and K-complexes appear	No eye movements apparent	Tonic	Higher arousal stimulus required; threshold may be lower if meaning is added to stimulus
Stage 3	Slow waves comprise greater than 20% but less than 50% of 30-sec epoch	No eye movements apparent	Tonic	High arousal threshold; significant stimulus required for arousal to occur
Stage 4	Slow waves comprise greater than 50% of 30-sec epoch	No eye movements apparent	Tonic	High arousal threshold; significant stimulus required for arousal to occur
Stage REM	RLVMF background with notched theta (sawtooth) activity	Clear rapid and conjugate eye movements present	Hypotonic	Threshold similar to Stage 2; if stimulus is incorporated into dream content, arousal is less likely

EEG, Electroencephalogram; *EOG*, electrooculogram; *EMG*, electromyogram; RLVMF, relatively low-voltage, mixed-frequency.

mature infants exhibit a lack of concordance between electrophysiological parameters of sleep and behavioral variables. This may also be true in some term infants.[7,8] There has been significant lack of agreement regarding definitions of sleep and waking states in infants, since criteria recognized for adults often do not apply to infants. A number of investigators have suggested solutions to this problem. Prechtl and Beintema suggested state definition based on observable behaviors[9]; Anders, Emde, and Parmelee suggested utilization of behavioral and polygraphic features[10]; and Hoppenbrouwers suggested state definition based on polygraphic features, with observational criteria used only as supplemental information.[11] Despite intense debate regarding state definition, it is clear that sleep in infants and children differs significantly from that in adults and probably serves a different function.

FETUSES AND PREMATURE INFANTS

Rhythmical cycling of periods of activity and quiescence can be identified in the human fetus by 28 to 32 weeks of gestation.[7] Neither quiet nor active sleep can be identified in premature neonates between 24 and 26 weeks of gestation,[12] but by 28 to 30 weeks, active sleep can be identified by the presence of eye movements, body movements, and irregular respiratory movements. Chin muscle hypotonia is difficult to evaluate in fetuses and premature infants because few periods of tonic activity accur before 36 weeks of gestation.[7] Quiet sleep, on the other hand, cannot be clearly identified at this time and active sleep comprises most of the sleep period. Quiet sleep does not become significant until approximately 36 weeks of gestation,[7] but once present it continues to increase in volume until it becomes the dominant sleep state at approximately 3 months of postnatal life.

Spontaneous fetal movements can be identified at approximately 10 weeks of gestation, and rhythmical cycling of activity can be recorded in utero by 20 weeks.[13] At 28 to 30 weeks, brief quiet periods begin to appear, although their periodicity is unstable.[14] By 32 weeks' conceptual age, body movements are absent in 53% of 20-second epochs during 2- to 3-hour sleep recordings.[7] The number of no-movement epochs increases to 60% at term.

Maturational patterns are apparent in EEG recordings of normal premature infants as early as 24 weeks of gestation. Conflicting evidence exists concerning the independence of the maturation of sleep and the EEG with respect to intrauterine stage. Very young premature infants and full-term neonates have similar EEG patterns when compared at the same conceptual age. On the other hand, when the premature infant reaches 40 weeks' conceptual age, it still has not attained a degree of organization as high as that of the full-term newborn.[8] Premature infants show spindle development that is approximately 4 weeks in advance of that seen in full-term infants, and a statistical difference in length of quiet sleep exists between term and premature infants when measured at the same conceptual age.[15] Some conflict in reports, however, may be the result of differences in the definition and calculation of gestational age and conceptual age, or may be actual differences precipitated by development in an extrauterine environment significantly different from the normal intrauterine milieu. Extrauterine development of the premature infant occurs either in a 24-hour lighted environment or under cycled lights, rather than in the 24-hour darkness of the uterus. In addition, significantly preterm newborns often have significant medical and developmental problems that require continual medical interventions. The effect of constant light and frequent medical treatment on the development of the nervous system and sleep cycling has not yet been elucidated.

Term Infants: Birth to 12 Months

Three distinct sleep states can be identified in the term newborn: active sleep (REM), quiet sleep (NREM), and indeterminant sleep. Indeterminant sleep is defined as a state in which criteria for neither REM nor NREM can be identified.[10] Sucking movements are common during active sleep.[16] During this state fine twitches are almost continuous and grimaces, smiles, and tremors also occur. Intermittent large athetoid limb movements, stretching of the torso, and occasional vocalizations take place. Bursts of muscle movement and irregular respiration occur concomitantly with phasic eye movements. Quiet sleep, on the other hand, is characterized by minimal movement.[7] Muscle tone is increased above the level seen in active sleep.

During the first 3 months of life, striking changes occur in many physiological functions. Ten to 12 weeks of age appears to be a critical period of reorganization, when infantile sleep behavior and physiology shifts to a more mature form. Sleep-wake patterns change significantly. In a newborn infant, total sleep time is about 16 to 17 of 24 hours.[7] Total sleep time slowly decreases, reaching 14 to 15 hours by 16 weeks of age and 13 to 14 hours by 6 to 8 months of age (Fig. 2–7).

Development of attentive behaviors occurs concomitantly with the development of quiet sleep and sustained sleep patterns. These

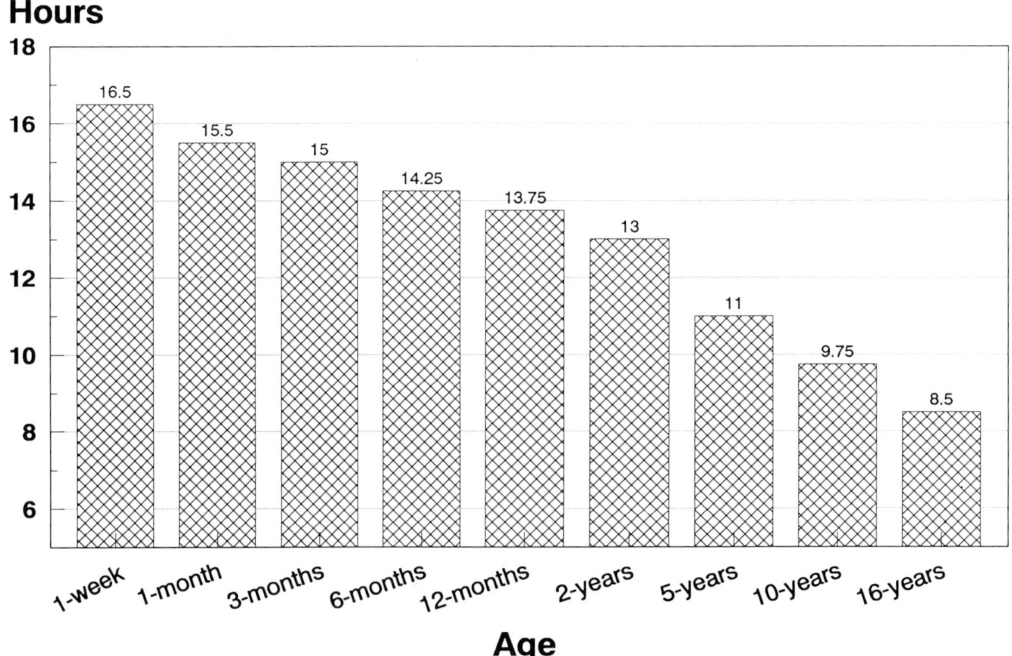

FIGURE 2–7. Total sleep time (per 24 hours clock time) across age groups. (Modified from Ferber R: Solve your child's sleep problems. New York, Simon & Schuster, 1985, p 19. Copyright © 1985 by Richard Ferber, M.D. Reprinted by permission of Simon & Schuster, Inc.)

changes suggest continued development of inhibitory and controlling feedback mechanisms secondary to the increasing complexity of neural networks and neurochemical maturation.[7] By 3 months of age, maturation of these systems produces a relatively stable diurnal distribution of sleep and wake. There is also a remarkably regular alternation of active and quiet sleep.[11] Before 3 months of age, concordance between physiological variables is remarkably high.[17] Sleep state organization appears to be "locked in." One explanation may be a lack of maturation of essential feedback control. A lack of variability is occasionally seen in cardiac function when the conductive tissue of the heart fails to respond to regulatory input, resulting in a fixed rate, with almost equal beat-to-beat intervals. Periodic respiration, common in NREM sleep until 3 weeks of age, becomes rare after 7 weeks.[18]

During the first 6 months of life, consolidation and entrainment of sleep at night develop. Major changes occur in the duration of single sleep periods and their placement in the 24-hour day (Fig. 2–8). Coons has impressively described this progression.[19] Her study revealed that at 3 weeks of age the mean length of the longest sleep period was 211.7 minutes, or 23.2% of the total sleep time during the 24-hour period. By 6 months of age the longest sleep period was 358 minutes, or 48% of the total sleep time. Between 3 weeks and 6 weeks sleep periods lengthened considerably, and by 6 weeks of age the longest sleep period was no longer randomly distributed throughout the day. At 3 months the pattern had become more consistent. Although sleep had begun to consolidate and establish its relation with the light-dark cycle by 6 weeks of age, the longest wake period was still randomly distributed at 3 months, becoming acceptably nonrandom at 4.5 months of age. Long sleep periods of 5 to 6 hours at 6 weeks of age gradually lengthen to 8 to 9 hours and shift to nighttime, so that a diurnal pattern is relatively well established by 12 to 16 weeks of age.[7] At 6 months of age the long sleep period immediately follows the longest wake period.[19] After 12 weeks of age the diurnal cycle continues to develop and daytime sleep becomes consolidated into well-defined daytime naps.[20] Waking patterns change only slightly in comparison with sleep patterns. Neonates awaken about every 4 hours and stay awake for 1 to 2 hours. The longest sustained wake period

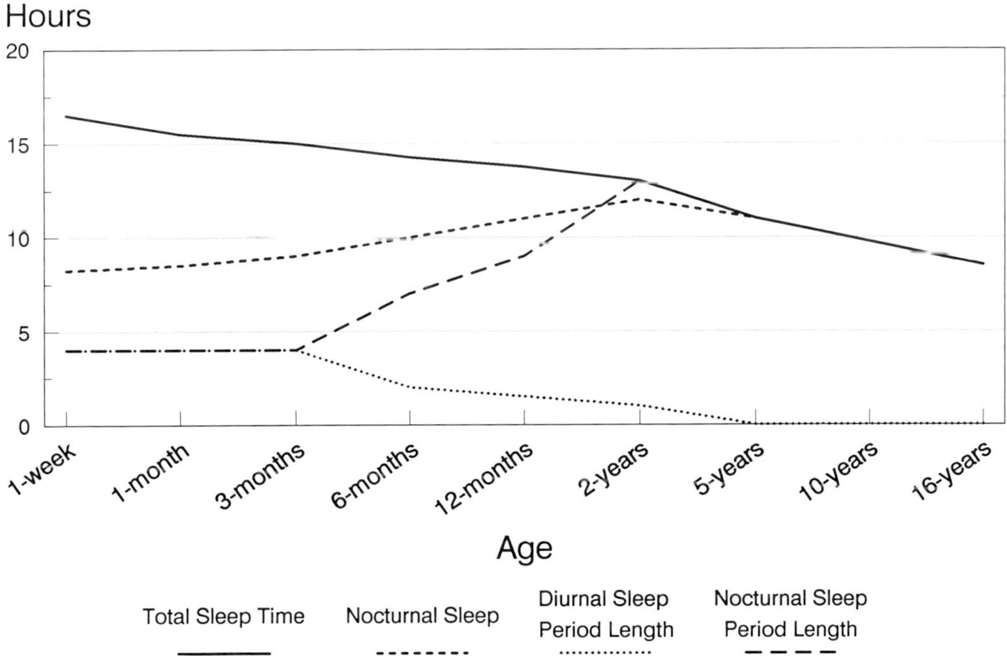

FIGURE 2–8. Development of the sleep-wake cycle in children. In infants sleep periods lengthen at night and shorten during the day until the longest sleep period appears at night at approximately 12 weeks of age. Total sleep time gradually decreases. Daytime sleep also decreases throughout the first 3 years of life, until the total sleep for 24 hours is consolidated into a single nocturnal sleep period.

increases slowly to 3 to 4 hours by 16 weeks of age.

Brief awakenings from sleep are more frequent during the first 2 months of life than at older ages.[11] In addition, infants 1 to 2 months of age are more likely to awaken from active sleep than from quiet sleep. Bowe and Anders reported that this variable helped discriminate between infant sleep at 2 and 9 months of age.[21] Good sleepers rarely woke from quiet sleep, whereas poor sleepers typically did. Sleep onset latencies in infants at 2 months were approximately 30 minutes. This was almost halved by 9 months of age. Anders and Keener have shown that 44% of 2-month-old infants and 78% of 9-month-old infants slept through the night.[22]

Striking changes occur in the EEG during this period of development. The *tracé alternant* pattern of quiet sleep can be first identified at 32 to 34 weeks of gestation.[23] This pattern is fully developed at 37 to 38 weeks, and mature neonates show this characteristic EEG pattern during quiet sleep (Fig. 2–9). Tracé alternant pattern gradually disappears over the first month of life. Sleep spindles appear almost simultaneously with the disappearance of tracé alternant pattern of quiet sleep at 4 to 6 weeks of age. Spindles are initially rudimentary, showing two spectral bands at 12 to 14 cps and 18 cps.[18] The 18 cps spindles disappear in approximately 7 days, but the 12 to 14 cps spindles remain. The shape of these spindles changes impressively early in development. At 2 months of age the spindles contrast so slightly with background EEG activity that no reliable measurements are possible.[24] Long spindles (lasting 1.8 to 3.4 seconds) are seen in the tracings of 3- to 4-month-old infants. This duration decreases continuously to an average of 0.5 to 0.7 second at the end of the second year. Spindle intervals become greater with increasing age, with a mean of 9 to 11 seconds at 6 months and 19 to 28 seconds at 24 months. After this time the spindle interval decreases with increasing age.

True slow waves with delta activity appear at approximately 8 to 12 weeks of age,[19] and quiet sleep becomes differentiated into four distinct stages, characteristic of the more mature electrophysiological pattern. At 3 months the proportion of quiet sleep is twice as great as active sleep.[15] By 8 months of age active sleep occupies approximately 30% of the total sleep time. After that age a continuous but significantly slower decline occurs until the adult volume is reached at approximately 5 years.[11]

Sleep onset is characteristically through REM

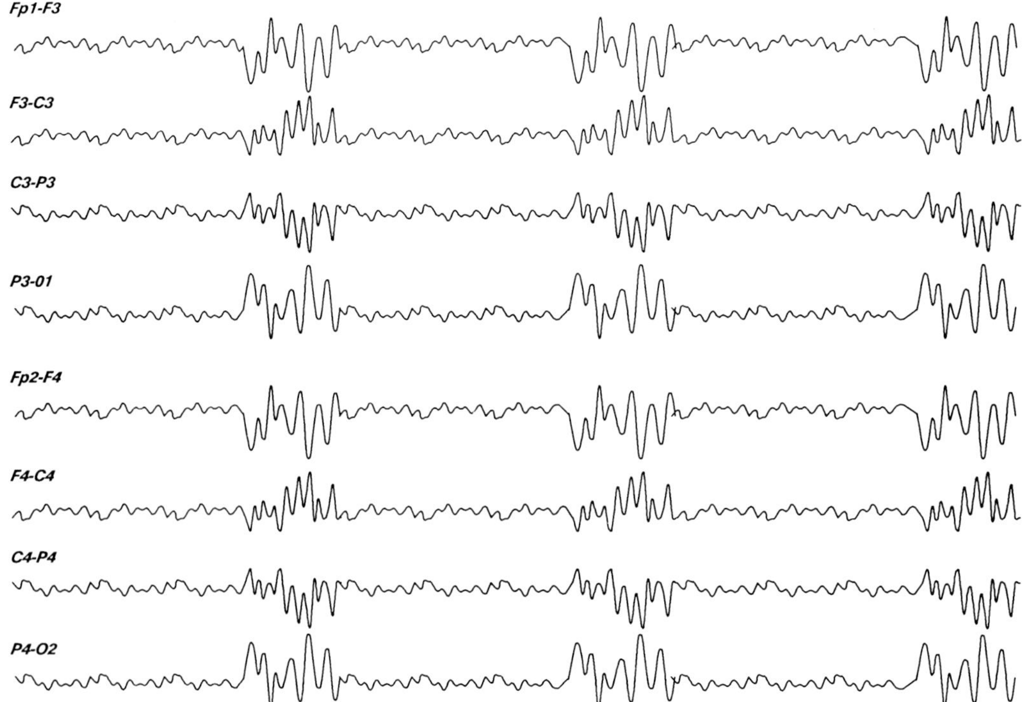

FIGURE 2–9. Schematic representation of tracé alternant EEG pattern in a 3-day-old infant. This EEG pattern is characteristic of quiet sleep during this period of development.

sleep in the newborn infant (i.e., the first REM period occurs within the first 15 minutes after sleep onset). During the first 12 weeks of life this gradually changes to sleep onset through NREM. At 3 weeks of age an infant is likely to have 64% of sleep periods beginning with REM sleep.[19] Younger infants (less than 3 months of age) manifest REM latencies that are predominantly shorter than 8 minutes.[25] Older infants produce a mixed distribution of short and long REM latencies. By 6 months the percentage of sleep onset REM periods (SOREMPs) is approximately 18%.[19] At 3 weeks of age the longest sleep period is as likely to have sleep onset through REM as through NREM. Between 4 and 13 months of age the total distribution of REM latencies appears to be bimodal, with latencies either shorter than 8 minutes or longer than 16 minutes.[25] Among older infants the temporal distribution of latencies constitutes a diurnal rhythm, with the longest latencies appearing between noon and 4 PM and a tendency of short latencies to occur between 4 AM and 8 AM hours. In the older infants REM latency also depends on the length of prior wakefulness. Long REM latencies are significantly more often preceded by long episodes of wakefulness than are short REM latencies. By 6 months of age the longest sleep period is only 20% more likely to be through REM.[19] The ratio of active sleep to quiet sleep is sometimes considered an indicator of maturation.[11] Active sleep time exceeds quiet sleep time during the first months of life. A reversal of this relationship is noted in 60% of infants at 3 months and 90% of infants at 6 months of age.

Specific changes in REM volume occur during the first year of life. During the first 6 months the total REM sleep volume decreases markedly. This represents a redistribution of sleep stages, since only a relatively small decrease in the total sleep time occurs during the first year. This change is considered an important indicator of central nervous system maturation.[15] Interestingly, the reduction in REM sleep is balanced by an increased proportion of the 24-hour day spent in wakefulness.

2 Years to 5 Years

Normative data and controlled studies of children in the preschool age group and in the early school years are surprisingly few. In contrast to the dramatic changes that take place during the first year of life, transformations during this period are more gradual. Growth and development continue in a steady manner. Sleep becomes consolidated into a long nocturnal period of approximately 10 hours.[26-29] During the first 2 to 3 years, daytime sleep continues but in discrete, short daytime naps. The first nap is usually in midmorning and the second early in the afternoon. Gradually the morning nap is given up, and by 3 to 5 years of age sleep is consolidated into a single nocturnal period.

During the latter half of the first year of life, REM sleep averages about 30% of the total sleep time. Small and large body movements associated with REM sleep during infancy become less frequent. REM periods are of approximately uniform length, despite daytime naps. As the child continues to develop, a gradual change is seen in the uniformity and duration of these REM periods. The first REM period of the night becomes quite short, whereas succeeding periods tend to become longer and more intense as morning approaches. The overall cycle length also increases slightly.[16] At 2 to 3 years of age children still show a cycle length of about 60 minutes, with the first REM period occurring 1 hour after sleep onset. By 4 to 5 years of age the cycle has lengthened gradually to 60 to 90 minutes. When monitoring in the laboratory, the first REM period, however, may be missed on the EEG in the younger age groups. In young children, after lightening of the EEG tracing occurs, it again deepens without an intervening REM period. Only after another cycle of about 60 to 90 minutes can the first REM period actually be documented.

Between 2 and 5 years of age, REM percentage gradually decreases from 30% of the total sleep time to the adult level of 20% to 25% (Fig. 2–10). These changes appear to be closely related to the augmented periods of wakefulness during the daytime. Diminution of REM volume progresses until about 3 to 4½ years when daytime napping has terminated. By this age, distinct differences between early and late portions of the sleep period have emerged.[16]

Typically children in this age range have approximately seven cycles during each nocturnal sleep period.[29] Sleep onset latency averages about 15 minutes in the younger children but lengthens to between 15 and 30 minutes in the older children in this developmental group. SWS predominantly occurs during the first third of the night,[28] and as much as 2 hours may be spent in Stages 3 and 4. EEG voltage is also high during this period. Stage 2 first appears from 3 to 4 minutes after the child falls to sleep, Stage 3 appears about 11 minutes after sleep onset, and Stage 4 appears about 4 minutes later.[29]

Unique characteristics of sleep occurring in

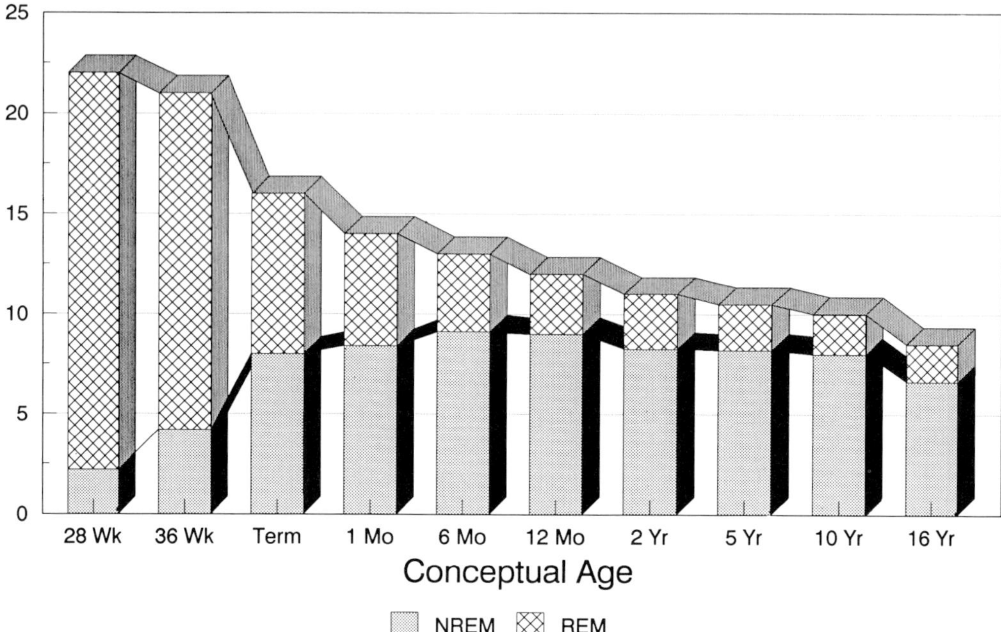

FIGURE 2–10. Ontogeny of REM and non-REM sleep. Total time spent in REM sleep decreases considerably throughout infancy and early childhood. By 3 to 5 years of age the adult level of about 25% of the total sleep time is reached.

this age range may signify stabilization and maturation of the sleep state. A relatively small number of sleep stage changes is a striking feature.[27] Approximately 3½ stage shifts per hour occur, which is significantly different from changes of the young adult; EEG voltage is consistently higher; and NREM Stage 4 is consistently longer. Another outstanding difference of sleep in this age group is the smooth progression of stages, whether moving deeper (toward Stage 4) or lighter (toward wake). Transition is regular and consistent, whereas adults often move abruptly across several stages at a time as the EEG progresses toward lighter or deeper sleep.[27,28]

5 TO 10 YEARS

Growth and development remain constant, steady, and gradual during middle childhood. This time, however, is not a latent period. It is characterized by activation and change, searching, exploring, and increasingly sophisticated decision making. It is a period of preparation and rehearsal, trials and errors.[30]

Sleep continues to coalesce into an adult pattern. Sleep patterns of children during middle childhood resemble those of older individuals. Although considerable individual variability exists, there is an orderly sequence of sleep stages, spontaneously shifting from one stage to another. Individuals have a certain stability of the pattern, and the amount of time spent in each sleep stage and the number of sleep stages are fairly consistent from night to night.[28] When compared with adult sleep patterns, total sleep time in middle childhood is approximately 2½ hours longer, with the added time unequally distributed among the sleep stages. Stages in children of this age group tend to be longer than in adults, but the sleep architecture seems to be as stable.

Middle childhood is also a time of transition. After an initially long NREM period, some children exhibit regularly spaced REM periods of similar duration (the pattern seen in infancy), while others reveal a more mature pattern of progressively longer REM periods as sleep progresses.[16] The volume of REM sleep approximates the adult level, which is considerably less than in infants and younger children.

Although body movements during sleep decrease in frequency, they are seen more often in this age group than in adolescents and young adults. Stage 4 volume decreases from approximately 2 hours in the preschool child to 75 to 80 minutes in the latter portion of middle childhood.[16] Males tend to exhibit a significantly greater volume of SWS than females of comparable age.[28,31,32]

Naps during this period of development are rare. The tendency to sleep during the day seems to be lowest in this age group, and consistent daytime napping during middle childhood often represents a pathological process. Prepubescent children are generally alert throughout the entire day. Carskadon and co-workers have shown mean sleep onset latencies of preadolescent (Tanner Stage 1) children to be greater than 15 minutes,[31,33] which is an extremely alert and vigilant level.

Adolescence

Gradual and consistent maturation during middle childhood gives way to a second period of rapid change during adolescence. Not since infancy are there such quantum leaps and striking changes in physical growth, hormonal alterations, and psychological, social, and cognitive development. Stability yields to the upheaval of navigating into adulthood. These dramatic changes are important in assessing sleep and sleep disorders of adolescents.

By early adolescence, electrophysiological variables of sleep have approximated normal young adult values (Fig. 2–6). Certain elements of less mature patterns may, however, be observed occasionally.[16] For example, body movements during sleep are usually at adult levels but at times may be as frequent as in younger children. Total REM volume is at adult levels, and REM periods clearly lengthen as the sleep period progresses. Stage 4 sleep time is at an adult level of approximately 45 to 60 minutes. Total sleep time decreases from 10 hours during middle childhood to approximately 8½ hours by 16 years of age.[34,35]

Carskadon, Dement, and co-workers have intensively studied sleep habits and sleep patterns of adolescents.[33,36,37] These observations have revealed a number of interesting trends in the sleep of teenagers. Significant differences can be seen in patterns between school nights and nonschool nights. Whereas total sleep time for children 10 years of age tends to be the same on school nights and nonschool nights (approximately 587 minutes), young adolescents sleep less on school nights than nonschool nights (522 minutes versus 560 minutes, respectively). Bedtimes and wake times are generally more controlled by outside influences on school nights. Limits are set by parents, homework, starting time of classes in the morning, and alarm clocks. These observations have led to the conclusion that sleep on nonschool nights is more natural than sleep on school nights and that the greater sleep time on nonschool nights reflects recovery from sleep deprivation during the week.

Observations by Webb and Agnew[38] and Williams and co-workers,[29] have revealed a continuous decrease in total sleep time through middle and late adolescence of approximately 2 hours. If this sleep restriction is cumulative, subjective and objective evidence of increased daytime sleepiness should appear. In fact, older adolescents report greater difficulty with daytime sleepiness and nocturnal sleep than do younger adolescents.[36] Among the methods used to assess sleepiness and alertness are pupillometry,[39,40] the Stanford Sleepiness Scale (a validated seven-point Likert scale measuring subjective sleepiness),[41,42] brainstem evoked potentials,[43] and the Multiple Sleep Latency Test (MSLT).[44,45] The MSLT, developed in the mid-1970s at the Stanford University Sleep Research Center, is the most widely used procedure for objective measurement of daytime sleep tendency. This test consists of a series of opportunities to sleep, administered at 2-hour intervals across a day using a standard procedure.[45] Sleepiness is measured as the speed of falling asleep (average sleep onset latency) across these nap opportunities. The presence of REM sleep during these naps is also noted. MSLT scores are related to a number of variables that range from the amount of sleep on one (or several) nights preceding the study[46-49] to pathological states such as narcolepsy.[50,51] An average sleep onset latency of less than 5 minutes was found to be associated with performance decrements and unintentional episodes of sleep.[45]

In a series of exquisite experiments by Carskadon and co-workers, manifest sleepiness during adolescence was dramatically demonstrated.[46-49] Twelve girls and fifteen boys were observed longitudinally over 7 years to determine sleep tendency changes during puberty. When subjects were given the opportunity to sleep for 10 hours, total sleep time did not vary significantly with adolescent maturational state and all groups slept for a little more than 9 hours per night. One conclusion drawn from these data was that *adolescents do not have a reduced need for sleep as they mature*. Time spent in REM sleep also remained constant between developmental stages in these subjects. SWS, on the other hand, decreased dramatically (by approximately 35%) between Tanner Stage 1 and Tanner Stage 5. A concomitant fall in the mean sleep onset latency occurred in midadolescence, indicating reduced daytime alertness despite a constant total sleep time. This finding also suggested that *sleep requirements do not decrease, and may in fact increase, as the adolescent ages.*

Time in bed and total sleep time decrease as the adolescent ages, resulting in a cumulative sleep debt. This sleep debt becomes significant during late adolescence and is accompanied by a continued fall in daytime alertness (as measured by the MSLT) to levels that are close to pathological.[49] The impact on daytime functioning may be significant. A number of normal adolescents therefore have significant disturbances in daytime alertness because of a normal pubertal increase in daytime sleepiness, as well as a cumulative or additive restriction of nocturnal sleep to meet expectations and obligations. Though there is considerable variability between individuals, many adolescents (particularly in the older age groups) have some degree of daytime impairment due to sleepiness.

REFERENCES

1. Agnew HW and Webb WB: Measurement of sleep onset by EEG criteria. Am J EEG Technol 1972;12:127.
2. Carskadon MA and Dement WC: Normal human sleep: an overview. In Kryger MH, Roth T, and Dement WC (eds): Principles and practice of sleep medicine. Philadelphia, WB Saunders, 1989.
3. Guilleminault C, Phillips R, and Dement WC: A syndrome of hypersomnia with automatic behavior. Electroencephalogr Clin Neurophysiol 1975;38:403.
4. Ogilvie RD and Wilkinson RT: The detection of sleep onset: behavioral and physiological convergence. Psychophysiology 1984;21:510.
5. Oswald I, Taylor AM, and Treisman M: Discriminative responses to stimulation during human sleep. Brain 1960;83:440.
6. Guilleminault C and Dement WC: Amnesia and disorders of excessive daytime sleepiness. In Drucker-Colin RR and McGaugh JL (eds): Neurobiology of sleep and memory. New York, Academic Press, 1977.
7. Parmelee AH and Stern E: Development of states in infants. In Clemente CD, Purpura DP, and Mayer FE (eds): Sleep and the maturing nervous system. New York, Academic Press, 1972.
8. Dreyfus-Brisac C: Ontogenesis of sleep in human prematures after 32 weeks of conceptual age. Dev Psychobiol 1970;3:91.
9. Prechtl HFR and Beintema D: The neurological examination of the full term newborn infant. In Clinics in developmental medicine, 12. London, Spastics Society and Heinemann, 1964.
10. Anders T, Emde R, and Parmelee AH (eds): A manual of standardized terminology, techniques and criteria for scoring of states of sleep and wakefulness in newborn infants. UCLA Brain Information Service, NINDS Neurological Information Network, Los Angeles, 1971.
11. Hoppenbrouwers T: Sleep in infants. In Guilleminault C: Sleep and its disorders in children. New York, Raven Press, 1987.
12. Dreyfus-Brisac C: Sleep ontogenesis in early human prematurity from 24 to 27 weeks of conceptual age. Dev Psychobiol 1968;1:62.
13. Sterman MB: The basic rest-activity cycle and sleep: developmental considerations in man and cats. In Clemente CD, Purpura DP, and Mayer FE (eds): Sleep and the maturing nervous system. New York, Academic Press, 1972.
14. Dreyfus-Brisac C: Ontogenèse du sommeil chez le premature humain: étude polygraphique. In Minokowski A (ed): Regional development of the brain in early life. Oxford, Eng, Blackwell, 1967.
15. Stern E et al: Sleep cycle characteristics in infants. Pediatrics 1969;43:65.
16. Roffwarg HP, Dement WC, and Fisher C: Preliminary observations of the sleep-dream pattern in neonates, infants, children, and adults. In Harms E (ed): Problems of sleep and dreams in children. New York, Macmillan, 1964.
17. Harper RM et al: Development of ultradian periodicity and coalescence at 1 cycle per hour in electroencephalographic activity. Exp Neurol 1981;73:127.
18. Metcalf D: The ontogenesis of sleep-awake states from birth to 3 months. Electroencephalogr Clin Neurophysiol 1979;28:421.
19. Coons S: Development of sleep and wakefulness during the first 6 months of life. In Guilleminault C (ed): Sleep and its disorders in children. New York, Raven Press, 1987.
20. Parmelee A et al: Infant sleep patterns from birth to 16 weeks of age. J Pediatr 1964;65:576.
21. Bowe TR and Anders TF: The use of semi-Markof model in the study of the development of sleep-wake states in infants. Psychophysiology 1979;16:41.
22. Anders TF and Keener M: Developmental course of nighttime sleep-wake patterns in full term and premature infants during the first years of life. Sleep 1985;8:173.
23. Nolte R et al: The "tracé alternant" of the sleeping EEG in full-term premature and hypotrophic neonates. Electroencephalogr Clin Neurophysiol 1969;27:625.
24. Lenard HG: The development of sleep spindles during the first two years of life. Electroencephalogr Clin Neurophysiol 1970;29:217.
25. Schulz H et al: REM latency: development in the first year of life. Electroencephalogr Clin Neurophysiol 1983;56:316.
26. Mattison RE, Handford HA, and Vela-Bueno A: Sleep disorders in children. Psychiatr Med 1987;4:149.
27. Kohler WC, Coddington D, and Agnew HW: Sleep patterns in 2-year-old children. J Pediatr 1968;72:228.
28. Ross JJ et al: Sleep patterns in pre-adolescent children: an EEG-EOG study. Pediatrics 1968;42:324.
29. Williams RL, Karacan I, and Hursch CJ: Electroencephalography (EEG) of human sleep: clinical applications. New York, Wiley, 1975.
30. Levine ME: Middle childhood. In Levine ME et al (eds): Developmental-behavioral pediatrics. Philadelphia, WB Saunders, 1983.
31. Carskadon MA, Keenan S, and Dement WC: Nighttime sleep and daytime sleep tendency in preadolescents. In Guilleminault C (ed): Sleep and its disorders in children. New York, Raven Press, 1987.
32. Coble PA et al: EEG sleep of normal healthy children.

I. Findings using standard measurement methods. Sleep 1984;7:289.

33. Carskadon MA et al: Pubertal changes in daytime sleepiness. Sleep 1980;2:453.
34. Ames LB: Sleep and dreams in childhood. In Harms E (ed): Problems of sleep and dreams in children. New York, Macmillan, 1964.
35. Carskadon MA: The second decade. In Guilleminault C (ed): Sleeping and waking disorders: indications and techniques. Boston, Butterworths, 1982.
36. Carskadon MA and Dement WC: Sleepiness in the normal adolescent. In Guilleminault C (ed): Sleep and its disorders in children. New York, Raven Press, 1987.
37. Carskadon MA, Orav EJ, and Dement WC: Evolution of sleep and daytime sleepiness in adolescents. In Guilleminault C and Lugaresi E (eds): Sleep/wake disorders: natural history, epidemiology, and long-term evolution. New York, Raven Press, 1983.
38. Webb WB and Agnew HW: Sleep and dreams. Dubuque, Ia, William C Brown, 1973.
39. Lowenstein O and Loewenfeld IE: Electronic pupillography—a new instrument and some clinical applications. Arch Ophthalmol 1958;59:352.
40. Lowenstein O, Feinberg R, and Loewenfeld IE: Pupullary movements during acute and chronic fatigue: a new test for the objective evaluation of tiredness. Invest Ophthalmol 1963;2:138.
41. Hoddes E, Dement W, and Zarcone V: The development and use of the Stanford Sleepiness Scale (SSS). Psychophysiology 1972;9:150.
42. Herscovitch J and Broughton R: Sensitivity of the Stanford Sleepiness Scale to the effects of cumulative partial sleep deprivation and recovery oversleeping. Sleep 1981;4:83.
43. Broughton R: Performance and evoked potential measures of various states of daytime sleepiness. Sleep 1982;5:S135.
44. Carskadon MA and Dement WC: Sleep tendency: an objective measure of sleep loss. Sleep Res 1977;6:200.
45. Carskadon MA et al: Guidelines for the Multiple Sleep Latency Test (MSLT): a standard measure of sleepiness. Sleep 1986;9:519.
46. Carskadon MA and Dement WC: Effects of total sleep loss on sleep tendency. Percept Mot Skills 1979;48:495.
47. Carskadon MA, Harvey K, and Dement WC: Acute restriction of nocturnal sleep in children. Percept Mot Skills 1981;53:103.
48. Carskadon MA, Harvey K, and Dement WC: Sleep loss in young adolescents. Sleep 1981;4:299.
49. Carskadon MA and Dement WC: Cumulative effects of sleep restriction on daytime sleepiness. Psychophysiology 1981;18:107.
50. Guilleminault C, Dement WC, and Passouant P: Narcolepsy. In Weitzman ED (ed): Advances in sleep research, vol 3. New York, Spectrum, 1976.
51. Wilson R et al: REM latencies in daytime sleep recordings of narcoleptics. Sleep Res 1972;2:166.

3

Sleep, Wake, and Chronobiological Considerations

A striking characteristic of all nucleated organisms involves the cycling of physical and biological processes in a predictably recurring fashion. Although on the surface these rhythms appear simple and linked to the light-dark cycle, complex mechanisms inherently control these patterns. Over 200 years ago deMairan observed activity of plant blossoms opening and closing independent of the light-dark cycle.[1] In a series of exquisite observations he showed that plant leaves continued their predictable movement despite being placed in a box under 24-hour dark conditions. These observations led to the conclusion that daily sequencing of many biological activities does not depend on exposure to the day-night cycle. Aschoff has described over 100 biological rhythms that cycle in a circadian manner.[2] Rhythmical fluctuations affect the function of all biological processes from cellular activity to mental alertness and human behavior, provide a temporal niche for protection of the organism, and permit the organism to perform certain vital functions.

Comprehension of biological rhythms is of great importance in understanding health maintenance and disease processes. Recent evidence has shown that strokes and myocardial infarctions tend to occur in the morning, during sleep or just a few hours after awakening.[3,4] The median lethal dose (LD50) of medications varies over the course of 24 hours.[5] In addition, biological clocks may be reset by certain medications resulting in a phase delay or a phase advance or having no effect depending on the phase of the circadian cycle in which they are ingested.[6] Methylxanthines such as theophylline and caffeine, as well as alcohol, are effective in this regard.

Human performance is also affected significantly by circadian phases. Alterations in work efficiency and somatic symptoms accompany rapid sleep-wake phase shifts.[7,8] Delays may occur in the reestablishment of normal sleep patterns, indicating the possible importance of correlating sleep-wake cycles and sleep stage changes to specific work-rest cycle rotations. Bonnet has reported that significant memory loss may occur during brief awakenings from sleep.[9] Both short-term and long-term memory are significantly less when subjects are awakened from Stage 4 sleep than with awakenings from Stage 2 sleep. When learning occurs immediately after a person is awakened, significant loss of information also occurs. When subjects are permitted to remain awake for at least 8 minutes, learning significantly improves and is not different from information retention after a longer period of wake. Busby and Broughton studied the waking ultradian rhythms in visual performance and in motility in groups of non-medicated hyperkinetic children.[10] With regard to ultradian rhythmicity, some subjects showed clear ultradian peaks in performance, which were present across a wide range of frequencies in one or more variables. It seems therefore that a comprehensive appreciation of circadian rhythms and their effect on behavior, performance, and health is important for child health care professionals.

POLYPHASIC NATURE OF THE SLEEP-WAKE CYCLE

In 1975 Broughton proposed a circasemidian (approximately 12 hours) sleep-wake biorhythm.[11] He suggested that two sleep periods exist, a major period at night and a minor period in the midafternoon. He also proposed that this 12-hour sleep tendency was a reflection of a bimodal rhythm of slow-wave sleep. Evidence for this bimodal sleep tendency has been documented by many independent studies.[12]

Children generally give up naps by age 5 years. The last nap that is abandoned generally occurs in the afternoon, and sleep becomes monophasic by the time school is entered.[13] Naps taken by adults generally occur at times similar to those taken by preschool children, most often midday, and approximately 12 hours from midnocturnal sleep.[14] Objective sleepiness when measured by the Multiple Sleep Latency Test (MSLT) reveals a significant decrease in the mean sleep onset latency during the midafternoon period.[15] Indeed, sleep onset latency during this afternoon period is almost as short as the time it takes to return to sleep in the middle of the night. This increase in sleep tendency is demonstrable even in the presence of altered sleep-wake schedules, as in individuals on shift work.[16] In addition, the well-known after lunch dip of performance has been shown to occur in almost all individuals,[17] is exacerbated by prior sleep loss, and appears to be related more to time of day than to food intake.[18] This postprandial somnolence is expressed in some cultures by a midafternoon siesta.[19] The siesta naptime may be a societal or cultural response to the normal circasemidian sleep-wake rhythm of the known decreased work performance at these times.[20,21]

Occupational and automotive accidents attributable to sleepiness occur at times similar to the proposed circasemidian sleep tendency (middle of the night and 12 hours later at midday).[22] In fact, the timing of all these accidental deaths clusters about the midnight and secondary midafternoon peaks.[23] Patients with disorders of excessive somnolence (e.g., patients with narcolepsy, sleep apnea, and idiopathic central nervous sytem hypersomnia; see Chapter 8) also show midafternoon privileged periods for sleep. These observations clearly show that a circasemidian sleep-wake rhythm is as powerful as the circadian rhythm and is most likely stronger than an ultradian waking rhythm.

Although sleep tendency appears to occur in a circasemidian pattern, the converse, a circasemidian rhythm of wakefulness, may take priority.[24] Since sleep can be consciously suppressed by an increased state of arousal, wakefulness most likely holds a hierarchical priority position. Sleep cannot suppress wakefulness to a similar extent except in certain pathological states. Essential functions of wakefulness are clear. Broughton proclaims that "it makes greater biological sense that the brain be programmed for two daily prolonged periods of wakefulness than for two of sleep."

Because of consolidation of sleep and wake into single long periods within the 24-hour light-dark cycle, it has been assumed in the past that sleep was a unitary event. Studies had emphasized the temporal relationship of the sleep-wake cycle to other rhythmical physiological and chemical operations.[25] More recent data, however, refute this assumption and clearly show that the sleep period is composed of recurring short-term physiological events characterized by a sequence of four to five regularly recurring 90-minute cycles.[26,27] A daytime ultradian variation in sleepiness with a periodicity of approximately 90 minutes was predicted by Kleitman's basic rest activity cycle (BRAC) hypothesis.[13,28,29] Evidence is growing that the sleep-wake cycle itself is polyphasic and ultradian in nature rather than circadian. The monophasic nature of sleep in our society therefore appears to be purely social in origin.[24]

Evidence exists for sleep-wake biorhythms of periods falling between 12 hours and 1½ hours, with clusters around periods of approximately 3 and 6 hours.[24] This polyphasic nature of the sleep-wake cycle is prominently exemplified during infancy. Newborns and young infants who are fed on demand display a remarkably stable sleep-wake rhythm with a period lasting 3 to 4 hours.[13,30] Strikingly similar periods of sleep probability have been found in adult subjects recorded for 24 hours under continuous bed rest conditions.[31] Further support was provided by Zulley, who described an approximately 4-hour rhythmicity of sleep in the disentrained state[32] and some evidence that slow-wave sleep exhibits a periodicity of 3 to 4 hours.[33] Significant evidence supports the existence of this ultradian rhythm throughout the 24-hour day, manifested by alterations in non–rapid eye movement (NREM) and REM states during sleep and in somnolence and alertness during wakefulness.[24]

CENTRAL CONTROL OF BIOLOGICAL RHYTHMS: THE SUPRACHIASMATIC NUCLEI

Rhythmical biological phenomena with periods ranging from 1½ hours to about 24 hours persist in the absence of external environmental periodicities.[34] An inherent "clock" exists at the cellular level, endogenously regulating the waxing and waning of various physiological events.[35] Most human behavioral and physiological processes reveal a temporal structure that matches the 24-hour light-dark cycle. This 24-hour time frame confines a wide variety of functions, from endocrine secretions and temperature regulation to sensory processing and cognitive performance.[1] Persistence of cycling of these functions under constant conditions suggests internal generation rather than a passive response to exogenous stimuli. Rhythms appear to be generated by one or more master oscillating clocks, located in the central nervous system and synchronized by various environmental time cues called *zeitgebers* (literal translation "time givers").

The first concerted effort to identify the location of the primary circadian pacemaker in mammals was conducted by Richter[36] in a series of experiments involving creation of lesions and dissections of various organ systems. Circadian rhythms were preserved after removal of endocrine tissues and focal destruction of numerous areas of the central nervous system. These rhythms, however, were abolished when large lesions were placed ventromedially in the hypothalamus. In simultaneous experiments Moore and Eichler[37] and Stephan and Zucker[38] identified a loss of circadian rhythmicity in rats after bilateral ablation of the suprachiasmatic nuclei (SCN) of the hypothalamus. It was proposed from these data that the SCN represented a primary biological clock. Subsequent experimental work sought to test the hypothesis that the SCN acted autonomously as a circadian pacemaker. Inouye and Kawamura simultaneously recorded multiple unit activity from two sites in the brains of rats, one at or near the SCN and the second in one of many other central nervous system locations.[39] Initially both sites displayed clear circadian rhythmicity. After dissection creating an "island" of hypothalamus containing the SCN, and ocular enucleation to remove visual stimuli, circadian rhythmicity was lost at all brain locations outside the island but persisted within the isolated tissue that contained the SCN. Inouye and Kawamura concluded that rhythmicity of this island was independent of afferent inputs from elsewhere in the brain. Rusak and Groos showed that stimulation of the SCN altered the period and phase of the circadian rhythms of feeding and locomotor activity in experimental animals.[40] Evidence implicating the suprachiasmatic nuclei as the biological pacemaker is compelling. In addition to abolition of the circadian rhythms of drinking and locomotor activity, rhythmical activity of other physiological activities is eradicated after destruction of the SCN, including (but not limited to) adrenal corticosterone secretion,[37] pineal serotonin *N*-acetyltransferase activity,[41] photoperiodic gonadal response,[42] and the sleep-wakefulness cycle.[43]

The SCN are dorsal to the optic chiasm and lateral to the third ventricle in the rat and hamster. They consist of small, densely packed neurons subdivided into at least three separate regions.[44] The existence of the SCN in humans has only recently been discovered.[45] The presence of a single master biological clock, however, has come into question. Two independent pacemakers, designated X and Y, were proposed by Moore-Ede in 1983.[46] According to this theory, the SCN function as the Y oscillator and are the controlling center for such physiological processes as growth hormone secretion, urine calcium excretion, skin temperature, and the sleep-wake cycle.[47] This oscillator is relatively labile (the weaker of the two major oscillators), and its control of processes varies considerably during *free-running* (the natural endogenous period of a biological rhythm when time cues are removed) conditions. The location of the X oscillator is as yet unknown but is probably outside the SCN.[46] The X oscillator appears to control core body temperature, plasma cortisol levels, urine excretion of potassium, and REM sleep. It is highly stable (when compared with the Y oscillator), and under free-running conditions these physiological rhythms cycle in a manner similar to the normal entrained state. These two main oscillating systems are coupled under normal entrained conditions but can function independently. It is postulated that the X and Y pacemakers control secondary oscillators in a multioscillator system.

Existence of two circadian clocks is supported by animal experiments. Pickard and Turek made unilateral lesions of the paired SCN in hamsters maintained in constant light conditions.[48] Before surgery, circadian rhythm of locomotor activity was dissociated into two distinct components. Following destruction of 50% to 100% of a single SCN, a single bout of activity returned. Lesions affecting less than 50% of the unilateral SCN did not abolish the dissociated pattern of two periods of activity. Bilateral destruction eliminated the circadian pattern of activity in all animals under both dissociated and consolidated conditions. Pickard and Turek concluded that these data demonstrated that each SCN is capable of maintaining circadian rhythmicity by itself and that at least two circadian oscillators (or systems) exist within the SCN.

Pathways by which environmental influences affect biological cycles and physiological rhythms have been elusive. Autoradiographic studies have identified a retinal projection exiting the optic chiasm and terminating in the SCN.[49] These connections of the SCN to the retina are separate from the primary visual pathway[50] and are termed the *retinohypothalamic tract* (RHT). Transection accomplished by ablation of the SCN has the dramatic effect of eliminating circadian rhythms altogether.[37,38]

The functional role of the direct and indirect retinal afferents to the SCN in the entrainment process has been difficult to evaluate. The SCN receives primary and secondary photic input via the RHT and a *geniculohypothalamic tract* originating from the retinorecepient neurons in and near the intrageniculate leaflet of the lateral geniculate nucleus.[51] The RHT alone, however, appears sufficient to mediate entrainment.[52] Bilateral lateral geniculate nucleus lesions destroying the intrageniculate leaflet in animals do not eliminate entrainment.

Secondary oscillators exist outside the SCN, but how the SCN communicates with these oscillators and directly driven processes is relatively unknown.[1] Hormones may have a coupling or modulating influence. A hierarchy of oscillators appears to be present. The circadian system of oscillators appears to be present. The circadian system is exquisitely sensitive to photic cues from the environment and probably directly influences the dominant pacemaker. Other cues, however, may exert significant effects on the system by directly or indirectly influencing other elements of the multioscillatory system.

SYNCHRONIZATION OF BIOLOGICAL FUNCTIONS AND PACEMAKER RHYTHMS

Entrainment of biological rhythms to a particular cycle is influenced by environmental cues, the most recognizable of which is the light-dark cycle. Environmental cues tend to regulate, couple, and set the phase relation between organism and environment.[53] In the entrained state, sleep has a fairly precise 24-hour periodicity. Entrainment to this circadian cycle is directly related to the timing of morning waking by available zeitgebers, and to a lesser extent by the timing of going to bed.

Core body temperature shows a rhythm parallel to the sleep-wake cycle. It peaks in the early to middle evening, begins to fall approximately 1 to 1½ hours before sleep onset, reaches its nadir during the last third of the sleep period, begins to rise about 30 minutes to 2 hours before waking, and increases throughout the day to the next evening maximum.[24] This temperature rhythm is extremely stable and is considered to be the best marker of human circadian rhythms.[47] The length of sleep, as well as its internal structure, seems to depend primarily on the phase of the averaged temperature cycle.[54] In free-running subjects, bedtime is most frequently chosen just after the nadir of the temperature cycle.[55]

In the absence of zeitgebers, rhythms free run and demonstrate a persistent periodicity. This supports the presence of a biological clock controlling these events. These rhythms, however, are not necessarily the same as the normal entrained rhythm.[56] Without environmental cues most individuals operate on a greater than 24-hour day. Although the sleep-wake rhythm is normally highly correlated with body temperature, in the absence of zeitgebers they become dissociated (uncoupled) and seem to be controlled by different clocks.[53]

Environmental cues regulate or set the phase relationship between independent rhythms. Synchronization of the human circadian system to a 24-hour day therefore implies that the biological clocks are reset daily. These clocks must adjust their periods in each cycle to compensate for the difference between their intrinsic periods and the 24-hour light-dark cycle and become coupled so that overt rhythms occur at the appropriate daily phases.[1]

Light appears to be a universal zeitgeber for the circadian rest-activity cycle. Human circadian rhythms, however, were once thought to be insensitive to light stimuli, with synchronization to the 24-hour day accomplished through social contacts or the sleep-wake schedule. The demonstration of an intensity-dependent neuroendocrine response to bright light led to renewed consideration of light as the synchronizer of the human circadian pacemaker. In 1986 Czeisler documented that simple bright light exposure resets the human circadian pacemaker independent of the timing of the sleep-wake cycle.[57] Exposure to bright light in the evening for a period of 4 hours over seven consecutive evenings resulted in a 6-hour delay shift of a laboratory subject's circadian pacemaker, as indicated by continuous recordings of body temperature and cortisol secretion. The magnitude, rapidity, and stability of the shift were unexpected and suggest that exposure to bright light can indeed reset the human circadian pacemaker controlling variations in physiological, behavioral, and cognitive function. A hierarchical model exists in which the external light-dark cycle ordinarily synchronizes the endogenous circadian oscillator, which in turn governs the internal organization and spontaneous duration of sleep.[58] Environmental factors may act together or separately on a given physiological variable. Lewy and co-workers have shown that high-intensity artificial light (as well as sunlight) suppresses melatonin secretion, which suggests a possible role for sunlight to entrain human circadian and circannual rhythms.[59] As previously discussed, the complex mechanism by which light effects circadian rhythmicity and couples it to the external 24-hour periodicity of ambient light is mediated from receptors in the retina via the RHT to the SCN. Congenitally blind or enucleated mammals are virtually unresponsive to light-dark cycles.

There is ample evidence that prolonged exposure to light throughout the day is not necessary for photic entrainment of biological rhythms. Brief exposures to light at dawn and dusk may fully account for entrainment.[60] Stable entrainment of rhythms under "skeleton" photoperiods has been documented in several species of animals. An organism can be entrained to a photoperiod normally lasting about 8 to 16 hours with brief pulses of light at two circadian phases corresponding to normal dawn and dusk.[61] In the free-running state, brief light pulses cause phase shifts of rhythms, the magnitude and direction of which depend on the time within the circadian cycle at which the light pulse is presented.[62] In nocturnal animals light pulses presented at the beginning of the daily active period produce phase delays, whereas pulses presented toward the end of the active period produce phase advances. During most of the rest period, light pulses have little effect, which results in a so-called dead zone on a phase response curve. The shape of the phase response curve for light pulses for these experimental animals suggests that entrainment may be accomplished by a combination of phase delays and advances, producing a net daily shift equal to the difference between the period of an oscillator and 24 hours.

The intrinsic period of an oscillator and its phase response characteristics should determine whether it will entrain to a light-dark cycle of a given periodicity.[1] Entrainment occurs only when the difference between the intrinsic period of the oscillator and the extrinsic cycle does not exceed the maximal phase shift that can be induced by light. However, limits of entrainment appear somewhat flexible. It has been shown that individuals can be entrained only to periods approximating 24 hours. The *range of entrainment* is approximately 22 to 26 hours, depending on the strength of the zeitgeber. Beyond this range the individual is out of synchrony with the demands of the environment.[53] The dichotomy between "night owls" and "morning larks" probably reflects individual differences in the intrinsic periodicities of the circadian clocks.[1]

Environmental stimuli may have diverse effects on rhythmical physiological and behavorial processes. Certain rhythms may become entrained while intrinsic rhythms may be masked. Mistlberger and Rusak have described criteria for distinguishing masking from entrainment.[1] An entrained rhythm should follow an environmental cycle over a limited range of periods; the phase relationship between an entrained rhythm and an environmental cycle should vary depending on their periods; the phase relationship should be reestablished if the environmental cycle is abruptly shifted; the rhythm should persist in the absence of the periodic stimulus; and the initial phase of the free run should reflect the apparent phase of the rhythm during entrainment.

A hierarchical model exists in which the external light-dark cycle synchronizes the endogenous oscillator.[53] The oscillator then regulates the timing and duration of the sleep-wake cycle.

Certain nonphotic stimuli also appear to entrain rather than mask rhythms. These include food,[63] environmental temperature,[64] state of arousal,[65] and specific social cues.[66]

UNCOUPLING AND DESYNCHRONIZATION OF BIOLOGICAL RHYTHMS

Studies of various physiological cycles have relied on uncoupling rhythms and observing them in the free-running state. Without zeitgebers, internal desynchronization occurs.[67] This is dramatically exemplified by changes in the sleep-wake cycle and core temperature during free-running states. The typical free-running sleep-wake cycle and core body temperature experience a shift in cycle length with a mean period duration of 25.1 hours.[55,68] In a group of subjects studied by Czeisler and associates, the free-running non-24-hour rhythms of sleep-wake, body temperature, and neuroendocrine cycles remained internally synchronized with nearly identical periods, although their wave shapes and phase relationships were different from those during entrainment to a 24-hour day.[55] The duration of polygraphically recorded sleep episodes was highly correlated with the circadian phase of the body temperature rhythm at bedtime and not with the length of prior wakefulness. The rate of REM sleep accumulation, REM latency, bedtime selection, and self-rated alertness assessments were also correlated with the body temperature rhythm. Not only was the sleep length dependent primarily on its phase within the averaged temperature cycle, but also Czeisler and co-workers found that all free-running subjects chose to go to bed at certain phases of that temperature cycle much more frequently than at others. The greatest bedtime frequency was just after the circadian temperature cycle minimum, corresponding to the nadir of the subjective alertness assessment curve.

After a while in the free-running state, the sleep-wake cycle lengthens and in most subjects reaches an extraordinary duration of up to 50 hours. On the other hand, the temperature cycle remains remarkably stable at about 25 hours, regardless of the sleep-wake cycle length. Miles and co-workers studied the circadian rhythms of a blind individual who lived and worked in normal society and suffered from a severe cyclical sleep-wake disorder.[69] Investigations showed that he had circadian rhythms of body temperature, alertness, performance, cortisol secretion, and urinary electrolyte excretion that were desynchronized from the 24-hour societal schedule. These rhythms all had periods longer than 24 hours and indistinguishable from the period of the lunar day.

ORGANIZATION AND COUPLING OF SLEEP STAGES: INTERNAL ORGANIZATION

Although sleep is consolidated into an apparently unitary event, temporal isolation experiments and numerous observations of displaced sleep periods have clearly shown that the various components of sleep are controlled by different oscillators. In the free-running state, sleep organization becomes desynchronized. REM sleep advances to an earlier period of the night, the REM latency decreases significantly, and an increased volume of REM sleep is noted in the first 3 hours of the sleep period.[53] Although the total amount of REM sleep increases early in the sleep period, the total volume for the entire sleep period remains constant. REM sleep tends to occur preferentially during a specific phase of the circadian temperature cycle. The distribution of slow-wave sleep remains essentially the same.

DeKoninck and co-workers evaluated the timing of REM onset episodes in narcoleptic subjects to evaluate rhythms that appear to govern REM episodes.[70] They observed that the number of night cycles falling within a projected grid occurred significantly higher than chance, indicating that nighttime REM episodes tended to fall within the same periodicity as their preceding daytime episodes. This observation supports the hypothesis that an underlying basic rest-activity cycle governs REM sleep episodes in narcoleptic subjects.

Sleep, when it occurs at times out of phase with the normal nocturnal sleep period, shows different internal organization. When the sleep period is shifted 180 degrees out of phase, three specific effects are seen: (1) the proportion of time spent in certain sleep stages alters; (2) hourly distribution of certain stages within the sleep period changes; and (3) the usual sequence of stages is disturbed, with the mean duration of continuous intervals of each stage decreasing.[71] A significant increase in waking and decrease in REM sleep time occur during inverted sleep periods. The time spent in NREM stages does not change significantly. After sleep period reversal, REM and Stage 2 sleep shift toward the early part of the sleep period, and waking shifts toward the latter part. The duration of all stages of sleep decreases, and the number of changes of sleep stage increases. Despite these changes in duration, amount, stability, and timing of the sleep stages, the basic 90- to 100-minute cycling is preserved following acute inversion to day sleep. Thus the ultradian REM-NREM cycle persists without any proportional lengthening or any obvious subharmonic synchronization to the circadian cycle, revealing an autonomy between rhythms.[54] These variations may have significant effects on individuals subjected to changing shift work and study periods.

The time of day exerts a preferential influence on the distribution of the stages of sleep, with *REM sleep occurring more frequently during the morning hours, while slow-wave sleep occurs as a function of the amount of prior wakefulness*. Thus REM sleep appears to show circadian effects, while the amount of prior wakefulness appears to determine the volume of slow-wave sleep.[72] The latency to REM is related more to the amount of total sleep before the last REM onset than to awake time since the last sleep. While slow-wave sleep is a more awake-dependent process, REM sleep appears to be a more sleep-dependent rhythm.[73]

Age, length of prior wakefulness, length of time asleep, and a circadian influence all affect slow-wave sleep.[74] The volume of Stage 4 sleep decreases as an individual ages and as time asleep increases. Longer periods of wakefulness before sleep result in greater amounts of Stage 4 sleep in the first 3 hours of sleep. Sleep periods that begin at times other than the regular onset time tend to produce less Stage 4 sleep.

Consistent subjective, behavioral, and electroencephalographic sleep stage differences also occur during afternoon naps. Evans and coworkers have described differences between appetitive naps (light naps taken for psychological reasons) and replacement naps (those taken in response to temporary sleep deficits) and compared them with naps taken by habitual non-nappers.[75] Sleep onset latency is significantly shorter in those who nap regularly. One important characteristic of nappers appears to be their voluntary control over sleep: they can fall asleep easily in a wide variety of circumstances, whenever they choose to do so. Virtually no REM sleep occurs in afternoon naps. The amounts of NREM Stages 2, 3, and 4 are similar between nappers and non-nappers. With the exception of sleep onset latency, afternoon naps of nappers and non-nappers are similar to periods of consolidated sleep at the beginning of the night. Afternoon sleep of appetitive nappers is quite different from that of replacement nappers and non-nappers. Although the amount of time spent in the various stages is similar, the distribution of these stages differs from the other two groups. The appetitive napper has significantly more epochs of Stage 1 sleep and also significantly more changes in sleep stages than the other two.

The internal structure of sleep also varies with the phase of the temperature cycle. The first 50 minutes of REM sleep is accumulated an average of 2 hours earlier when sleep begins just after the trough of the temperature cycle than when it begins just after the temperature cycle maximum. This is not the case of with NREM Stages 3 and 4. Variation in REM sleep with the time of day is based on a close relation between a rhythm in REM sleep propensity and the body temperature rhythm and on the ability of both to oscillate together at a period different from that of the sleep-wake cycle.[55]

During the free-running state, other rhythms become uncoupled from the circadian body temperature rhythm.[76] The timing of growth hormone secretion, peripheral skin temperature, and slow-wave sleep is more closely linked to the sleep-wake cycle itself than to the core temperature rhythm. In addition, a component of the cortisol secretion rhythm has been shown to be related to the sleep-wake pattern, whereas other components of the cortisol rhythm remain coupled to the body temperature.

REFERENCES

1. Mistlberger R and Rusak B: Mechanisms and models of the circadian timekeeping system. In Kryger MH, Roth T, and Dement WC (eds): Principles and practices of sleep medicine. Philadelphia, WB Saunders, 1989, pp 141-152.
2. Aschoff J: Exogenous and endogenous components in circadian rhythms. Cold Spring Harbor Symp Quant Biol 1960;25:11-28.
3. Kolata G: Heart attacks at 9:00 a.m. Science 1986; 233:417-418.
4. Wingard DL and Berkman LF: Mortality risk associated with sleeping pattern among adults. Sleep 1983;6:102-107.
5. Halberg F: Temporal coordination of physiological function. Cold Spring Harbor Symp Quant Biol 1960;25:289-310.
6. Anch AM et al: Sleep: a scientific perspective. Englewood Cliffs, NJ, Prentice Hall, 1988, pp 59-86.
7. Hauty GT and Adams T: Phase shifts of the human circadian system and performance deficit during the periods of transition. II. West-East flight. Aerospace Med 1966;37:1027-1033.
8. Sollberger A: Biological rhythm research. Amsterdam, Elsevier/North Holland, 1966.
9. Bonnet MH: Memory for events occurring during arousal from sleep. Psychophysiology 1983;20:81-87.

10. Busby KA and Broughton RJ: Waking ultradian rhythms of performance and motility in hyperkinetic and normal children. J Abnorm Child Psychol 1983; 11:431-442.
11. Broughton RJ: Biorhythmic variations in consciousness and psychological functions. Can Psychol Rev 1975;16:217-230.
12. Montplaisir J and Godbout B (eds): Sleep and biological rhythms: basic mechanisms and application to psychiatry. Oxford University Press, New York, 1990.
13. Kleitman N: Sleep and wakefulness. Chicago, University of Chicago Press, 1963, pp 131-194.
14. Evans FJ and Orne MT: Recovery from fatigue. U.S. Army Medical Research and Performance Command, Fort Detrick, Frederick, Md (NTIS No. A100347).
15. Richardson GS et al: Circadian variation of sleep tendency in elderly and young adult subjects. Sleep 1982;5(suppl 2):S82-S94.
16. Akerstedt C and Gillberg M: Experimentally displaced sleep: effects on sleepiness. Electroencephalogr Clin Neurophysiol 1982;54:220-226.
17. Blake MJF: Time of day effects on performance in a range of tasks. Psychosom Sci 1967;9:349-350.
18. Angus RG and Heslegrave RJ: Effects of sleep loss on sustained cognitive performance during a command and control stimulation. Behav Res Meth Instr Comput 1985;17:55-67.
19. Broughton RJ: The siesta: social or biological phenomenon? Sleep Res 1983;12:28.
20. Browne RC: The day and night performance of teleprinter switchboard operators. Occup Psychol 1949; 23:121-126.
21. Hildebrandt G, Rohmert W, and Rutenfranz J: 12 and 24 h rhythms in error frequency of locomotive drivers and the influence of tiredness. Int J Chronobiol 1974;2:175-180.
22. Lavie P, Wollman M, and Pollack J: Frequency of sleep related traffic accidents and hour of day. Sleep Res 1986;15:275.
23. Smolensky M, Halberg F, and Sargent F: Chronobiology of the life sequence. In Ito K, Ogata K, and Yoshimura Y (eds): Advances in Climatic Physiology. Tokyo, Igaku Shoin, 1972, pp 515-516.
24. Broughton RJ: Chronobiological aspects and models of sleep and napping. In Dinges DF and Broughton RJ (eds): Sleep and alertness: chronobiological, behavioral, and medical aspects of napping, New York, Raven Press, 1989, pp 71-98.
25. Mills JN: Human circadian rhythms. Physiol Rev 1966;46:128-171.
26. Jouvet M: Neurophysiology of the state of sleep. Physiol Rev 1967;47:117-177.
27. Kety SS, Evarts EV, and Williams HL (eds): Sleep and altered states of consciousness. Baltimore, Williams & Wilkins, 1967, p 45.
28. Kleitman N: The nature of dreaming. In Wolstenholme GEW and O'Connor MO (eds): The nature of sleep. London, Churchill, 1961, pp 349-364.
29. Kleitman N: Basic rest-activity cycle—22 years later. Sleep 1982;5:311-317.
30. Meier-Koll A et al: A biological oscillator system and the development of sleep-waking behavior during early infancy. Chronobiologia 1978;6:301-308.
31. Nakagawa Y: Continuous observations of EEG patterns at night and in daytime of normal subjects under restrained conditions. I. Quiescent state when lying down. Electroencephalogr Clin Neurophysiol 1980; 49:524-537.
32. Zulley J: The four-hour sleepwake cycle. Sleep Res 1988;17:403.
33. Broughton RJ et al: Chronobiological aspects of SWS and REM sleep in extended night sleep of normals. Sleep Res 1988;17:361.
34. Richter CP: Sleep and activity: their relation to the 24-hour clock. Proc Assoc Res Nerv Ment Dis 1967;45:8-27.
35. Schweiger EH, Wallraff HG, and Schweiger H: Endogenous circadian rhythm in cytoplasma of *Acetabularia*: influence of the nucleus. Science 1964; 146:658-659.
36. Richter CP: Sleep and activity: their relation to the 24-hour clock. In Kety S, Evarts E, and Williams H (eds): Sleep and altered states of consciousness. Baltimore, Williams & Wilkins, 1967, pp 8-28.
37. Moore RY and Eichler VB: Loss of a circadian adrenal corticosterone rhythm following suprachiasmatic lesion in the rat. Brain Res 1972;42:201-206.
38. Stephan FK and Zucker I: Circadian rhythms in drinking behavior and locomotor activity of rats are eliminated by hypothalamic lesion. Proc Natl Acad Sci USA 1972;69:1583-1586.
39. Inouye ST and Kawamura H: Persistance of circadian rhythmicity in mammalian hypothalamic "island" containing the suprachiasmatic nucleus. Proc Natl Acad Sci USA 1979;76:5962-5966.
40. Rusak B and Groos G: Suprachiasmatic stimulation phase shifts rodent circadian rhythms. Science 1982;215:1407-1409.
41. Moore RY and Klein DC: Visual pathways and the central neural control of a circadian rhythm in pineal serotonin *N*-acetyltransferase activity. Brain Res 1974;71:17-33.
42. Stetson MH and Watson-Whitmyre M: Nucleus suprachiasmaticus: the biological clock in the hamster? Science 1976;191:197-199.
43. Ibuka N and Kawamura H: Loss of circadian rhythm in sleep-wakefulness cycle in the rat by suprachiasmatic nucleus lesions. Brain Res 1975;96:76-81.
44. Moore RY: Organization and function of a central nervous system circadian oscillator: the suprachiasmatic hypothalamic nucleus. Fed Proc 1983;42:2783-2789.
45. Lydig R et al: Suprachiasmatic region of the human hypothalamus: homolog to the primate circadian pacemaker? Sleep 1980;2:355-361.
46. Moore-Ede MC: The circadian timing system in mammals: two pacemakers preside over many secondary oscillators. Fed Proc 1983;42:2802-2808.
47. Refresher course in sleep disorders medicine. Stanford University, Stanford, Calif, March 1986.
48. Pickard GE and Turek FW: The suprachiasmatic nuclei: two circadian clocks? Brain Res 1983;268:201-210.
49. Moore RY: The retinohypothalamic projection in the rat. J Comp Neurol 1972;146:1-14.
50. Moore RY: Retinohypothalamic projection in mammals: a comparative study. Brain Res 1973;49:403-409.
51. Pickard GE: The afferent connections of the suprachiasmatic nucleus of the golden hamster with emphasis on the retinohypothalamic projection. J Comp Neurol 1982;211:65-83.
52. Zucker I, Rusak B, and King RG Jr: Neural bases for circadian rhythms in rodent behavior. In Reisen AH and Thompson RF (eds): Advances in psychobiology. New York, Wiley, 1976, pp 35-74.
53. Anch AM et al: The rhythm of sleep. In Anch AM et al (eds): Sleep: a scientific perspective. Englewood Cliffs, NJ, Prentice Hall, 1988, pp 59-86.
54. Czeisler CA et al: Timing of REM sleep is coupled

to the circadian rhythm of body temperature in man. Sleep 1980;2:328-346.
55. Czeisler CA et al: Human sleep: its duration and organization depend on its circadian phase. Science 1980;210:1264-1267.
56. Webb WB and Agnew HW Jr: The effects of a chronic limitation of sleep length. Psychophysiology 1974; 11:265-274.
57. Czeisler CA et al: Bright light resets the human circadian pacemaker independent of the timing of the sleep-wake cycle. Science 1986;233:667-671.
58. Czeisler CA et al: Entrainment of human circadian rhythm by light-dark cycles: a reassessment. Photochem Photobiol 1981;34:239.
59. Lewy AJ et al: Light suppresses melatonin secretion in humans. Science 1980;210:1267-1269.
60. Nelson RJ and Zucker I: Absence of extraocular photoreception in diurnal and nocturnal rodents exposed to direct sunlight. Comp Biochem Physiol 1981; 69:145-148.
61. Pittendrigh CS and Daan S: A functional analysis of circadian pacemakers in nocturnal rodents. IV. Entrainment: pacemaker as clock. J Comp Physiol 1976;106:291-331.
62. Takahashi JS and Zatz M: Regulation of circadian rhythmicity. Science 1982;217:1104-1111.
63. Boulos Z and Terman M: Food availability and daily biological rhythms. Neurosci Biobehav Rev 1980; 4:119-131.
64. Aschoff J and Tokura H: Circadian activity rhythms in squirrel monkeys: entrainment by temperature cycles. J Biol Rhythms 1986;1:91-100.
65. Rawson KS: Effects of tissue temperature on mammalian activity rhythms. Cold Spring Harbor Symp Quant Biol 1960;25:105-113.
66. Weaver RA: The circadian system of man. New York, Springer-Verlag, 1979.
67. Aschoff J: Circadian rhythms in man. Science 1965;148:1427-1432.
68. Aschoff J and Wever R: Spontanperiodik des menschen bei asschluss aller zeitgeber. Naturwissenschaften 1962;49:337-342.
69. Miles LEM, Raynal DM, and Wilson MA: Blind man living in normal society has circadian rhythms of 24.9 hours. Science 1977;198:421-423.
70. DeKoninck J et al: Are REM cycles in narcoleptic patients governed by an ultradian rhythm? Sleep 1986;9:162-166.
71. Weitzman ED et al: Acute reversal of the sleep-waking cycle in man: effect on sleep stage patterns. Arch Neurol 1970;22:483-489.
72. Karacan I et al: Changes in stage 1-REM and stage 4 sleep during naps. Biol Psychiatry 1970;2:261-265.
73. Moses JM et al: Rapid eye movement cycle is a sleep dependent rhythm. Nature 1977;265:360-361.
74. Webb WB and Agnew HW: Stage 4 sleep: influence of time course variables. Science 1971;174:1354-1356.
75. Evans FJ et al: Appetitive and replacement naps: EEG and behavior. Science 1977;197:687-689.
76. Weitzman ED, Czeisler CA, and Moore-Ede MC: Sleep-wake, neuroendocrine and body temperature circadian rhythms under entrained and non-entrained (free-running) conditions in man. In Suda O, Hayaishi H, and Nakagawa H (eds): Biological rhythms and their central mechanism. Amsterdam, Elsevier/North Holland, 1979, pp 199-227.

4

Anatomy of Sleep

The sleeping and waking states depend on activity of the entire brain and not on particular or independent regions. In general, neural activity in the brainstem-diencephalic ascending reticular activating system is responsible for the maintenance of alertness and the waking state.

Sleep is a complex, active phenomenon. Sleep is composed of physiologically distinct, but highly synchronized, states that cycle at regular intervals. It stands to reason that sleep is generated and maintained by many different regions of the central nervous system working together rather than simply by a reduction in activity of the reticular activating system.

This chapter focuses on the various anatomical centers of the central nervous system and their known or proposed function within the sleep-wake cycle. Most of the data delineating these anatomical areas have been derived from animal lesion experiments. Other data come from observations of signs and symptoms in humans who have disease or dysfunction of particular topological regions of the brain. It must be remembered, however, that in the normal human no single area of the central nervous system functions in isolation. Elucidation of all interrelationships is beyond the scope of this text.

CORTEX

Cyclical sleeping and waking behavior can occur in the absence of the cortex. This has been well documented in animal studies[1-3] and in observations of human newborns with anencephaly and holoprosencephaly.[4,5] The cortex is intimately involved with regulation and maintenance of wakefulness by directly stimulating the ascending reticular activating system (Fig. 4–1). Increased activity in the reticular activating system results in a general arousal response. There is some evidence that overstimulation of this cortex–reticular activating system–cortex (C-RAS-C) activation loop may be responsible for the hyperactivity and motor restlessness seen in many children with attention deficit–hyperactivity disorder, as well as children with syndromes associated with excessive daytime sleepiness. Objective signs of increased sleep pressure have been documented in a group of children with attention span problems, hyperactivity, motor restlessness, behavioral difficulties, and/or school failure.[6] Short mean sleep onset latencies, frequent sleep onsets, numerous microsleep episodes, and pathologically short sleep onset latencies in one or several Multiple Sleep Latency Test naps have been identified in this group of children. Reduction in excessive sleep pressure might explain the positive effect of stimulant medication on the symptoms of overactivity, motor restlessness, and at-

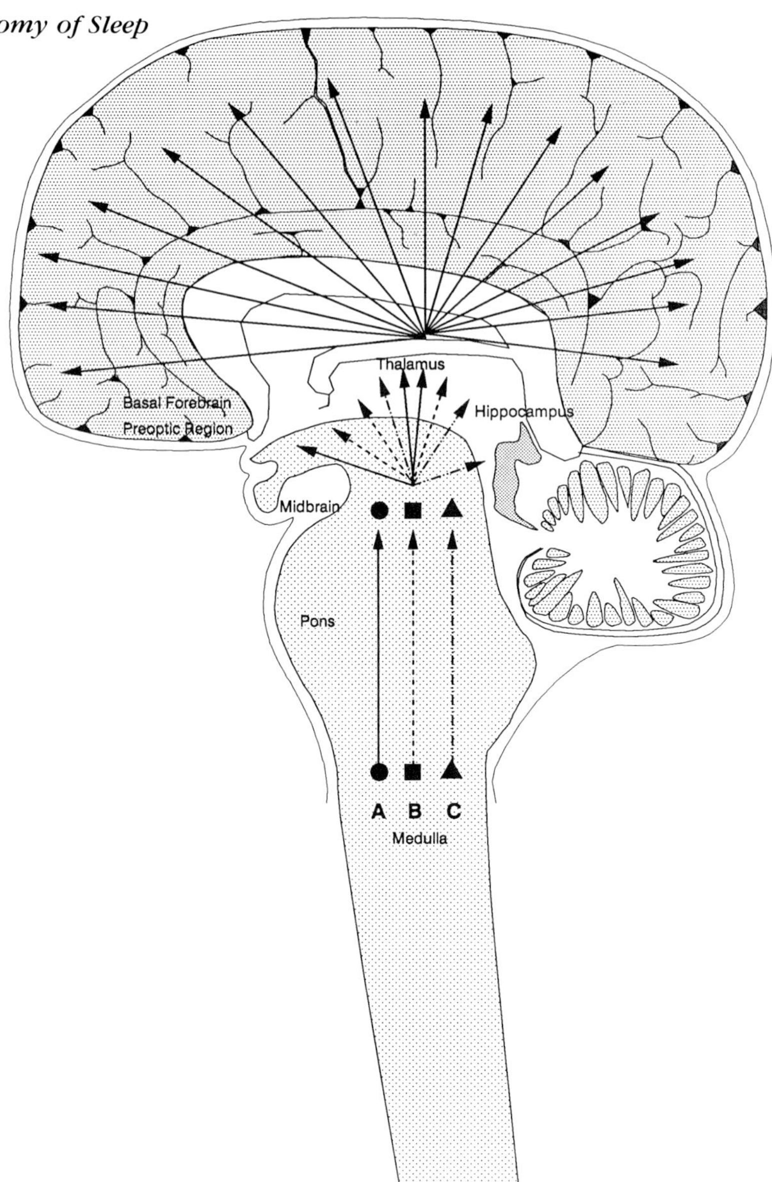

FIGURE 4–1. Schematic mechanism for generation of wakefulness. *Solid circles* represent the neurons of the reticular formation. Their major ascending projections into the forebrain proceed along two major routes. The dorsal route terminates in the nonspecific thalamic nuclei, which in turn project in a widespread manner to the cerebral cortex. The ventral route passes through and terminates in the subthalamus and hypothalamus and continues into the basal forebrain and septum, where neurons in turn project in a widespread manner to the cerebral cortex and hippocampus. *Solid squares* represent catecholamine neurons of the lower brainstem and locus ceruleus (dorsal pons), which contain norepinephrine, and of the substantia nigra and ventral tegmental area (ventral midbrain), which contain dopamine. The norepinephrine neurons are mainly implicated in processes of cortical activation and project directly and diffusely to the cerebral cortex, as well as to the subcortical way stations. The dopamine neurons are predominantly implicated in processes of behavioral activity and responsiveness and project heavily into the basal ganglia and frontal cortex. *Solid triangles* represent acetylcholine neurons of the brainstem reticular formation (including the laterodorsal and pedunculopontine tegmental nuclei in the dorsal pons and midbrain) and basal forebrain (substantia innominata, diagonal band nuclei, and septum). Cholinergic neurons are implicated in cortical activation and from the brainstem project predominantly to subcortical way stations, including the thalamus, subthalamus, hypothalamus, and basal forebrain and septum. The cholinergic basal forebrain neurons project in a widespread manner to the cerebral cortex and hippocampus. Not shown are other neuronal systems implicated in wakefulness, including histamine neurons located in the posterior hypothalamus, which also project directly to the cerebral cortex. Glutamate neurons located through subcortal structures and in the cerebral cortex are important in processes of cortical activation and wakefulness. Multiple peptides, such as substance P, corticotropin-releasing factor, thyrotropin-releasing factor, and vasoactive intestinal polypeptide, may be involved in wakefulness and are often co-localized with one of the other primary neurotransmitters, such as norepinephrine and acetylcholine. The neuronal systems implicated in the maintenance of wakefulness may be involved in primary processes of sensory transmission and attention, motor response and activity, and orthosympathetic and neuroendocrine (particularly adrenocorticotropic hormone and thyrotropin-releasing hormone) responses and regulation, by which they may enhance and prolong vigilance and arousal.

tention span deficits in *some* children with attention deficit–hyperactivity disorder. Reducing sleepiness, reducing microsleep episodes, and exogenously stimulating the cortex may break the C-RAS-C feedback loop, resulting in improvement of symptoms.

Behavioral components of sleep onset may also be under the control of cortical activity. Habits and rituals associated with sleep onset create a relaxed and practiced situation that may facilitate physiological sleep-onset mechanisms. Absence of appropriate and patterned sleep onset associations results in significant difficulties in sleep initiation and maintenance during early childhood.

Although sleep and wake cycling may be preserved in the absence of the cortex, sleep and wake are severely dysfunctional in many patients with generalized cortical disease. Although some recognizable EEG characteristics remain (e.g., sleep spindles, vertex sharp transients), architecture may be severely disrupted and in some cases no recognizable sleep stages can be seen.[7,8]

CEREBELLUM

The cerebellum is mainly responsible for the control of skeletal musculature, posture, and movement. During sleep, cerebellar activity and feedback may be involved with postural adjustments and body movements, accessory respiratory muscle movements, extraocular muscle movements, and alterations in muscle tone.[9] Although the cerebellum contributes to the generation of muscle atonia during sleep,[10,11] cerebellar activity seems to have little effect on the sleep-wake cycle itself. The cerebellar vermis may also be involved in the regulation (i.e., suppression) of sleep spindles. Lesions in this area result in the production of numerous sleep spindles on the electroencephalogram (EEG).[12]

BASAL GANGLIA

The role of the basal ganglia in the sleep-wake cycle appears to be peripheral. Dopaminergic neurons in the substantia nigra innervate with thousands of synaptic contacts in the striatum.[13] Neuronal activity shows little change during wakefulness and during the various stages of sleep (including rapid eye movement [REM] sleep).

THALAMUS

Animal experiments using low-frequency stimulation of the midline thalamic nuclei have resulted in presleep behavior followed by sleep.[14] The region causing this response is very limited, however. Low-frequency stimulation of the anterior thalamic nuclei of animals has resulted in similar findings. These results have not been obtained in humans. The thalamus does not appear to be essential for sleep[15] but is integral to the production of sleep spindles.[16] A thalamic "pacemaker" may exist that drives cortical neurons and controls EEG synchronization during non-REM (NREM) sleep.[17] Periodic bursts of high-amplitude cortical waves and spindles become more frequent as deeper stages of sleep are achieved and seem to be initiated by activity in nonspecific thalamic nuclei through diffuse thalamocortical projections. Areas responsible for driving spindle production appear to be midline and are closely associated to the region where low-frequency stimulation promotes sleep in animals.[18]

Sleep spindles and K-complexes are distinctive features of the sleeping state and are never seen during wakefulness.[19] The function of spindles and K-complexes is unknown, but they are thought to have an important function in the regulation of slow-wave sleep (Fig. 4–2).[20]

HYPOTHALAMUS

The posterior, lateral, and medial hypothalamus is the cephalad continuation of the brainstem reticular activating system. Transection of the brainstem at the level of the posterior hypothalamus completely abolishes wakefulness.[21] Posterior hypothalamic lesions generally produce lethargy and sleepiness.[22] Hypersomnia, coma, changes in circadian rhythmicity may be noted in humans, depending on the exact site and extent of hypothalamic disease or dysfunction.

ANTERIOR HYPOTHALAMUS AND FOREBRAIN

Basal forebrain areas appear to contain powerful inhibitory and sleep-promoting centers.[23] Lesions within the preoptic region have an effect that is opposite to those of posterior hypothalamic lesions.[24] Insomnia and terminal sleeplessness[25] have resulted from lesions of the

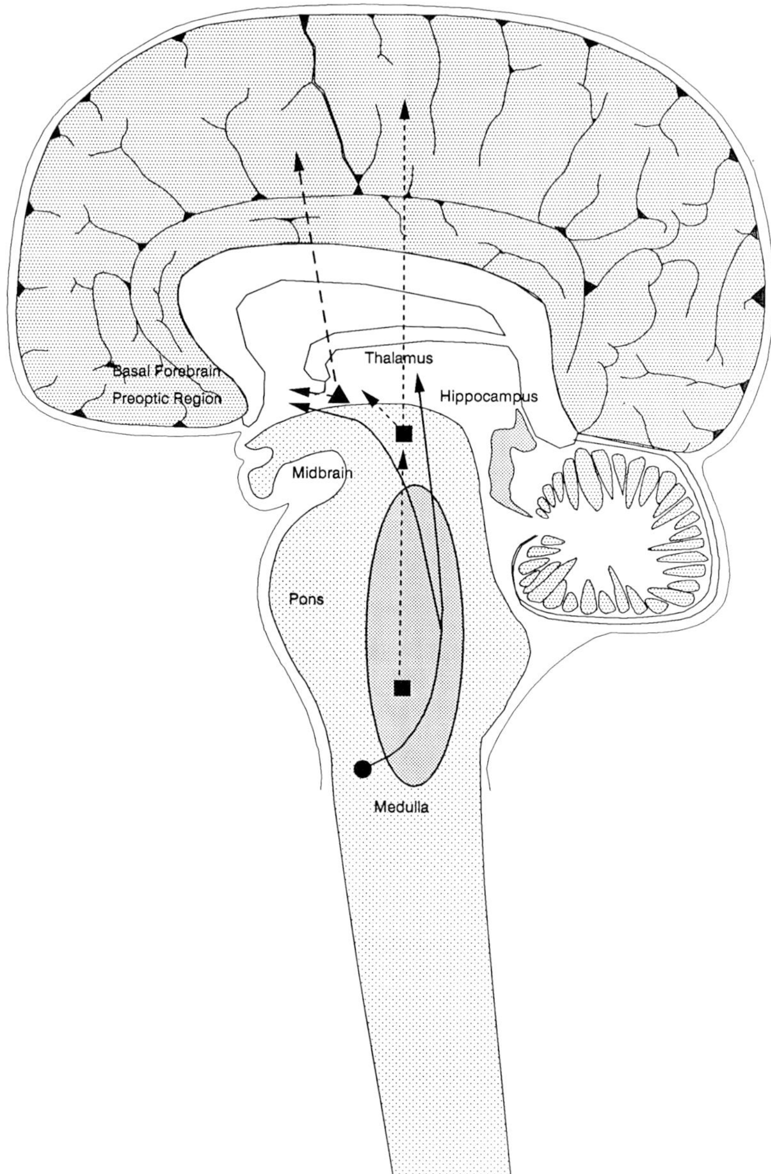

FIGURE 4–2. Schematic representation of mechanisms generating slow-wave sleep. *Solid circles* represent neurons of the solitary tract nucleus and adjacent tegmentum, implicated in slow-wave sleep regulation, which project forward into the visceral-limbic forebrain. *Solid squares* represent serotonergic neurons of the brainstem raphe nuclei, which may facilitate the onset of slow-wave sleep and which project forward into the rostral tegmentum, thalamus, subthalamus, hypothalamus, and basal forebrain and also from the midbrain directly to the cortex and hippocampus. *Solid diamonds* represent gamma-aminobutyric acid (GABA) neurons of the hypothalamus and septum of the basal forebrain, which project in a widespread manner to the cerebral cortex and hippocampus. These GABA neurons are also located in the cerebral cortex, where they are maximally active during slow-wave sleep. Not shown are other neuronal systems implicated in slow-wave sleep, including adenosine neurons located in the hypothalamus. Multiple peptides, such as the opiates, alpha-melanocyte-stimulating hormone, and somatostatin, may be involved in slow-wave sleep generation and are often co-localized with one of the other primary neurotransmitters, such as serotonin or GABA. The neuronal systems implicated in the maintenance of slow-wave sleep may be involved in primary processes of sensory inhibition and analgesia, behavioral inhibition, and parasympathetic and neuroendocrine (notably growth hormone) responses and regulation, by which they may facilitate the onset and maintenance of slow wave sleep.

anterior hypothalamus and basal forebrain, respectively.

When stimulated, the basal forebrain produces a short sleep onset latency, synchronization of the EEG, and involuntary sleep.[26-28] Lesions of this same area produce insomnia in animals. Identifying the cell bodies responsible for this phenomenon is difficult, since the region is quite dense and contains numerous transecting fiber tracts.[23] High-frequency stimulation of the thalamus, posterior hypothalamus, and brainstem produces arousal, whereas similar stimulation of the anterior hypothalamus produces rapid sleep onset. With high-frequency stimulation of the basal forebrain and low-frequency stimulation of the thalamus, presleep behavior occurs before EEG synchronization.[29]

BRAINSTEM RETICULAR ACTIVATING SYSTEM

In 1935 Bremer described the classic results of transection of the brainstem at two levels: first at the level of the midbrain just behind the third nerve (cerveau isolé) and second at the cervicomedullary junction (encephale isolé) in the cat.[30] The first transection isolates the cerebrum from the brainstem but leaves intact sensory input from the optic nerves and olfactory tracts, as well as motor output to the third nerve and preganglionic nerve cells of the oculomotor nuclei. The result is a picture of slow-wave sleep (but may be more that of coma than sleep), no alteration between sleep and wake, absence of REM sleep, absence of alerting response to sensory stimulation, and appearance of a monotonous sequence of spindles in the EEG. Wakefulness gradually returns, and after 7 to 15 days spontaneous periods of EEG desynchronization occur. REM sleep, however, does not reappear. Transection at the cervicomedullary junction results in a normal sleep-wake cycle. Bremer concluded that the junction between the diencephalon and the brainstem was crucial to sleep and wakefulness.

Rather than a single, isolated region in the brainstem, the reticular activating system appears to be diffusely distributed in the medulla and pons and extends into the posterior, medial, and lateral hypothalamic regions. Classic experiments by Moruzzi and Magoun[31] revealed that electrical stimulation of a portion of the brainstem resulted in EEG changes identical to those seen on awakening from sleep or during an arousal, alerting reaction. The area from which EEG synchronization occurs runs through most of the length of the brainstem in its central core. Electrical stimulation in these regions also changes the activity of cortical and thalamic neurons, abolishes thalamic recruiting potentials, has a marked effect on cortical evoked potentials, and significantly affects perception.[9]

Evidence exists that many reticular formation neurons have both cephalad and caudad projections.[32,33] This complex system also appears to have many interneuronal connections with the brainstem "deactivating" system located in the medullary raphe nuclei.

Ascending somatic and auditory pathways are laterally placed in the brainstem, while the ascending reticular activating system is located in its central core. This ascending pathway extends from the brainstem reticular formation through the mesencephalic tegmentum in the diencephalon, subthalamus, hypothalamus, and ventromedial thalamus to the internal capsule (diffuse thalamocortical projections).[34] Excitatory impulses from the brainstem core result in generalized desynchronization of the cortex via diffuse thalamocortical projections or via an extrathalamic route.

The reticular formation has received its name from the lacework appearance of fiber bundles subjected to myelin staining. A total of 98 nuclei have been identified in the lower brainstem.[35] Many of these nuclei are responsible for vegetative functioning of the organism (e.g., respiratory control, cardiovascular control). Cell bodies of this region are highly polymorphic and contain a wide variety of neurotransmitters, including serotonin in the midline raphe nuclei, noradrenalin in the locus ceruleus, and acetylcholine in the posterior hypothalamic regions. Nuclei that are highly involved in the sleep-wake cycle include the locus ceruleus, nucleus raphe pallidus, and nucleus cuneiformis. Lesions of the cephalic parts of the reticular formation generally result in a chronic loss of wakefulness, stupor, or coma, with hypersynchronous EEG activity not affected by peripheral stimulation.[36-41]

RAPHE NUCLEI

Midline raphe nuclei are two columns of cell bodies extending from the upper medulla to the pontomedullary junction.[42-43] The neurotransmitter of this area is primarily serotonin, is considered to work in opposition to the reticular activating system, and is essential for the initation of NREM sleep.

Raphe nuclei lesions produce partial or complete insomnia, depending on the extent of the lesion. In animal experiments complete destruction of the nuclei results in a complete inability to sleep.[44] On the other hand, slow-wave sleep can be selectively abolished by partial lesions.

Dorsal raphe nuclei appear to be important in the control of phasic events during REM sleep. Increased activity of neurons in the nucleus raphe pallidus results in a decrease in phasic activity similar to the suppression of ponto-geniculo-occipital wave activity by electrical stimulation of the raphe nuclei in animals.[45,46]

LOCUS COERULEUS

The locus coeruleus is located in the dorsolateral portion of the rostral and caudal mesencephalic tegmentum and is closely related to the trigeminal complex. Noradrenalin-containing locus coeruleus neurons within the pons appear to be key elements in the control and organization of EEG desynchronization, tonic and phasic components of REM sleep, hippocampal theta activity, saccadic eye movements, postural atonia, and phasic twitching. Major activity in this region, however, results in sleep atonia. Lesions of the locus coeruleus abolish REM atonia as do lesions of the pontine gigantocellular tegmental field.[9]

SUPRACHIASMATIC NUCLEI

The suprachiasmatic nuclei are paired nuclei in the anterior hypothalamic region adjacent to the optic chiasm, just lateral to the third ventricle. Lesions in the suprachiasmatic region disrupt the rhythmicity and entrainment of the sleep-wake cycle to the 24-hour day, but major alterations in the rhythmicity of the NREM-REM cycles within sleep itself may not occur initially.

The suprachiasmatic nuclei are linked to the retina by the retinohypothalamic tracts, and bilateral lesions of these pathways abolish light entrainment of circadian rhythms. Monosynaptic pathways have been identified, and rhythm-controlling function appears to depend primarily on neuronal activity and not on neurosecretory functions.

Neurons of the suprachiasmatic nuclei are sensitive to overall levels of illumination. Light sensitivity of entrainment appears to be related to the secretion of melatonin. In addition to light-imposed rhythms of activity, neurons in this region possess an inherent rhythm of their own.[9] Ontogenetic development of the suprachiasmatic nuclei connections via the retinohypothalamic tracts during infancy parallels the changes from ultradian to circadian rhythms in the sleep-wake cycle.

Although the suprachiasmatic nuclei appear to be the central pacemaker, a single "clock" does not appear to exist or has yet to be identified. A central, powerful deep oscillator and a more diffuse, weaker oscillator function in synchrony during periods of entrainment. Core body temperature and the sleep-wake cycle are normally coupled. These two systems, however, uncouple and run independently during periods of temporal isolation. Under these "free-running" conditions, core body temperature, REM sleep, plasma cortisol secretion, and urinary potassium excretion remain stable. The sleep-wake cycle, plasma growth hormone secretion, and urinary calcium excretion rhythm become labile and cycle with a different period.

RAPID EYE MOVEMENT SLEEP: HOBSON-McCARLEY MODEL

In 1974 Hobson and McCarley proposed a mechanism that may explain the NREM-REM cycling within sleep (Fig. 4–3).[47] Their model postulates two classes of neuronal systems within the upper pons, which they identified as "REM-on" and "REM-off" systems.

The REM-off system is a collection of aminergic neurons located in the serotonergic dorsal raphe nuclei, noradrenergic locus coeruleus, and noradrenergic nucleus peribrachialis lateralis. Highest neuronal activity in these areas is noted during wakefulness. Discharge rates decline during NREM sleep and reach their lowest levels during REM sleep. The system appears to be both self-inhibitory and inhibitory to postsynaptic neurons.

REM-on cells are a collection of excitatory cholinergic neurons principally located in the mesencephalic, pontine, and medullary gigantocellular tegmental fields. Unit activity in these regions is lowest during wakefulness, increased during NREM sleep, and highest during REM sleep.

According to this model, discharges from the gigantocellular tegmental field activate the cortex via the ascending reticular activating system, cause conjugate eye movements through interconnections with the oculomotor nuclei, and decrease muscle tone via direct inhibitory postsynaptic potentials generated in the brainstem inhibitory reticular formation. Muscle twitches

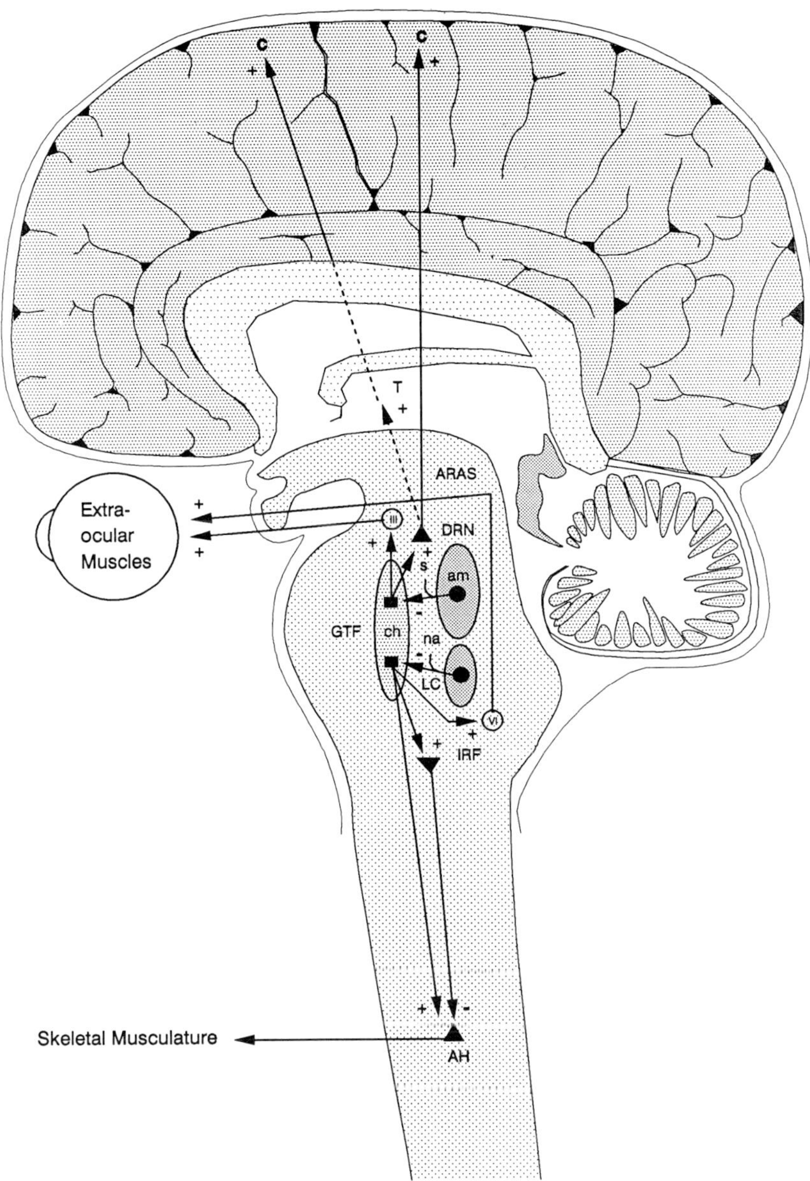

FIGURE 4–3. Schematic mechanism for the generation of REM sleep. Aminergic ("REM-off") neurons in the dorsal raphe nuclei (serotonergic) and the locus ceruleus (noradrenergic) produce inhibitory postsynaptic potentials on cholinergic ("REM-on") neurons in the mesencephalic, medullary, and pontine gigantocellular tegmental fields. These two systems of neurons continuously interact to produce the alteration between NREM and REM sleep. Neurons in the gigantocellular tegmental fields produce stimulating postsynaptic potentials to cause the epiphenomena seen during REM sleep. Positive postsynaptic potentials result in conjugate extraocular muscle movement through stimulation of the nuclei of the oculomotor, trochlear, and abducens nuclei. Cortical desynchronization occurs via projections to the thalamus and cortex through the ascending reticular activating system. Muscle atonia is produced by direct stimulation of neurons that produce inhibitory postsynaptic potentials at the level of the anterior horn cell. Intermittent muscle twitches occur through direct stimulation of the anterior horn cells. Not shown are interconnections with the autonomic nervous system, which result in the cardiac and respiratory irregularities noted during REM sleep. *C,* Cortex; *T,* thalamus; *ARAS,* ascending reticular activating system; *DRN,* dorsal raphe nuclei; *LC,* locus ceruleus; *GTF,* gigantocellular tegmental fields; *IRF,* inhibitory reticular formation; *AH,* anterior horn cells; *am,* aminergic neurons; *s,* serotonin; *na,* noradrenalin; *ch,* acetylcholine; +, stimulating postsynaptic potential; −, inhibitory postsynaptic potential. (Modified and reproduced with permission from Hobson JA: The cellular basis of sleep cycle control. Adv Sleep Res 1974;1:217-250; and Hauri P: Current concepts: the sleep disorders, Kalamazoo, Mich, The Upjohn Company, 1982, p 13.)

during REM sleep are caused by direct positive postsynaptic potentials at the level of the anterior horn cells, and irregularities in the cardiac and respiratory systems occur via influences on the autonomic nervous system.

SUMMARY

Control of sleep and the sleep-wake cycle is profoundly complex and for all practical purposes involves the whole brain. The following is a highly simplified summary of regions of the central nervous system involved in sleep and the sleep-wake cycle:

1. *Wakefulness*. Wakefulness and alertness appear to be maintained through activity of neurons in the brainstem reticular activating system, with feedback stimulation from a cortex–reticular activating system–cortex loop.
2. *Sleep onset*. Sleep onset involves a complex series of events that includes a decrease in activity of the neurons of the ascending reticular activating system; increase in activity in the preoptic region of the basal forebrain; possibly activity in the anterior thalamic nuclei; and possibly cortical influences associated with presleep behavior.
3. *NREM sleep*. Synchronization of the neocortex appears to be a result of activity in the midline raphe nuclei (and possibly the thalamus through diffuse thalamocortical projections). Thalamic nuclei are responsible for the generation of sleep spindles.
4. *REM sleep*. The locus ceruleus appears to be vital in generation of REM sleep. EEG desynchronization, phasic activity, and other REM-associated epiphenomena occur through multiple interconnections with the gigantocellular tegmental fields, a portion of the dorsal raphe nuclei, cerebellum, vestibular nuclei, and the cortex.

REFERENCES

1. Barret R, Merritt HH, and Wolf A: Depression of consciousness as a result of cerebral lesions. Res Publ Assoc Nerv Ment Dis 1967;45:241-276.
2. Kleitman N: Sleep and wakefulness. Chicago, University of Chicago Press, 1963, pp 241-242.
3. Oswald I: Sleeping and waking: physiology and psychology. Amsterdam, Elsevier/North Holland, 1962, p 232.
4. Nielson JM and Sedgwick RP: Instincts and emotions in an anencephalic monster. J Nerv Ment Dis 1949; 110:387-394.
5. Puech P et al: Un cas d'anencephalie hydrocephalique: etude electroencephalographique. Rev Neurol 1947; 79:116-124.
6. Sheldon SH et al: Sleep pressure in children with attentional deficits. Sleep Res 1991;204:443.
7. Wilkus RJ and Farrell DF: Electrophysiological observations in the classical form of Pelizaeus-Merzbacher disease. Neurology (Minneap) 1976;26:1042-1045.
8. Karacan I, Schneck L, and Hinterbuchner LP: The sleep-dream pattern in Tay-Sachs disease (preliminary observations). In Aronson SM and Volk BW (eds): Inborn errors of sphingolipid metabolism, Elmsford, NY, Pergamon Press, 1967, pp 413-421.
9. Parkes JD: Sleep and its disorders. Eastbourne, East Sussex, Eng, WB Saunders, 1985, pp 73-118.
10. Guglielmino S and Strata P: Cerebellum and atonia of the desynchronized phase of sleep. Arch Ital Biol 1971:109:210-217.
11. Marchesi GF and Strata P: Climbing fibers of rat cerebellum: modulation of activity during sleep. Brain Res 1970;17:145-148.
12. Marchesi GF, Scarpino O, and y Mauro AM: Studio poligrafico del sonno notturno in pazienti con sindrome cerebellare. Arch Psicol Neurol Psichiat 1977;4:455-472.
13. Anden NE et al: A quantitative study on the nigrostriatal dopamine neuron system in the rat. Acta Physiol Scand 1966;67:306-312.
14. Koella WA: Sleep: its nature and physiological organization. Springfield, Ill, Charles C Thomas, 1967, p 199.
15. Naquet R, Denavit M, and Albe-Fessard D: Comparaison entre le rôle du subthalamus et celui des differentes structures bulbo-mésencephaliques dans le maintien de la vigilance. Electroencephalogr Clin Neurophysiol 1966;20:149-164.
16. Bricolo A: Sleep abnormalities following thalamic stereotactic lesions in man. In Gastaut H et al (eds): The abnormalities of sleep in man. Proceedings of the XVth European Meeting on Electrophysiology, Bologna, 1967, Bologna, Auto Gaggi, 1968, pp 135-138.
17. Purpura DP and Yahr MD (eds): The thalamus. New York, Columbia University Press, 1966, p 438.
18. Eyzaguirre C and Fidone SJ: Physiology of the nervous system. Chicago, Year Book, 1975, pp 343-371.
19. Naitoh P et al: Dynamic relation of sleep spindles and K-complexes to spontaneous phasic arousal in sleeping human subjects. Sleep 1982;5:58-72.
20. Whitlock DG, Aruini A, and Moruzzi G: Microelectrode analysis of pyramidal system during transition from sleep to wakefulness. J Neurophysiol 1953;16:414-429.
21. Rossi GF: Electrophysiology of sleep. In Gastaut H et al (eds): The abnormalities of sleep in man. Proceedings of the XVth European Meeting on Electrophysiology, Bologna, 1967, Bologna, Auto Gaggi, 1968, pp 13-23.
22. Ranson SW: Somnolence caused by hypothalamic lesions in the monkey. Arch Neurol Psychiatry 1939;41:1-23.
23. Mitler MM: Toward an animal model of narcolepsy-cataplexy. In Guilleminault C, Dement WC, and Passouant P (eds): Narcolepsy. New York, Spectrum, 1976, pp 387-409.
24. von Economo C: Sleep as a problem of localization. J Nerv Ment Dis 1930;71:249-259.

25. McGinty D and Sterman M: Sleep suppression after basal forebrain lesions in the cat. Science 1968; 160:1253-1255.
26. Moruzzi G: The sleep-waking cycle. Ergebn Physiol 1972;64:1-165.
27. Sterman M and Fairchild M: Modification of locomotor performance by reticular formation and basal forebrain stimulation in the cat: evidence for reciprocal systems. Brain Res 1966;2:205-217.
28. Sterman MB and Clemente CD: Forebrain inhibitory mechanisms: cortical synchronization induced by basal forebrain stimulation. Exp Neurol 1962;6:91-102.
29. Clemente CD, Sterman MB, and Wyrwicka W: Forebrain inhibitory mechanisms: conditioning of basal forebrain induced EEG synchronization and sleep. Exp Neurol 1963;7:404-417.
30. Bremer F: Cerveau isolé et physiologie du sommeil. C R Soc Biol 1935;118:1235-1241.
31. Moruzzi G and Magoun HW: Brain stem reticular formation and activation of EEG. Electroencephalogr Clin Neurophysiol 1949;1:455-473.
32. McKeough DM: The coloring review of neuroscience. Boston, Little, Brown, 1982, pp 30-32.
33. Magni F and Willis WD: Identification of reticular formation neurons by intracellular recording. Arch Ital Biol 1963;101:681-702.
34. Jasper HH: Diffuse projection systems: the integrative action of the thalamic reticular system. Electroencephalogr Clin Neurophysiol 1949;1:405-409.
35. Olszewski J and Baxter D: The cytoarchitecture of the human brain stem. Philadelphia, Lippincott, 1954.
36. Cairns H: Disturbances of consciousness with lesions of the brain stem and diencephalon. Brain 1952; 75:109-146.
37. French JD: Brain lesions associated with prolonged unconsciousness. Arch Neurol Psychiatry 1952; 68:727-740.
38. Jefferson M: Altered consciousness associated with brain stem lesions. Brain 1952;75:55-67.
39. Jefferson G and Johnson RT: The cause of loss of consciousness in posterior fossa compression. Folia Psychiatry (Amsterdam) 1950;53:306-319.
40. Penfield W: The cerebral cortex in man. 1. The cerebral cortex and consciousness. Arch Neurol Psychiatry 1938;40:417-442.
41. Thompson GN and Nielson JM: Area essential to consciousness: cerebral localization of consciousness as established by neuropathological studies. J Am Med Assoc 1948;137:285.
42. Jouvet M: Neurophysiology of the states of sleep. Physiol Rev 1967;47:117-177.
43. Jouvet M: Biogenic amines and the states of sleep. Science 1969;163:32-41.
44. Morgane PJ and Stern WC: Monoaminergic systems in the brain and their role in the sleep states. In Barchas J and Usdin E (eds): Serotonin and behaviour, New York, Academic Press, 1973, pp 427-442.
45. Jacobs BL, Asher R, and Dement WC: Electrophysiological and behavioural effects of electrical stimulation of the raphe nuclei in cats. Physiol Behav 1973;11:489-495.
46. Simon RP, Gershon MD, and Brooks DC: The role of raphe nuclei in the regulation of ponto-geniculo-occipital wave activity. Brain Res 1973;58:313-330.
47. Hobson JA: The cellular basis of sleep cycle control. Adv Sleep Res 1974;1:217-250.

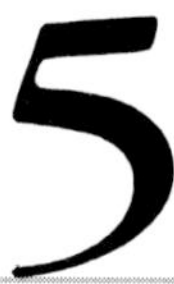

Physiological Variations During Sleep

Physiology of the human organism has been extensively studied, and many functions are clearly understood. Organ system responses in awake persons during various states of health and disease are well known. For many years function during the sleeping state has been assumed to parallel that of waking. In 1963 Nathaniel Kleitman published his historic volume *Sleep and Wakefulness*.[1] Kleitman proposed that physiological processes vary according to state; that is, organ systems function and interrelate differently when a person is asleep and awake. Since then several major texts describing human physiology during sleep have been published.[2] Over the past 25 years it has become clear that knowledge of functioning of the human organism in health and disease states only during periods of wakefulness provides limited insight on which to base many therapeutic regimens. If organ systems function differently during the sleeping state, it stands to reason that response to disease processes will vary between states. Principles of health maintenance should also follow this principle.

This chapter focuses on specific variations in function of organ systems during the sleeping state that may affect the response to disease processes and the efficacy of therapeutic regimens. Specific changes in the central nervous system (CNS), endocrine system, temperature regulation, cardiovascular system, and respiratory system are discussed.

CEREBRAL BLOOD FLOW DURING SLEEP

Consistency of cerebral blood flow (CBF) during sleep depends on alterations in cerebral vascular resistance. Upper and lower limits of autoregulation are not fixed but vary with the chemical environment, metabolic needs, and neurogenic input.[3] Data regarding CBF in sleeping humans are few because of difficulties in measurement. However, in 1981 Meyer and coworkers developed a noninvasive method for estimating local and regional blood flow in the brain[4] and opened the door for other investigators to study the effect of blood flow variations in the intact human CNS.

Animal experiments have revealed marked variations in CBF during sleep. There appears to be a significant decrease in CBF during NREM sleep and a profound increase during REM sleep. In general, cerebral vasodilatation occurs during sleep.[5] Response to state change is, however, heterogeneous, with different regions of the brain exhibiting different magnitudes of alteration. In addition, differences exist in blood flow between slow-wave sleep (SWS) and paradoxical, or rapid eye movement (REM), sleep.[6] Townsend found in humans a consistent decrease in CBF during SWS with an overall average decrease of 10%.[7] During REM sleep CBF increased significantly (overall increase of approximately 8% over the baseline state).

The exact mechanisms responsible for variations in CBF during sleep are unknown. However, changes may be in response to transformation in metabolic rates of cerebral tissue during various stages of sleep. Brain temperature decreases in non-REM (NREM) sleep and increases in REM sleep.[8] This REM-related increase is attributed to increased blood flow and increased metabolic rate during this stage. Neuronal activity in many CNS regions is higher during REM than during NREM sleep, and this increased activity may be responsible for the increased metabolic rate.[9] In addition, the control of CBF during sleep appears to have a neurogenic component.[10] Meyer and Toyoda have suggested that the variation in CBF during different stages of sleep is a function of neurogenic control.[11]

During REM sleep, local blood flow has been shown to increase in the rhombencephalon, while blood flow in the mesencephalon decreases.[12] CBF has been noted to increase by 30% to 50% in REM sleep when compared with SWS.[8] Larger differences are seen in the brainstem. White matter and cortex show the least alteration. During REM sleep, phasic oscillations in blood flow have been observed and appear to correlate with bursts of phasic activity (e.g., twitches, eye movements). During SWS, oscillations are not as dramatic or consistent.[12]

Intrinsic regulation of CBF during wakefulness and sleep is significantly affected by the chemical environment. Although CBF is dramatically altered by changes in arterial carbon dioxide tension ($Paco_2$), moderate changes in $Paco_2$ do not appear to be associated with significant variation in cerebral circulation during sleep.[13] When $Paco_2$ disturbances occur, extravascular pH appears to be an important variable.[14]

Cerebral metabolic rate and CBF seem to be insensitive to alterations in the arterial oxygen tension (Pao_2) within the physiological range.[8] If the arterial Pao_2 is lowered below about 50 mm Hg, CBF begins to increase precipitously in response to the hypoxia.[15] Hypoventilation seen during sleep in normal subjects results in a progressive decrease in oxygen saturation (Sao_2). In a study reported by Doust and Schneider a decrease in Sao_2 from 96% during wakefulness to 87% during SWS was seen in normal subjects.[16]

Intracranial pressure (ICP) also reveals sleep-related changes (Fig. 5–1). There is little variation in ICP from the waking state as the subject enters NREM sleep.[17] During REM sleep, however, large ICP waves, almost double those of the steady-state pressure, occur. In most individuals these ICP waves are of little clinical

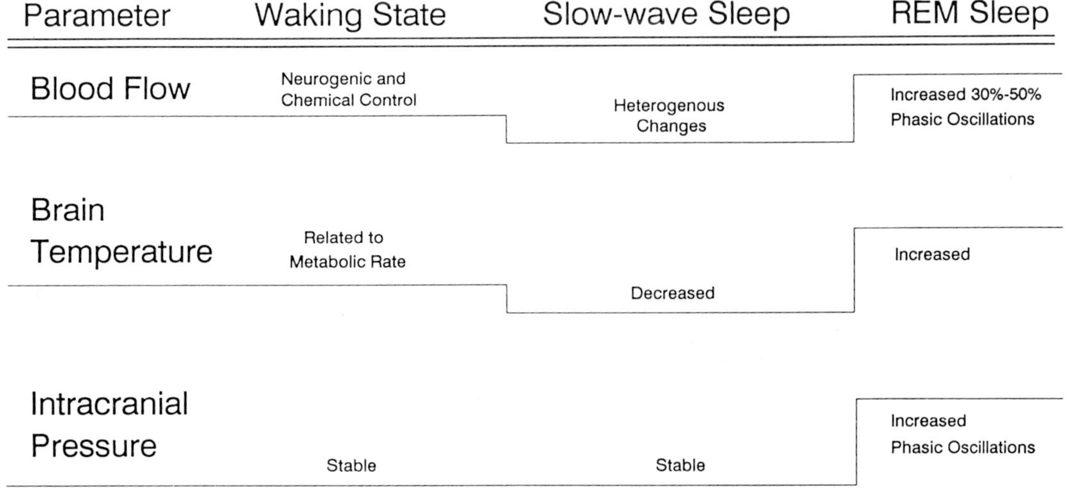

FIGURE 5–1. Central nervous system variations between waking and sleep states.

significance. However, in patients with little ICP reserve, small increases during sleep may result in depressed neuronal function.

BODY TEMPERATURE REGULATION DURING SLEEP

Core body temperature exhibits a highly stable circadian rhythmicity and has been used as a major marker for other endogenous rhythms (Fig. 5–2). As the night progresses, core body temperature falls and reaches its nadir during the early morning hours. During REM sleep, however, core temperature increases approximately 0.2° C.

Homeothermic temperature regulation is characteristic of mammals. Interestingly, animal experiments have shown that during REM sleep, body temperature follows environmental temperature, increasing as the ambient temperature increases and decreasing as the ambient temperature decreases. Return to NREM sleep is accompanied by a rise in core temperature to homeostatic levels. This positive correlation of variation of body temperature with environmental temperature during REM sleep suggests a shift toward poikilothermy (i.e., thermoregulatory mechanisms are depressed). On the other hand, a negative correlation exists during NREM sleep, indicating that thermoregulation remains intact during this state.[18]

Sweating and shivering are major temperature-regulating mechanisms during wakefulness. Significant variations are seen in both functions during sleep. Sweating remains intact during NREM sleep in neutral or warm environments[19] but is notably absent during REM sleep.[20] Similarly, shivering and thermoregulatory vasomotor activity, which occur during wakefulness and NREM sleep, are absent or significantly depressed during REM sleep. Absence of shivering during REM sleep results from mechanisms other than muscle atonia associated with this state. Animals with lesions created in the pontine tegmentum (which results in abolition of REM atonia) still do not shiver during REM sleep.[21]

The diaphragm is normally unaffected by generalized skeletal muscle inhibition during REM sleep but does not show increased activity (i.e., tachypnea) in response to warming or cooling. Cooling the hypothalamus during NREM sleep in animals increases oxygen consumption and metabolic heat production, but neither cooling nor heating of the hypothalamus during REM sleep results in a thermoregulatory response.[22] These data support the assumption that hypothalamic thermoregulation is significantly decreased or absent during REM sleep.

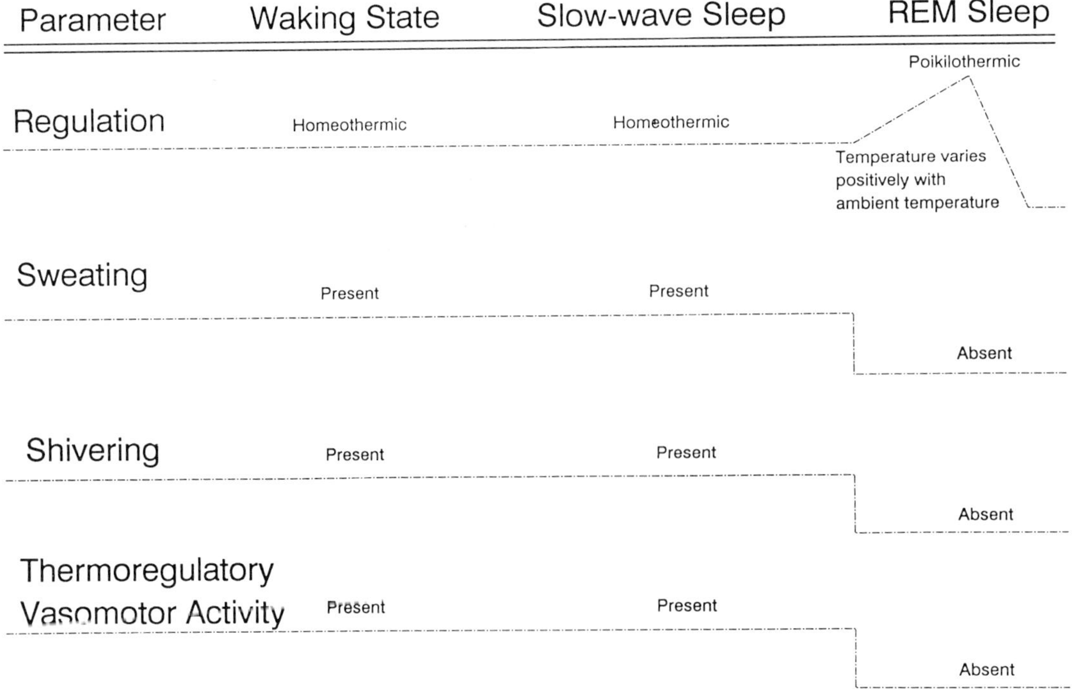

FIGURE 5–2. Variation in temperature regulation between waking and sleep states.

TABLE 5–1. Effects of Sleep on Hormone Secretion

Hormone	Normal Sleep Phase	Shifted Sleep Phase	Sleep Dependent
Growth hormone	Sleep onset secretion; peaks early in sleep period	Shift in secretion follows shift in phase	Yes
Prolactin	Secretion 30 to 90 min after sleep onset; peaks early morning	Shift in secretion follows shift in phase	Yes
Cortisol	Peaks at end of sleep; nadir early in sleep period	No significant change; sleep modulates (inhibits secretion)	No
Thyroid-stimulating hormone	Early evening peak; declines across sleep phase	No significant change; sleep modulates (inhibits secretion)	No
Luteinizing hormone	Rises during sleep in prepuberty; secondary waking peaks during puberty	Shift in secretion follows shift in phase	Yes
Follicle-stimulating hormone	Sleep-related rise in secretion	Shift in secretion follows shift in phase	Yes

ENDOCRINE VARIATIONS DURING SLEEP

The effects of the sleep cycle on hormone secretion are summarized in Table 5–1 and shown in Figure 5–3.

Growth Hormone

In prepubertal children, secretion of growth hormone (GH) is clearly coupled with sleep onset. GH is secreted exclusively during sleep,[23] with a peak early in the first third of the night during SWS. During puberty and throughout adolescence the pattern of GH secretion is modified from the prepubertal paradigm. Several minor peaks occur throughout the day, although GH still reaches its maximum concentration during sleep. Shifting of the sleep phase to times of day other than the normal sleep period is accompanied by shifts in the timing of GH secretion.[24,25] A 180-degree reversal of sleep phase results in a 180-degree shift in peak secretion

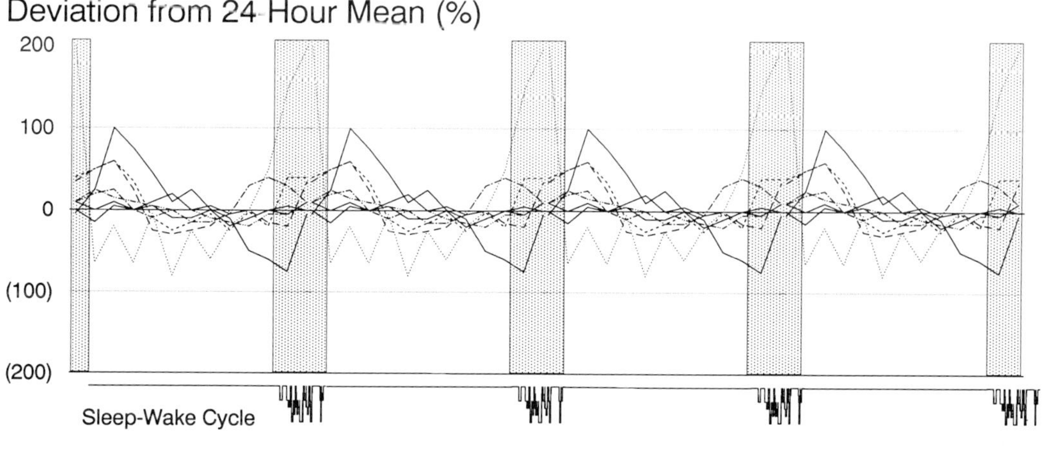

FIGURE 5–3. Circadian variations in endogenous hormone secretion. (Modified from Aschoff J: Circadian rhythms: general features of endocrinological aspects. In Kryger D [ed]: Endocrine rhythms. New York, Raven Press, 1979, pp 1-61. With permission.)

of GH. This sleep-associated release of GH has been related to Jouvet's theory of monoaminergic sleep systems. Agreement rests in observations that NREM sleep and hypothalamic releasing factors are both triggered by the same serotonergic neurons in the raphe nuclei of the brainstem.[26]

Prolactin

Under basal conditions, prolactin rhythmically peaks each night. As with GH, summits are almost entirely restricted to the sleep interval and are clearly coupled to the sleeping state.[27] Prolactin levels generally increase 30 to 90 minutes after sleep onset and reach maximal levels in the early morning hours.[19] Prolactin secretion also occurs during daytime naps and remains coupled to sleep after acute sleep-wake phase reversals. This sleep-related pattern of secretion is present from late puberty to old age and persists during pregnancy when greater amounts of prolactin are secreted. Although prolactin and GH secretion are both connected to the sleeping state, peaks of these two hormones are not coincident. In contrast to the adolescent and adult GH rhythm, the prolactin peak during sleep appears to be the only major aligned episode of release across 24 hours.[28]

Cortisol

Similar to core body temperature, cortisol follows a clear, well-established, and consistent circadian rhythm; it has also been used as a phase reference point for other endogenous rhythms.[29] Maximal cortisol secretion generally occurs at the end of the sleep period, and its nadir is reached early in the sleep period. Manipulating the timing of sleep does not dramatically change adrenocorticotropic hormone (ACTH) and cortisol secretion as it does with GH and prolactin, and its rhythm is probably independent of sleep itself, controlled by a different endogenous oscillator. A reduction in plasma cortisol concentration seems to occur regardless of the timing of the sleep period.[26] This suggests that cortisol secretion and the rhythm of the sleep-wake cycle are independent. Sleep appears only to modulate the release of cortisol, inhibiting rather than controlling secretion.

Thyroid-Stimulating Hormone

Daily maximums of thyroid-stimulating hormone (TSH) secretion occur rhythmically each evening before the onset of sleep.[30] TSH peak begins in the early evening and then declines across the sleep phase. This sleep-associated decline in TSH suggests that sleep is almost as important a determinant of the locus of the maximum TSH rhythm as it is for GH and prolactin. However, with shifts in the sleep phase, rise in TSH levels appears to be coupled to clock time rather than sleep period. Changing the timing of the sleep period reveals that inhibition of TSH secretion occurs with sleep, although the rise to peak of this hormone is still synchronized to clock time. Therefore sleep appears to truncate the circadian secretory episode of TSH.[26]

Luteinizing Hormone

Luteinizing hormone (LH) has been shown to drive male testosterone production by the Leydig cells of the testes and exhibits sleep-related rhythmicity during puberty.[31-33] However, these sleep-associated changes in LH secretion and testosterone production have been shown to occur before Tanner Stage 2.[34] LH increases during sleep seem to be responsible for initiation of pubertal changes. LH surges are followed momentarily by elevations in plasma testosterone levels, which in turn induce the changes in secondary sexual characteristics seen during this stage of development.[32,35] As young males pass through puberty, enhanced episodic release of LH and testosterone occurs during wakefulness until Tanner Stage 5 is reached. At this time an adult pattern of equivalent pulse height of LH secretion across the sleep cycle occurs.[32] Change of sleep phase results in a corresponding change in LH and testosterone activity. Testosterone levels peak during sleep in adults despite a weakened or absent nocturnal rise in LH activity.[19]

Follicle-Stimulating Hormone

Follicle-stimulating hormone (FSH) follows a pattern similar to LH. Increases in LH occur at sleep onset, and wakefulness appears to inhibit LH and FSH secretion. The delay of sleep or the acute reversal of the sleep-wake cycle results in corresponding changes in FSH activity patterns. Pubertal females show sleep-coupled release of LH and FSH during sleep.[19] Estradiol levels, however, do not increase until 10 to 14 hours later. Women having menstrual cycles do not show sleep-related release, but LH secretion may be inhibited 2 to 3 hours after sleep onset.

CARDIOVASCULAR VARIATIONS DURING SLEEP

The effects of the sleep cycle on the cardiovascular system are shown in Figure 5–4.

Heart Rate

Heart rate is generally reduced during natural sleep in most animal species. When compared with the heart rate during quiet wake (QW), the rate during synchronized (NREM) sleep is 4 to 8 beats slower per minute.[36] During REM sleep a decrease in rate of 17 beats per minute (approximately 8% less than the mean for QW) has been noted. Reduction in heart rate during sleep appears to parallel sleep-related alterations in blood pressure, in that the variation is more pronounced during REM sleep and that heart rate variability is clearly greater in REM sleep than in NREM-SWS.[37]

Heart rate is also significantly influenced by phasic phenomena of REM.[38] During bursts of rapid eye movements and body movements, there are clear episodes of short-lasting tachycardia followed occasionally by a rebound brief bradycardia before return to baseline levels.

Cardiac output is generally coupled to heart rate during wakefulness. During sleep, however, cardiac output has been shown to be only slightly reduced during SWS when compared with the waking state.[36,39] Reduction in cardiac output becomes more pronounced, however, during the tonic REM state, its average being about 9% less than during QW. Changes in cardiac output are not accompanied by changes in stroke volume, which tends to remain constant during QW, SWS, and REM cycles.

Blood Pressure

Extended studies of laboratory animals have revealed a moderate decrease (approximately 14 mm Hg) in blood pressure during NREM sleep when compared with QW.[37] A more significant fall (approximately 25 mm Hg) has been shown to occur during REM sleep. Changes in blood

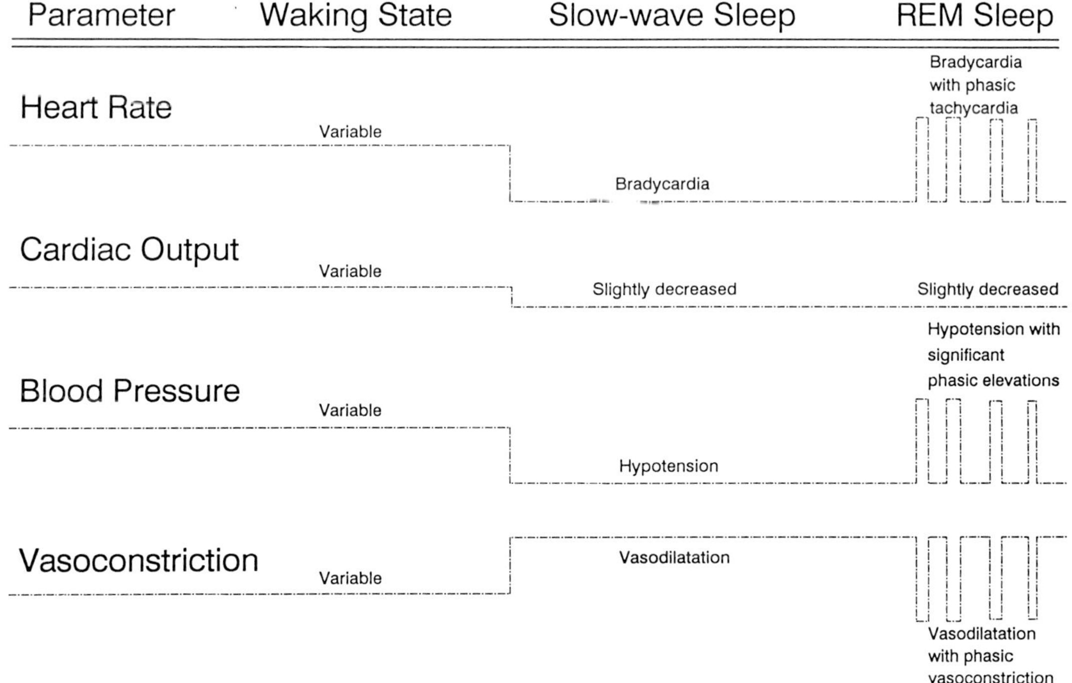

FIGURE 5–4. Cardiovascular variations between waking and sleep states.

pressure are more complex and variable during REM sleep than NREM sleep. Brief sharp increases in mean arterial pressure are superimposed on relatively hypotensive values. These oscillations in blood pressure appear to be related to brief excitatory somatomotor phenomena that are typical of REM sleep. Blood pressure rise begins with, or occurs shortly following, the onset of bursts of rapid eye movements and muscle twitches.[38]

Two types of blood pressure change in desynchronized sleep occur in the cat. First is a tonic blood pressure alteration, consisting of hypotension lasting throughout the desynchronized sleep episode. Second are frequent phasic pressure changes that consist of brief blood pressure rises simultaneously with other phasic phenomena.[40]

Marked, brief cutaneous vasoconstriction occurs concomitantly with phasic events during REM sleep.[19] Other regional vasoconstriction takes place as well. For example, urine volume production is significantly reduced during REM sleep, which is considered to be due to a reduced renal blood flow during this state. Central inhibitory influences on vasoconstriction present during REM sleep have been shown to be potentiated by sinoaortic denervation.[19] Vasoconstriction normally seen in the iliac artery during REM sleep is converted to vasodilatation. Surprisingly, the buffering action of the sinoaortic nerve depends more on chemoreceptive reflexes than on baroreceptor reflexes. The baroreflexes are diminished during REM sleep in the cat, a variation that may be necessary to maintain homeostasis.

Cardiovascular variations during sleep hold specific and significant clinical relevance. Phasic excitation of the heart and coronary circulation may precipitate decreased coronary artery blood flow and lead to myocardial infarction (or other myocardial dysfunction) during REM sleep. Nowling and co-workers have reported that nocturnal exacerbations of angina generally occur during REM sleep.[41] As early as 1923, MacWilliams reported that deaths from cardiac disorders were found to occur between 5 and 6 AM, a time when sleep is primarily in the REM state.

RESPIRATORY VARIATIONS DURING SLEEP

Well-defined changes in respiratory patterns occur during sleep. These alterations result in modification of ventilatory control, blood gas and respiratory patterns, and regulatory responses to changes that are significantly different from those in the waking state (Fig. 5–5).

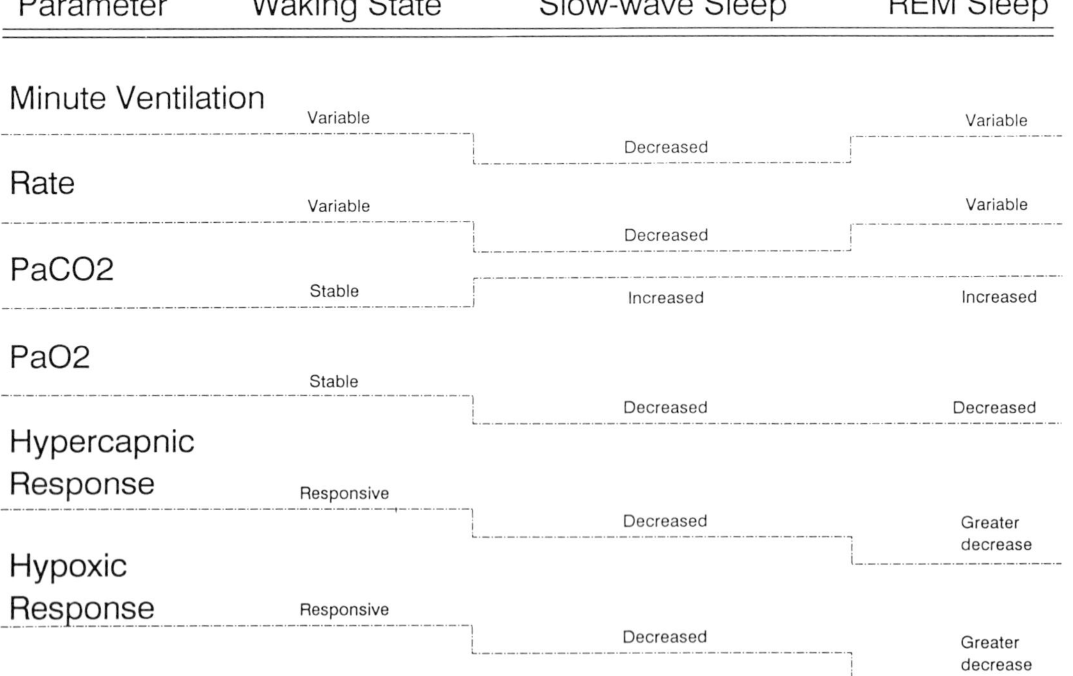

FIGURE 5–5. Respiratory variations between waking and sleep states.

In general, hypoventilation occurs during sleep in the normal individual. Minute ventilation decreases slightly during SWS. A change in metabolic rate is demonstrated by a decrease in oxygen uptake and an increase in carbon dioxide production of approximately 10% to 20%.[43] Subsequently a change in ventilatory control also occurs, since alveolar ventilation falls more than expected in response to these metabolic changes.[44] Consequently the Pa_{CO_2} increases during SWS.

One of the most striking features of breathing during SWS is its monotonous regularity and lack of breath-to-breath variability. Respiratory rate is slightly lower and tidal volume is slightly greater in SWS than in wakefulness.[45,46] All major indices of respiratory function appear to be in a stable state during this time. In contrast, significant irregularity is noted during REM sleep. Irregularities in respiratory patterns were part of the original description of REM sleep by Aserinsky and Kleitman in 1953.[47] These irregularities of respiration and rapid breathing patterns associated with REM sleep have been subsequently confirmed in studies of human infants, human adults, and other species.[48-50] As with cardiovascular changes, breathing patterns show a significant temporal relationship to the phasic components of REM sleep.[48,51,52]

Respiratory changes seen in REM sleep appear to be secondary to internally activated neural events.[53] This is consistent with the powerful REM sleep–coupled neural influences on other systems, which apparently arise from the brainstem.

The neonate (in particular the premature newborn) exhibits irregular breathing patterns. Breath-to-breath variability and long episodes of periodic breathing occur.[54,55] Periodic breathing patterns in premature infants occur during wake, quiet sleep, and active sleep. Although present during quiet sleep, periodic breathing is significantly increased during REM sleep.[56] During quiet sleep, periodic breathing appears to be quite regular: breathing and apneic intervals are of similar durations. These intervals are, on the other hand, quite irregular during active sleep.[57] The cause of periodic breathing is unknown, but many investigators believe that it depends on oscillations in blood gases during sleep.[58]

REM atonia, which affects almost all skeletal muscles, also affects muscles involved in respiration. The diaphragm, however, maintains its activity during REM sleep, but intercostal muscles and muscles of the upper airway are significantly hypotonic or atonic during this stage.[19] Decrease in muscle tone of the accessory muscles of respiration results in hypoventilation or upper airway occlusion. Neonates and infants appear particularly susceptible to intercostal muscle hypotonia resulting in rib cage collapse and "see-saw" respiratory efforts (paradoxical respiration).

Mucociliary clearance of pulmonary secretions is reduced during sleep. The cough reflex is significantly suppressed during NREM and REM sleep, and the presence of coughing appears to depend on arousal from sleep.[59] Decreased clearance of secretions becomes clinically significant in patients with pathological states in which mucus production is increased (e.g., asthma). Sleep is disrupted by numerous arousals, perhaps to assist in clearance of these pulmonary secretions. In addition, respiratory tract smooth muscle tone is affected by sleep. This tone is lower in NREM sleep than during wakefulness. Tone continues to decrease in tonic REM sleep, but a phasic increase is superimposed on this decrease during bursts of rapid eye movements.[19]

During wakefulness the newborn infant responds to hypoxia differently from older children and adults.[60] At lowered Pa_{O_2} a biphasic response is seen, with an initial period of hyperventilation followed by a fall in ventilation to a level below the baseline. A similar response curve is noted during REM sleep, but the initial hyperventilatory response is less dramatic. During NREM sleep, hyperventilation is noted and sustained, without the fall seen in the other two states.

Ventilatory response to hypoxemia is decreased during NREM sleep in adult men. In contrast, responses during NREM and wakefulness are similar in women. The reason for this sex differentiation is unknown.[61-63] During REM sleep the ventilatory response to hypoxia is below that of NREM sleep in both males and females.

Ventilatory response to hypercapnia is depressed during sleep in adult humans.[64] The slope of the ventilatory–carbon dioxide response curve falls during NREM sleep when compared with wakefulness.[65-67] This decrease in response from wakefulness to NREM sleep has been reported to be approximately 50%.[68,69] This change has not been observed in females.[70] Hypercapnic response appears to be lowest in REM sleep when compared with wakefulness and NREM. The mean hypercapnic response during REM sleep seems to be approximately 28% lower than in the other two states.[68,70,71]

In transient or semisteady state experiments

in human neonates, hypercapnic ventilatory response differs from that in adults. Studies indicate no difference in the ventilatory response to carbon dioxide between active and quiet sleep.[72-75] When rebreathing techniques are used, however, a lower response in REM sleep is suggested.[60,76] and the hypercapnic response is lower in preterm neonates than in term infants.[77]

SKELETAL MUSCLE ACTIVITY VARIATIONS DURING SLEEP

As early as 1894 a reduction in spinal reflexes and loss of patellar reflex activity during sleep were noted.[78] These observations have been systematically confirmed: Hodes and Dement have documented decrease in spinal reflexes during sleep,[79] and decrease in body motility associated with the progression into SWS has been corroborated by Rohmer and co-workers.[80]

Skeletal muscle activity and spinal cord reflex activity are diminished to their greatest extent during REM sleep.[79,81] Periodic twitches and muscular tremors of the face and limbs frequently occur during this stage of sleep.[82] Progressive relaxation of the skeletal musculature and attenuation of reflexes are most predominantly seen during REM sleep. During REM, periodic bursts of excitatory activity break through the generalized tonic inhibition. Hyperpolarization of the intracellular membrane is correlated with active inhibition of the motor neuron at the spinal level.[83] Stimulation of neurons in the pons (specifically in the nucleus pontis oralis) results in different peripheral effects depending on whether the subject is awake, in NREM sleep, or in REM sleep. During wakefulness, stimulation of these neurons results in excitatory postsynaptic potential generation. During REM sleep, however, inhibitory postsynaptic potentials are recognized. Thus membrane potentials are reversed depending on the state of arousal. There appears to be a neuronal gate that opens specifically during REM sleep. In addition, coactivation of facilitative and inhibitory neuronal activity explains the twitches and jerks accompanying REM sleep.

Major body movements are strongly related to the stage of sleep, with the rate of body movements progressively decreasing from waking, Stage 1, REM, Stage 2, and SWS.[84] Although body movements occur during all stages of sleep, they are most frequent during REM and least frequent during SWS.[85] Within a single night's sleep the number of body movements can vary from 70 to 200.[86]

VARIATIONS IN GENITOURINARY FUNCTION DURING SLEEP

Changes in renal function occur during sleep and are characterized by a decrease in urine volume and an increase in urine osmolality.[87] These changes generally occur in conjunction with REM sleep but appear to be more related to decrease in regional blood flow and not primarily mediated by REM-related antidiuretic hormone release (although a nocturnal peak in vasopressin secretion can be demonstrated).[88] In addition to renal conservation of water during sleep, excretion of sodium chloride is reduced during this state.

Penile tumescence occurs during REM sleep in male children and adults.[89-92] The most striking number of nocturnal penile tumescence episodes occurs in the prepubertal and pubertal years, gradually declining in frequency throughout the later years of life. A similar phenomenon appears to occur in females during REM sleep. Most evidence for this phenomenon stems from similarities between phasic shifts of vaginal vascular blood flow and penile blood flow during REM sleep. Karacan and co-workers have reported clitoral erections in three women during REM sleep.[93] Abel and co-workers have documented increases in relative pulse pressure within the vagina during REM sleep.[94]

VARIATIONS IN GASTROINTESTINAL FUNCTION DURING SLEEP

Physiological activity during sleep is not homogeneous. It varies as a function of the stage of sleep as well as the time of night. Parasympathetic activity seems to dominate NREM sleep, and sympathetic activity dominates REM sleep.[95]

Gastrointestinal function is extrinsically and intrinsically modified during sleep. Finch and co-workers have demonstrated that gastroduodenal motility during sleep shows a strong relationship with body movements as well as sleep stage changes.[96] Although there appears to be no statistically significant relationship between gastric acid secretion and stages of sleep,[97] a circadian variation of secretion is seen, with peaks occurring about 2 AM. Gastric acid secretion is not inhibited during sleep in patients with duodenal ulcers. However, epigastric pain during sleep in duodenal ulcer patients may be more related to the prolonged fast associated with sleep than to factors associated with gastric acid secretion.[98]

Swallowing and esophageal function are important determinants of gastroesophageal reflux during sleep. Swallowing is significantly suppressed during sleep.[99] This suppression is most noticeable during SWS, and refluxed gastric contents maintain mucosal contact for longer periods. Acid contact and prolonged acid clearance are considered the prime factors in the development of esophagitis in patients with gastroesophageal reflux.[100]

Salivary flow, another important determinant of acid clearance, nearly ceases during sleep.[101] Body position also appears to play an important role in acid clearance, with supine positions associated with markedly prolonged esophageal acid clearance.[100]

Orr and co-workers have documented that sleep impairs esophageal acid clearance in both normal subjects and patients with esophagitis.[99] However, in patients with esophagitis, acid clearance took significantly longer even during waking hours. This is especially noteworthy, since most gastroesophageal reflux occurred during arousals from sleep in this study, as well as in a study of spontaneous gastroesophageal reflux in normal subjects.[102] These data clearly implicate defective acid clearance as a major cause of esophageal inflammation in patients with gastroesophageal reflux. Little data are available regarding esophageal motility and acid clearance during sleep in infants with significant gastroesophageal reflux.

REFERENCES

1. Kleitman N: Sleep and wakefulness. Chicago, University of Chicago Press, 1963.
2. Orem J and Barnes CD: Physiology in sleep. New York, Academic Press, 1980.
3. Ekstrom-Jodal et al: Cerebral blood flow autoregulation at high arterial pressures and different levels of carbon dioxide tension in dogs. Eur Neurol 1972;6:6-10.
4. Meyer JS et al: Mapping local blood flow of human brain by CT scanning during stable xenon inhalation. Stroke 1981;12:426-436.
5. Bridges TH et al: Plethysmographic studies of the cerebral circulation: evidence for cranial nerve vasomotor activity. J Clin Invest 1958;37:763-772.
6. Reivich M et al: The effects of slow-wave sleep and REM sleep on regional blood flow in cats. J Neurochem 1968;15:301-306.
7. Townsend RE, Prinz PN, and Obrist WD: Human cerebral blood flow during sleep and waking. J Appl Physiol 1973;35:620-625.
8. Greenberg JH: Sleep and the cerebral circulation. In Orem J and Barnes CD (eds): Physiology in sleep. New York, Academic Press, 1980, pp 57-95.
9. Reivich M: Blood flow and metabolism couple in the brain. In Plum F (ed): Brain dysfunction in metabolic disorders. New York, Raven Press, 1974, pp 125-140.
10. Perves MJ: The physiology of the cerebral circulation. London, Cambridge University Press, 1972.
11. Meyer JS and Toyoda M: Studies of rapid changes in cerebral circulation and metabolism during arousal and rapid eye movement during sleep in human subjects with cerebrovascular disease. In Zulch KJ (ed): Cerebral circulation and stroke. New York, Springer-Verlag, 1971, pp 156-163.
12. Baust W: Local blood flow in different regions of the brain during natural sleep and arousal. Encephalogr Clin Neurophysiol 1967;22:365-372.
13. Alexander SC et al: Cerebral carbohydrate metabolism during hypocarbia in man. Anesthesiology 1965;26:624-632.
14. Wahl M et al: Micropuncture evaluation of importance of perivascular pH for the arteriolar diameter on the brain surface. Pfluegers Arch 1970;316:152-163.
15. Kogure K et al: Mechanism of cerebral vasodilatation in hypoxia. J Appl Physiol 1970;29:223-229.
16. Doust LJW and Schneider RA: Studies of the physiology of awareness: anoxia and the levels of sleep. Br Med J 1952;1:449-455.
17. Gucer G and Viernstein LJ: Intracranial pressure in the normal monkey while awake and asleep. J Neurosurg 1979;51:206-210.
18. Henane R et al: Variations in evaporation and body temperatures during sleep in man. J Appl Physiol 1977;42:50-55.
19. Orem J and Keeling J: A compendium of physiology in sleep. In Orem J and Barnes CD: Physiology in sleep. New York, Academic Press, 1980, pp 315-335.
20. Parmeggiani PL et al: Temperature changes in cats sleeping at different environmental temperatures. Brain Res 1971;33:397-404.
21. Hendricks JC, Bowker RM, and Morrison AR: Functional characteristics of cats with pontine lesions during sleep and wakefulness and their usefulness for sleep research. In Koella WP and Levin P (eds): Sleep 1976. Basel, S Karger, 1977, pp 207-210.
22. Parmeggiani PL et al: Hypothalamic temperature during sleep cycles at different ambient temperatures. Electroencephalogr Clin Neurophysiol 1975;38:589-596.
23. Parker DC et al: Rhythmicities in human growth hormone concentration in plasma. In Krieger DT (ed): Endocrine rhythms. New York, Raven Press, 1979, pp 143-173.
24. Parker DC and Rossman LG: Physiology of human growth hormone release in sleep. In Scow RO (ed): Endocrinology. Amsterdam, Excerpta Medica, 1973, pp 655-660.
25. Parker DC and Rossman LG: Sleep-wake cycle and human growth hormone, prolactin and luteinizing hormone. In Raiti S (ed): Advances in human growth hormone research, Washington, DC, US Government Printing Office, 1974, pp 294-312.
26. Parker DC et al: Endocrine rhythms across sleep-wake cycles in normal young men under basal state

conditions. In Orem J and Barnes CD (eds): Physiology in sleep. New York, Academic Press, 1980, pp 145-179.
27. Parker DC, Rossman LG, and VanderLaan EF: Sleep-related, nychtohemeral and briefly episodic variation in human plasma prolactin concentrations. J Clin Endocrinol Metab 1973;36:1119.
28. Sassin JF et al: Human prolactin: 24-hour pattern with increased release during sleep. Science 1972;177:1205-1207.
29. Aschoff J: Circadian rhythms: general features and endocrinological aspects. In Krieger D (ed): Endocrine rhythms. New York, Raven Press, 1979, pp 1-61.
30. Parker DC, Pekary AE, and Hershman JM: Effect of normal and reversed sleep-wake cycles upon nychtohemeral rhythmicity of plasma thyrotropin: evidence suggestive of an inhibitory influence in sleep. J Clin Endocrinol Metab 1976;43:318-329.
31. Boyar R et al: Synchronization of augmented luteinizing hormone with sleep during puberty. N Engl J Med 1972;287:582-586.
32. Parker DC et al: Pubertal sleep-wake patterns of episodic LH, FSH, and testosterone release in twin boys. J Clin Endocrinol Metab 1975;40:1099-1109.
33. Kapen S et al: Effect of sleep-wake cycle reversal on luteinizing hormone secretory pattern in puberty. J Clin Endocrinol Metab 1974;39:293-299.
34. Judd HL, Parker DC, and Yen SSC: Sleep-wake patterns of LH and testosterone release in prepubertal boys. J Clin Endocrinol Metab 1977;44:865-869.
35. Judd HL et al: The nocturnal rise of plasma testosterone in pubertal boys. J Clin Endocrinol Metab 1974;38:710-713.
36. Mancia G et al: Vasomotor regulation during sleep in the cat. Am J Physiol 1971;220:1086-1093.
37. Guazzi M and Zanchetti A: Blood pressure and heart rate during natural sleep of the cat and their regulation by carotid sinus and aortic reflexes. Arch Ital Biol 1965;103:789-817.
38. Gassel MM et al: Phasic changes in blood pressure and heart rate during the rapid eye movement episodes of desynchronized sleep in unrestrained cats. Arch Ital Biol 1964;102:530-544.
39. Kumazawa T et al: Haemodynamic patterns during desynchronized sleep in intact cats and cats with sinoatrial deafferentiation. Circ Res 1969;24:923-937.
40. Mancia G and Zanchetti A: Cardiovascular regulation during sleep. In Orem J and Barnes CD (eds): Physiology in sleep. New York, Academic Press, 1980, pp 1-55.
41. Nowlin JB et al: The association of nocturnal angina pectoris with dreaming. Ann Intern Med 1965;63:1040-1046.
42. MacWilliams JA: Blood pressure and heart action in sleep and dreams. Br Med J 1923, pp 1196-1200.
43. Phillipson EA, Murphy E, and Kozar LF: Regulation of respiration in sleeping dogs. J Appl Physiol 1976;40:688-693.
44. Sullivan CE: Breathing in sleep. In Orem J and Barnes CD (eds): Physiology in sleep. New York, Academic Press, 1980, pp 213-272.
45. Orem J, Netick A, and Dement WC: Breathing during sleep and wakefulness in the cat. Respir Physiol 1977;30:265-269.
46. Lugaresi E et al: Breathing during sleep in man in normal and pathological conditions. In Fitzgerald H, Gautier H, and Lahiri S (eds): The regulation of respiration during sleep and anesthesia. New York, Plenum, 1978, pp 35-45.
47. Aserinsky E and Kleitman N: Regularly occurring periods of eye motility, and concomitant phenomena, during sleep. Science 1953;118:273-274.
48. Phillipson EA, Kozar LF, and Murphy E: Respiratory load compensation in awake and sleeping dogs. J Appl Physiol 1976;40:895-902.
49. Snyder F et al: Changes in respiration, heart rate, and systolic blood pressure in human sleep. J Appl Physiol 1964;19:417-422.
50. Snyder F: Autonomic nervous system manifestations during sleep and dreaming. In Kety SS, Evarts EV, and Williams HL (eds): Sleep and altered states of consciousness. Baltimore, Williams & Wilkins, 1967, pp 469-487.
51. Aserinsky E: Periodic respiratory pattern occurring in conjunction with eye movements during sleep. Science 1965;150:763-766.
52. Baust W, Holzbach E, and Zechlin O: Phasic changes in heart rate and respiration correlated with PGO-spike activity during REM sleep. Pfleugers Arch 1972;331:113-123.
53. Pompeiano O: The neurophysiological mechanisms of the postural and motor events during desynchronized sleep. In Ketty SS, Evarts EV, and Williams HL (eds): Sleep and altered states of consciousness. Baltimore, Williams & Wilkins, 1967, pp 351-423.
54. Rigatto H and Brady JP: Periodic breathing and apnea in preterm infants. I. Evidence for hypoventilation possibly due to central respiratory depression. Pediatrics 1972;50:202.
55. Rigatto H and Brady JP: Periodic breathing and apnea in preterm infants. II. Hypoxia as a primary event. Pediatrics 1975;55:604.
56. Rigatto H et al: Ventilatory response to 100 per cent and 15 per cent O_2 during wakefulness and sleep in preterm infants. Early Hum Dev 1982;7:1.
57. Rigatto H: Control of breathing during sleep in the fetus and neonate. In Kryger MH, Roth T, and Dement WC (eds): Principles and practice of sleep medicine. Philadelphia, WB Saunders, 1989, pp 237-248.
58. Waggener J et al: Apnea duration is related to ventilatory oscillation characteristics in newborn infants. J Appl Physiol 1984;57:536.
59. Bateman JRM et al: Reduction in clearance of secretions from the human lung during sleep. J Physiol 1978;284:55P.
60. Rigatto H: Control of ventilation in the newborn. Annu Rev Physiol 1984;46:661-674.
61. White DP et al: Hypoxic ventilatory response during sleep in normal women. Am Rev Respir Dis 1982;126:530-533.
62. Douglas NJ et al: Hypoxic ventilatory response decreases during sleep in normal men. Am Rev Respir Dis 1982;125:286-289.
63. Hedemark LL and Kronenberg RS: Ventilatory and heart rate response to hypoxia and hypercapnia during sleep in adults. J Appl Physiol 1982;53:307-312.
64. Douglas NJ: Control of ventilation during sleep. Clin Chest Med 1985;6:563.
65. Birchfield RI, Sieker HO, and Heyman A: Alterations in respiratory functions during natural sleep. J Lab Clin Med 1959;54:216-222.
66. Douglas NJ et al: Respiration during sleep in normal man. Thorax 1982;37:840-844.
67. Gothe B et al: Effects of quiet sleep on resting and

CO_2 stimulating breathing in humans. J Appl Physiol 1981;50:724-730.

68. Bulow K: Respiration and wakefulness in man. Acta Physiol Scand 1963;59(suppl 209):1-110.
69. Douglas NJ et al: Hypercapnic ventilatory response in sleeping adults. Am Rev Respir Dis 1982;126:758-762.
70. Berthon-Jones M and Sullivan CE: Ventilation and arousal response to hypercapnia in normal sleeping adults. J Appl Physiol 1984;57:59-67.
71. White DP: Occlusion pressure and ventilation during sleep in normal humans. J Appl Physiol 1986; 61:1279-1287.
72. Anderson JY et al: Transient ventilatory response to CO_2 as a function of sleep state in full term infants. J Appl Physiol 1983;54:1482-1488.
73. Davi M et al: The effect of sleep state on chest distortion and on the ventilatory response to CO_2 in neonates. Pediatr Res 1979;13:982-986.
74. Haddad GG et al: CO_2-induced changes in ventilation and ventilatory pattern in normal sleeping infants. J Appl Physiol 1980;48:684-688.
75. Rigatto H, Kalapesi Z, and Leahy FN: Chemical control of respiratory frequency and tidal volume during sleep in preterm infants. Respir Physiol 1980;41:117-125.
76. Honma Y et al: Ribcage and abdominal contributions to ventilatory response to CO_2 in infants. J Appl Physiol 1984;56:1211-1216.
77. Moriette G et al: The effect of breathing CO_2 on ventilation and diaphragmatic electromyography in newborn infants. Respir Physiol 1985;62:387-397.
78. Tarchanoff J: Quelques observations sur le sommeil normal. Arch Ital Biol 1894;21:318-321.
79. Hodes R and Dement WC: Depression of electrically induced reflexes ("H" reflexes) in man during low voltage EEG sleep. Electroencephalogr Clin Neurophysiol 1964;17:617-629.
80. Rohmer F et al: La motilité spontanée, la fréquence cardiaque et la fréquence respiratoire au cours du sommeil chez l'homme normal: leurs relations avec les manifestations electroencephalographiques et la profondeur du sommeil. In La Société d'Electroencephalographie et de Neurophysiologie Clinique de Langue Française (eds): Le sommeil de nuit normal et pathologique, etudes electroencephalographiques Paris, The Society, 1965, pp 192-207.
81. Jacobson A et al: Muscle tonus in human subjects during sleep and dreaming. Exp Neurol 1964:10:418-424.
82. Baldridge BJ, Whitman RM, and Kramer M: The concurrence of fine muscle activity and rapid eye movements during sleep. Psychosom Med 1965; 27:19-26.
83. Chandler SH, Nakamura Y, and Chase MH: Intracellular analysis of synaptic potentials induced in trigeminal jaw-closer motoneurons by pontomesencephalic reticular stimulation during sleep and wakefulness. J Neurophysiol 1980;44:372-382.
84. Wilde-Frenz J and Schulz H: Rate and distribution of body movements during sleep in humans. Percept Mot Skills 1983;56:275-283.
85. Oswald I et al: Melancholia and barbiturates: a controlled EEG and eye-movement study of sleep. Br J Psychiatry 1963;109:66-78.
86. Gardner R and Grossman WL: Normal motor patterns in sleep in man. In Weitzman ED (ed): Advances in sleep research, Vol 2. New York, Spectrum, 1975, pp 67-107.
87. Mandell A et al: Dreaming sleep in man: changes in urine volume and osmolality. Science 1966;151: 1558-1560.
88. Rubin RT et al: Secretion of hormones influencing water and electrolyte balance (antidiuretic hormone, aldosterone, prolactin) during sleep in normal adult men. Psychosom Med 1978;40:44-59.
89. Halverson H: Genital and sphincter behavior on the male infant. J Gen Psychol 1940;56:95-136.
90. Ohlmeyer P, Brilmayer H, and Hullstrung H: Periodische vorgange im Schlaf. Pfleugers Arch 1944;248:559-560.
91. Fisher C, Gross J, and Zuch J: Cycle of penile erections synchronous with dreaming (REM) sleep: preliminary report. Arch Gen Psychiatry 1965;12:29-45.
92. Karacan I et al: Sleep-related penile tumescence as a function of age. Am J Psychiatry 1975;132:932-937.
93. Karacan I, Rosenblum A, and Williams R: The clitoral erection cycle during sleep. Psychophysiology 1970;7:338.
94. Abel GG et al: Women's vaginal responses during REM sleep. J Sex Marital Ther 1979;5:5-14.
95. Snyder F et al: Changes in respiration, heart rate, and systolic pressure in human sleep. J Appl Physiol 1964;19:417.
96. Finch P et al: Relationship of fasting gastroduodenal motility to the sleep cycle. Gastroenterology 1982; 83:605-612.
97. Orr W et al: Sleep patterns and gastric acid secretion in duodenal ulcer disease. Arch Intern Med 1976;136:655-660.
98. Orr W and Robinson M: The sleeping gut. Med Clin North Am 1981;65:1359-1376.
99. Orr W, Robinson M, and Johnson L: Acid clearance during sleep in the pathogenesis of reflux esophagitis. Dig Dis Sci 1981;26:423-427.
100. Johnson LF, DeMeester TR, and Haggitt RC: Esophageal epithelial response to gastroesophageal reflux: a quantitative study. Am J Dig Dis 1978;23:498-509.
101. Helm JF et al: Determinants of esophageal acid clearance in normal subjects. Gastroenterology 1980; 78:1181.
102. Dent J et al: Mechanism of gastroesophageal reflux in recumbent asymptomatic human subjects. J Clin Invest 1980;65:256-257.

6

Dreams

In 1953 Aserinsky and Kleitman published their historic discovery of rapid eye movement (REM) sleep.[1] Dement and Kleitman subsequently published evidence that the REM sleep state was associated with dreaming.[2] Sigmund Freud proposed that dream content was a mirror to underlying psychological and psychopathological processes.[3] These works opened the door to study of dreams, their perceptual content, and physiological events as important considerations in clinical practice. Despite rapid advances in the understanding of sleep physiology and the impetus given to the study of the dream sleep state, there is still no consensus regarding the meaning of dreams.[4] Research into the biological and psychological meaning of dreams continues.

Dreams, as defined by Hobson and McCarley, are mental experiences that occur in sleep and are characterized by hallucinoid imagery, predominantly visual and often vivid. The bizarre elements in dreams are due to spatiotemporal distortions, such as condensation, discontinuity, and acceleration, and to delusional acceptance of these phenomena as "real" at the time they occur.[5] Distinct formal properties of the dream may or may not be associated with strong emotions. Subsequent recall of these mental events is usually poor unless an immediate arousal from the REM sleep state occurs.

Sensory errors and hypnagogic hallucinations of sleep onset differ significantly from typical dreams. *Hypnagogic hallucinations* occur at sleep onset and involve reworking of scenes from events that have occurred during the previous few hours. Despite their fanciful appearance, hypnagogic hallucinations lack an essential dreamlike quality.[6] Sensory errors are frequently accompanied by a feeling of weightlessness, loss of balance, falling, or floating, perhaps caused by partial sensory deafferentation from vestibular and muscle proprioceptive input. Imagery of hypnagogic hallucinations may be interrupted by a *hypnic jerk,* a massive myoclonic event resulting in arousal (see Chapter 9). *Hypnopompic hallucinations* (dreams) are qualitatively different from hypnagogic hallucinations in that intense imagery is accompanied by perceptual release. They occur during REM sleep and are most intense late in the sleep period.

FUNCTION OF DREAMS AND REM SLEEP

Interpretation of dreams significantly predates the scientific study of sleep.[7] Dreams have interested humans throughout history. The very existence of dreams as part of every individual's life has demanded experimentation and explanation.

Psychodynamic Theory

Freud's psychodynamic theory relies heavily on subconscious mechanisms. Freud considered dream mentation to be a direct reflection of the subconscious mind. He regarded the dream as a "window" and the symbols as representing an individual's wishes and deep-seated desires that are fulfilled by the dream. According to Freud, the foundation for understanding and interpreting dreams lies in understanding the significance of each symbol for the dreamer.

Decades of dream research have, however, failed to establish a unified, systematic, or widely accepted theory of the meaning of dreams. The clinical usefulness of dream interpretation is also widely debated. The psychoanalytical position that dream interpretation is central and at times crucial to the therapeutic process contrasts dramatically with many current theories.

Salley has described dream content in a patient with multiple personalities and categorized the dreams as *internal self-helpers*.[8] These internal self-helper personalities were interpreted as underlying synthetic programs that regulated unconscious information processing. Dreaming was seen as having the restorative function of providing a mechanism for communication across separate levels of cognitive organization and assimilation and for accommodation of new data into memory systems.

Physiological Determination of Dreams

Recent research into the neurobiology of dream sleep provides new evidence for possible structural and functional substrates of formal aspects of the dream process. Data suggest that dream sleep is physiologically determined and shaped by a brainstem neuronal mechanism that can be modeled physiologically and mathematically.[5] Formal features of the dream generator process having strong implications for dream theory include periodicity and automaticity of forebrain activation during dreams. This suggests a preprogrammed neural basis for dream mentation during sleep. In addition, intense and sporadic activation of the brainstem sensorimotor circuits including reticular, oculomotor, and vestibular neurons possibly determines spatiotemporal aspects of dream imagery. Shifts in transmitter ratios also occur during this state and may account for dream amnesia. Hobson and McCarley suggest that the automatically activated forebrain synthesizes the dream by comparing information generated in specific brainstem circuits with information stored in memory.[5]

Information Processing and Learning Theory

Information-processing and computer model theories view dreaming as a mechanism that reprograms information-processing structures within the central nervous system and links recently acquired data with old memory systems.[9-12] These models of dream function fit well into a direct clinical use of dreams in facilitating cognitive restructuring.

In 1968 Dewan and Greenberg proposed that REM sleep was involved in consolidating material learned during wakefulness.[13,14] This hypothesis proposes that an individual (or laboratory animal) would have a greater volume of REM sleep following periods of wakefulness during which there is significant stimulation and learning than after periods when there is little novel stimulation and acquisition of new knowledge or behaviors. Many compelling observations on the relationship between learning, forgetting, and REM sleep have subsequently been published.

Hobson and McCarley's activation-synthesis hypothesis proposes that dreams result from the stimulation of the rhombencephalon, which excites various cortical areas.[5] This biologically determined activation is seen as motivationally neutral and unrelated to the past history of the individual. The activation-synthesis hypothesis allows for the projective use of dream content in assessment of the individual; however, the biological determination of dream content suggests that dreams are of no greater (or lesser) clinical value than any other mental activity.

After a comprehensive review of the literature, Horne and McGrath have concluded that acquisition of new material may be directly related to the volume of REM sleep.[15] When laboratory animals are exposed to learning algorithms, their subsequent sleep has a greater proportion of REM sleep than is observed in control animals. The disruption of sleep after learning activities has lead to "forgetting" of the newly acquired material.[16,17]

Protein Synthesis Theory

Other lines of inquiry have linked REM sleep, and presumably protein synthesis, to various aspects of learning and memory.[18] Many have theorized that synthesis and metabolism of new proteins are a major mechanism responsible for retention of learned material. Ample data suggest that inhibition of REM sleep by protein synthesis blockers or other agents impairs retention of learned material.[19] REM sleep in animals, and presumably also in humans, is a time of increased protein synthesis.[20]

Literature on protein synthesis and learning persuasively indicates that protein synthesis is involved in the retention of newly acquired information. The mechanism is apparently related to a protein buildup on the surface of the neuron between the sites of a strong synapse to the neuron and a weak synapse to that neuron.[21] The protein strengthens the weaker synapse, increasing the influence on the postsynaptic neuron. In this way, protein synthesis alters the synaptic structure of the brain and may participate in the retention of newly learned material. This hypothesis has been supported by Drucker-Colin, Bowersox, and McGinty, who have shown that medications that block or inhibit protein synthesis also block or inhibit REM sleep.[22]

Unlearning Theory

Crick and Mitchison proposed a model for REM sleep function in which dreaming is an attempt to "unlearn" maladaptive mental connections among brain programs. According to this hypothesis, dreaming results in "forgetting" faulty central processing and programming. As a result, dream analysis is viewed as psychologically deleterious, since the patient attempts to recall dream material that he or she is trying to eliminate.[23]

Developmental Theory

Dream activity associated with REM sleep may have a developmental function. Roffwarg, Muzio, and Dement have hypothesized that REM sleep serves a crucial developmental function by providing endogenous stimulation for normal sensorimotor development.[24] Infants who are too immature to acquire intense stimulation from interactions with the environment require this endogenous stimulation for appropriate neural development. Anch and Tepas have supported this hypothesis from a neurophysiological perspective.[25] Their data revealed that early blinding of experimental animals was associated with significantly greater REM sleep than late blinding, presumably because animals blinded early needed more supplemental endogenous input to the visual system owing to the lack of external visual stimulation.

CENTRAL ORIGIN OF REM SLEEP EVENTS AND DREAM MENTATION

From the time REM sleep was differentiated into tonic and phasic components, there have been speculation and experimentation on the possibility that phasic events may be the building blocks of dreams.[19] Phasic events, such as rapid eye movements and muscle twitches, may be the polygraphically recordable manifestations of activity of some central source of endogenous stimulation or "dream generator."

To better understand possible relationships between phasic physiological activity and mentation during sleep, Rechtschaffen and co-workers focused on non-REM (NREM) sleep, in which phasic activity is more rare.[26] The relationship between mentation and the occurrence of the phasic integrated potential from electromyographic (EMG) activity of the extrinsic eye muscles was studied. NREM sleep periods containing much phasic activity of the eye muscles were likely to contain bizarre, dreamlike mentation. Periods with tonic EMG activity were less likely to contain similar dreamlike mentation.

Roffwarg and colleagues have tried to relate dream content to middle ear EMG activity,[27] and several attempts have been made to connect the direction and amount of eye movements during REM sleep with visual scanning of dreams.[28] Other studies have correlated limb movements and small muscle jerking with dream activity.[29] Wolpert found an association between dreamed movements of the arms and action potentials in the wrist muscles.[30] Dement and Kleitman hypothesized that during REM sleep the motor system controlling eye movements does not generate movements at random.[31] Eye movements appear to follow visual activity during the dream. This hypothesis has been tested by examining the oculomotor activity during dreams in which there were fairly distinct and stereotypic eye movements, for example, when the dream involved watching a tennis match or climbing stairs. When these types of dreams were examined and eye movements were evaluated by objective measurements of electrooculographic activity, movements frequently conformed to the ongoing activity of mentation (e.g., regularly recurring left and right movements during a dream of watching a tennis match).[32] These findings strongly support the contention that the eyes do scan scenes (or move with the scene) occurring in dreams. Specific correlations have also been reported between eye movement direction and orientation of the hallucinated gaze during dreams. The dreamer may be "scanning" the visual field, which might imply cortical control of the eye movements while dreaming.[33]

An alternative hypothesis relates to the generation of oculomotor activity at the brainstem level.[34] The cortex is then provided with "feed-forward" information about the direction of the eye movements. According to this hypothesis, the dreamer does not so much scan dream imagery as synthesize visual imagery appropriate to the dream. A similar mechanism might form the basis of dream imagery by inhibition and excitation of neurons of the lateral geniculate body[35] and the visual cortex[36] during REM sleep, when retinal input is reduced and unformed.

Eye movement–related inhibition of sensory relays, as well as the possible exclusion of exogenous inputs by internally generated mechanisms, may also contribute to the maintenance of sleep during periods of intense central activation of the brain.[37] According to this hypothesis the dream may have a sleep maintenance mechanism built into its physiological substrate rather than functioning at a psychological level. In the waking state, a corollary discharge of the oculomotor system has been shown to suppress visual transmission during saccadic eye movements, possibly contributing to the stability of the visual field during that state.[38] The possibility that oculomotor impulses trigger visual imagery is fascinating in view of the demonstrated quantitative correlation between eye movement intensity and dream intensity.[39]

Across different species, as vision becomes more binocular, REM sleep volume increases. Berger and Walker theorized that this trend reflects a role of REM sleep in the development of the neurological ability to perform binocularly coordinated eye movements.[40] The ability for conjugate binocular eye movements is thus preserved during sleep.

McCarley has pointed out that pharmacological compounds that intensify and increase the duration of REM sleep also intensify and increase dreaming. Compounds inhibiting REM sleep also inhibit dreaming.[41] Acetylcholine agonists promote REM sleep and dreaming. All clinically effective antidepressants suppress REM and dreaming. Antidepressants particularly suppress a short REM latency, high REM intensity, and long duration of the first REM period characteristic of depression. Antidepressants probably function by increasing norepinephrine and serotonin in the central nervous system. Use of these compounds to suppress overly vigorous or disturbing dream activity and nightmares is based on this REM sleep–suppressant action.

In the laboratory, pontine reticular neurons isolated from synaptic input by tetrodotoxin respond to cholinergic agents with intense, prolonged depolarization and increased excitability.[42] Similar phenomena are seen during REM sleep. This pharmacological action is the likely mechanism for REM sleep–promoting effects of cholinergic compounds. Interestingly, paroxysms of REM sleep and dreaming are symptoms of intoxication with insecticides compounded with acetylcholine agonists.

Questions remain regarding cortical localization of the dreaming process. Some evidence supports the contention that the right cerebral hemisphere shows increased activation or efficiency during REM sleep and dreaming.[43] Meyer and co-workers investigated the question of hemispheric lateralization during dreaming and REM sleep by measuring cerebral blood flow in four right-handed narcoleptic subjects.[44] Sleep onset REM periods (SOREMPs) were associated with recall of dreams in three subjects and with hypnagogic hallucinations in one patient. During sleep with dreaming, mean gray matter blood flow was significantly greater in the right hemisphere than in the left. Increases were found in the right parietal, occipital, and posterotemporal regions. These data suggest that representation of visuospatial perceptions during dreaming may be greater in the right than the left hemisphere for these right-handed individuals. Several other studies using electrophysiological data and psychometric-behavioral assessments in the immediate postwaking period have suggested that the REM-NREM cycle may reflect an alternation in relative right and left cerebral hemispheric activation or efficiency, respectively, or an increase in the right hemispheric activity during REM sleep.[45,46] Other studies on cerebral hemispheric specialization suggest that the right and left hemispheres process information in different and sometimes conflicting ways. REM and NREM sleep may reflect relatively greater activation of efficiency of the right and left hemispheres, respectively. Mentation during wakefulness is dominated by the left hemisphere and its heavy language orientation. Theories of dreaming suggest that new solutions or adaptations to existing problems may be enhanced by REM sleep and reflected in dreams.[47]

Conflicting evidence does exist.[48,49] Two experiments were conducted to evaluate interhemispheric differences in late auditory evoked potentials during REM sleep, Stage 2 sleep, and Stage 4 sleep. Examination of these data indicated relative hemispheric balance in REM and Stage 2 with the largest asymmetries appearing in Stage 4. The results do not support the hypothesis that REM sleep and NREM sleep are associated with differential activation of the two cerebral hemispheres. Rather, they suggest that the sleep cycle is characterized by variations in degrees of asymmetry. In addition, asymmetries noted during slow-wave sleep were not consistently in favor of the left hemisphere.[50] Gabel found no conclusive evidence that dreaming is localized exclusively to the right hemisphere.[47] Data based on measurement of cerebral blood flow have shown that right hemispheric blood flow is increased during REM sleep at sleep onset in narcoleptic patients. Clearly, however, there is not a complete equivalence between right hemispheric activation or enhanced efficiency and states such as REM sleep or dreaming.[43]

CHARACTERISTICS OF DREAMS AND DREAM SLEEP

During REM sleep the sensorium and the motor centers of the central nervous system are stimulated. The nature and content of this activation are probably the result of structural and biochemical factors related to genetic and anatomical determinants.[19] The major difference between REM sleep and wakefulness is that during REM sleep, stimuli entering the sensorium are endogenous in origin and must be processed with deeply inhibited locomotor function.

Dreams in REM sleep are typically more visual than auditory.[51] In the dreams of adults, the dreamer is usually the central character. Scenes shift suddenly. Dreams are most often short, but appreciation of the real-time content may be absent or significantly distorted.

Adults wake spontaneously with dream recall about once every three or four nights. The most vivid and best remembered dreams occur at the end of the night, coincident with the longest and most intense REM period. Some form of mentation occurs throughout the night in all stages of sleep, although there are vivid and consistent differences in the nature and frequency of dream reports from the different stages of sleep in laboratory subjects.[51] In general, self-centered, hallucinatory images are reported in 60% to 80% of awakenings from REM sleep. Vague, fragmentary, poorly described thoughts are noted in 30% to 50% of wakings from NREM sleep.

When subjects are awakened from REM sleep, they generally relate a vivid, sequential story line that is identified as the dream. Reports are filled with complex, multisensory experiences. If awakened from NREM sleep, on the other hand, subjects generally report more abstract mentation, lacking a storylike quality. Most often, reports following awakenings from NREM sleep are of thoughts or stationary scenes. They are less elaborate and vivid than REM sleep content. Nevertheless, mentation readily judged to be dreaming, with complex story and action, can occur in NREM sleep, although not as frequently.[52-55] Independent (blinded) judges usually can easily distinguish REM from NREM reported mental activity. No content at all is reported from a majority of Stage 2 awakenings. Gaillard has found that mental content is reported after only about 30% of awakenings from this stage of sleep.[56] Mental activity in slow-wave sleep is even less frequent than in Stage 2 and is often completely absent. It seems most likely that dreaming is not exclusively a right hemispheric phenomenon but rather reflects a greater influence or efficiency of right hemispheric processes than of left hemispheric processes.

Cartwright and Ratzel studied 10 subjects who were REM sleep deprived for three consecutive nights by being awakened at the onset of each REM period and asked for a report of what was on their minds.[57] Two groups were formed by dividing these reports at the median on the Dream-like Fantasy Scale. All subjects underwent psychological tests before deprivation, which were repeated after deprivation but before the recovery night of uninterrupted sleep. In this experiment subjects low in REM onset fantasy showed more postdeprivation changes in waking test behavior than subjects high in REM onset fantasy. Psychological testing revealed that moderate REM deprivation was accompanied by more positive changes in waking subjects whose fantasy tended to be REM state specific than in those whose fantasy mentation was generally more available throughout sleep and waking states.

The literature gives some indication that representation of the "self" is a cardinal aspect of the dream experience. Self-participation is much more common in dreams reported after wakings from phasic REM periods than in those occurring in the tonic REM phase. Weinstein, Schwartz, and Ellman used five scales specifically designed to measure absorption in dreaming and compared the results with three scales previously shown to discriminate phasic from tonic awakenings within REM sleep.[58] Two REM stage and six Stage 2 dream reports were collected from each of 20 subjects on four baseline nights. Scales developed to measure self-participation could accurately discriminate phasic from tonic awakenings.

Additional evidence has been presented that dream content and character differ according to sleep stage and state, as well as normal and pathological characteristics of individuals. Kramer and co-workers asked three independent judges to sort randomly selected dreams of normal college students and schizophrenic patients according to the dreamer, night of occurrence, and sequential order within a night.[59] Sorting was successful at statistically significant levels for all but determination of the sequence of dreams within a night. Kramer and associates concluded that dreams are orderly, nonrandom events reflecting day-to-day changes in an individual's life. Further work is needed to determine whether there is order among dreams of a given night.

Historically, most interest in dreaming has focused on the psychological meaning of dreams. Several investigations have been instrumental in the development of an alternative hypothesis relating dreams to biological states, that is, suggesting that dreams have a biological rather than a psychological meaning.[60,61] Other investigations have noted an association of dreams of death with serious organic disease, especially cardiovascular disease.[62]

Smith has prospectively evaluated this question of dreams reflecting biological states.[63] Dreams were evaluated for the predicted correlations of the number of dream references to death and separation in men and women, respectively, with various levels of severity of cardiovascular disease. All subjects were inpatients on a nonacute cardiology service. Severity of heart disease was evaluated with anatomical and physiological measurements obtained during cardiac catheterization. A six-point scale was developed to identify increasing severity of disease reflected by coronary angiography and measurement of ejection fraction. No correlation was found between the number of dream references to death or separation and the severity of abnormalities identified by coronary angiography. The number of dream references did correlate with the severity of cardiac dysfunction as measured by the ejection fraction, a more sensitive indicator of disease severity. These data provide prospective support for the theory that dreams may reflect biological states and suggest a possible biological meaning of dreams.

Although the meaning of dreams is still open to significant debate, dreams clearly differ greatly during different stages of sleep. The reason for this difference is presumed to be a profound increase in firing (or profoundly altered firing patterns) of certain brainstem neurons during REM sleep.[19] This increase in neuronal activity is thought to be related to the properties of REM sleep, such as motor inhibition, rapid eye movements, muscular twitching, cardiovascular irregularities, respiratory irregularities, and other phasic phenomena.

DREAMS DURING CHILDHOOD

Dreams during childhood are often thought to be frightening to the child. This nightmarish reputation has been obtained from the few dreams that are so extreme in affect that they awaken children, who in turn awaken their parents.[64] Between the ages of 3 and 5 years, children spend a significant portion of their sleep time in REM sleep and have as many as eight or nine REM periods each night. These REM periods vary from approximately 18 minutes early in the night to about 30 minutes at the end of the night. Out of all these periods, very few dreams are frightening.

Children's dreams tend to be briefer than adults' dreams, even though children spend more time in REM sleep and their dreams center on the interpersonal concerns about which they are most emotionally aroused.[65] During dreams emotional material from the child's present waking life is blended with related material from the past. These "fantasy programs" may permit new and potentially creative programs to emerge. To some extent a child's age influences the subject matter of dreams [66] Ames points out that the child's personality and life experiences must always be considered in trying to understand dreams. But it seems likely that age should also be considered, at least in the early years of life. This factor has been often overlooked. Studies of children's dreams suggest a definite developmental trend in the kinds of things dreamed about. Possibly confirming this proposal is the observation that dreams appear to be close to the sequence of fears in waking life, with subjects appearing in dreams about 16 months to 1 year after they have been prominent waking fears. Foulkes and Breger have reported studies confirming Ames' contention of a developmental trend in dream content.[65,66]

Foulkes, Breger, and Ames have independently reported significant data regarding the content of dreams during childhood.[65-68] The following descriptions are based on their significant works.

First 2 Years

As discussed in Chapter 2, REM sleep occupies a much more significant percentage of the total sleep time during early years of life. Activation of the cerebral cortex during REM sleep appears to be vital for development of the central nervous system. Since dream reports are difficult to obtain from infants and toddlers, however, evaluation of dream content during this period is limited. Nonetheless, dreams probably play a significant biologic and psychological role in normal childhood development.

3 to 5 Years

At 3 years of age children begin to report occasional dreams. Their descriptions are most often brief, averaging 14 words. These dreams may wake the child, but they generally lack emotion, possess few feelings or little affect, and are static and nonnarrative. Slightly more than one third of the dreams are about animals or contain representations of humans (usually the parents and self) as animal figures. Few dreams are specifically about parents. Dreams are reported from approximately one fourth of REM awakenings and 10% of NREM awakenings, although at this age the reports are similar in content and affect regardless of the sleep stage. Little interpersonal action is described. Most reports reflect self needs such as hunger and thirst.

By 4 years of age dreams cause less wakefulness. Reports are more frequent and fairly reliable, although they may be confused with fanciful tales. Dreams of parents and playmates occur more often.

5 to 7 Years

Between 5 and 7 years of age dreams and their reports are longer (70 words for girls; 48 words for boys) and near adult levels in length. The dreamer has more participation as the central character. Dream reports occur in almost half of awakenings from REM sleep and slightly less than one fourth of awakenings from NREM sleep. A capacity for generating small-scale scenarios occurs. Reliable claims of affective dream experiences appear. Troublesome dreams reported by boys become less frequent. Children of both sexes dream about adult male strangers substantially more often than during previous developmental levels. Dreams of being chased, threatened, and unable to move are commonly reported. Dreams of ghosts and the supernatural appear; and characters from movies and television programs may be figures in dreams. Personal difficulties and worries are reported, but the dreams are mostly pleasant. There is great variability from child to child in dream reports. During this period many children like to dream and to report their dreams. At times they do not want to be awakened from a dream and may try to go back to sleep to "finish" the dream.

8 to 11 Years

From 8 to 11 years of age dream reports can be elicited after approximately two thirds of awakenings from REM sleep. Dream report length remains stable. Dreams are often voluntarily reported by the child. Self-participation by the dreamer significantly increases. Act-specific aptitude begins to play a role in the selection of the dreamer's activities. Dreams are mostly pleasant during this time but may be significantly affected by television and movie content and characters. Children are often aware that this might happen and may say "This will give me a bad dream." Nightmares occur in at least one third of all dream reports. Dreams of animals become infrequent during this developmental period, and there is more variety in dream settings, reflecting an expanded waking environment. School and sports events appear in places where the action had occurred.

11 to 13 Years

Percentages of dream reports from REM and NREM sleep remain at about the same level as in the prior developmental period. During prior stages the family was the main focus of dreams. They now are generally replaced in dreams by peers. The ratio of dreams with verbal acts to dreams with locomotor acts reaches a new high.

Seventy-two percent of dreams contain mentalistic acts, and a minority of dream reports include feelings.

A great deal of dreaming occurs during this period. Good dreams predominate, but nightmares are still strong. By 12 years nightmares have decreased in frequency. Dreams of daily activities are common. Dream locations may be confused. Many children report that their dreams are "crazy," "strange," or "funny."

13 to 15 Years

Between 60% and 80% of REM awakenings lead to dream reports in 13- to 15-year-olds. Dream characters are usually peers of the same sex, rather than adults or family members. Ratio of verbal acts to locomotor acts during dreams reaches its developmental maximum. A significant portrayal of symbolic activity occurs at this time. Dreams are less often about everyday things and are more apt to be reported as "weird" and "confusing." Some youngsters become interested in the psychological implications of their dreams. Although young adolescents may sleep restlessly, they generally do not wake or frequently report nightmares.

DREAM MENTATION

Responsiveness during sleep is considerably reduced from the awake state. One factor that may be related to reduced responsiveness is mentation during sleep. For example, Foulkes has suggested that reduced responsiveness to external stimuli during sleep may be related to the sleeper's preoccupation with ongoing cognitive activity.[68] Foulkes hypothesized that the vivid mental activity of REM sleep excludes other sources of stimulation. This might explain why REM sleep appears electroencephalographically and subjectively similar to light sleep, while behavioral responsivity appears more closely related to deeper stages of sleep.

Variables that distinguish waking from sleeping (REM) thought have been described.[69] Mentation reports from the waking state tend to have more topic shifts than those from the REM state, which often have a single theme and storylike quality. Heightened response thresholds to sensory stimuli, in conjunction with the state of high cortical activation typical of REM sleep, have been thought to account for the storylike quality of REM dream imagery. Wollman and Antrobus described an experiment in which an intermittent auditory stimulus was the model for environmental influence on waking mentation. The major factor distinguishing mentation reports of waking subjects from those of subjects awakened from REM sleep was the number of thought-units per report, with waking subjects changing topics more frequently. Removal of the intermittent auditory stimulus reduced the number of topic shifts in waking subjects.[69]

Using a technique of free association in an experimental setting, Cavallero found differences in the quality of memory traces involved in the production of REM and sleep onset dreams.[70] Free associations with a dream collected immediately after an experimental awakening were compared with those recalled 2 months later. A first group of results supported the hypothesis that free associations are sensitive to the proximity of the amount of dream production. A second group showed that differences between sleep onset dreams and REM dreams do not appear to be due to differences in formal characteristics of the dream report.

Cognitive dream psychology on one hand regards dreaming as higher symbolic activity but on the other hand sees its organizational and functional characteristics as derivative of or inferior to those of waking consciousness. Purcell and co-workers have studied the degree of self-reflective metacognition in dreams from different sleep stages.[71] They found that greater self-reflectiveness occurred in REM dreams than in those from Stages 2 and 4, which did not differ. High-frequency dream recallers showed more dream self-reflectiveness than did low-frequency recallers. Continuation of the experiment assessed the extent to which self-reflectiveness and lucid dreaming could be learned as a cognitive skill by varying levels of intention and attention paid to dreaming. Three weeks of home dream reports were collected. Results revealed that the four experimental groups had greater dream self-reflectiveness than did a baseline control group. The most effective treatment to improve self-reflectiveness during dreams was the mnemonic. Attention patterning schemas learned during the waking state resulted in more self-reflectiveness and lucid dreaming than occurred in the baseline group or an attention control condition. Therefore dreaming may not be single minded but rather variable along a continuum of self-reflectiveness, suggesting functional and organizational levels that are consistent with the concept of dreaming as high-order cognitive activity.

Burton, Harsh, and Badia assessed the relationship between responsiveness to auditory stimuli presented during sleep and cognitive activity during sleep.[72] Subjects were instructed while awake to turn off a tone by taking a deep breath. The same tone was then presented during Stage 2 and REM sleep. Subjects were awakened to assess the relationship between responding and reports of ongoing cognitive activity. Consistent with the view that cognitive activity reduces responsiveness, significantly fewer appropriate responses were found when cognitive activity was reported than when no cognitive activity was reported. Trained judges rated the subjects' reports of cognitive activity as incorporation of the tone or the breathing response or both into the cognitive content. Incorporation was associated with a reduced likelihood of responding relative to no incorporation. These data suggest that reduced responsiveness is associated with cognitive activity only when incorporation occurs. The findings support the hypothesis that the reduced responsiveness to external stimulation during sleep is, at least in part, due to ongoing cognitive activity.

Clearly, cognitive activity occurs during sleep, and this cognitive activity appears more lucid, intense, and storylike during REM sleep than other states. Behavioral response to cognition is attenuated during these periods of intense central activation by the inhibition of alpha-motor neurons. Physiological evidence shows that the profound EMG suppression during REM sleep is a consequence of the direct inhibition of spinal cord motor neurons.[73] As a result, any organized motor pattern that might be generated during the intense brain activation of REM sleep cannot be expressed. This inhibition appears to be greater during phasic REM sleep than tonic REM sleep. Brylowski, Levitan, and LaBerge have shown that the mean spinal reflex suppression is greater during lucid REM sleep than during nonlucid REM. This reflex suppression appears to be correlated with increased eye movements, heart rate, and respiratory rate.[74] Results of these experiments support previous findings that lucid REM sleep is not a state closer to wake than nonlucid REM. Rather, lucid dreaming occurs during unequivocal REM sleep and is characteristically associated with phasic REM activity.

Certain central nervous system lesions and disorders can affect motor inhibition during REM sleep and result in bizarre (and sometimes violent) motoric behaviors. Schenck described four men with histories of injuring themselves or their spouses by aggressive behaviors during sleep, often during attempted dream enactment.[75] A fifth subject, a woman, described disruptive, nonviolent sleep and dream behaviors. Polysomnography did not detect seizures but did document a REM sleep disorder with variable loss of chin atonia, extraordinarily increased limb twitch activity, and increased REM ocular activity and density. A broad range of REM sleep behaviors were recorded, including stereotypical hand motions, reaching and searching gestures, punches, kicks, and verified dream movements. Slow-wave sleep was elevated for age in all patients. Harmful behaviors were absent in NREM sleep. There were no associated psychiatric disorders, although four of the patients had serious neurological disorders, ranging from Guillain-Barré syndrome to atypical dementia. The authors believe that this phenomenon of REM sleep neurobehavioral disorder is another category of parasomnia (see Chapter 10). Further evaluation of this disorder may increase understanding of the neurophysiology, behavior, and cognition during dream (REM) sleep.

REFERENCES

1. Aserinsky E and Kleitman N: Regularly occurring periods of eye motility and concomitant phenomena during sleep. Science 1953;118:273-274.
2. Dement W and Kleitman N: The relation of eye movements during sleep to dream activity: an objective method of the study of dreaming. J Exp Psychol 1957;53:339-346.
3. Freud S: The interpretation of dreams. New York, Basic Books, 1953.
4. Foulkes D: A grammar of dreams. New York, Basic Books, 1978.
5. Hobson JA and McCarley RW: The brain as a dream state generator: an activation-synthesis hypothesis of the dream process. Am J Psychiatry 1977;134:1335-1348.
6. Parkes JD: Sleep and its disorders. Philadelphia, WB Saunders, 1985, pp 23-26.
7. Anch AM et al (eds): Sleep: a scientific perspective. Englewood Cliffs, NJ, Prentice Hall, 1988.
8. Salley RD: Subpersonalities with dreaming functions in a patient with multiple personalities. J Nerv Ment Dis 1988;176:112-115.
9. Greenberg R and Pearlman C: REM sleep and the analytic process: a psychophysiological bridge. Psychoanal Q 1975;44:392-403.
10. Evans C: Landscapes of the night: how and why we dream. New York, Viking Press, 1984.
11. Palombo SR: Dreaming and memory: a new information processing model. New York, Basic Books, 1978.
12. Winson J: Brain and psyche. Garden City, NY, Doubleday, 1985.
13. Dewan EM: The P (programming) hypothesis for REMS. Psychophysiology 1968;5:365-366.
14. Greenberg R and Dewan E: Aphasia and dreaming: a test of the P-hypothesis. Psychophysiology 1968; 5:203-204.
15. Horne J and McGrath M: The consolidation hypothesis

for REM sleep function: stress and other confounding factors—a review. Biol Psychol 1984;18:165-184.

16. Fishbein W: Disruptive effects of rapid-eye-movement sleep deprivation on long-term memory. Physiol and Behav 1971;6:279-282.
17. Fishbein W, McGaugh JL, and Swarz JR: Retrograde amnesia—electroconvulsive shock effects after termination of rapid-eye-movement sleep deprivation. Science 1971;172:80-82.
18. Mirmiran M et al: Effects of experimental suppression of active (REM) sleep during early development upon adult brain and behavior in the rat. Brain Res 1983;283:277-286.
19. Anch AM et al (eds): Sleep: a scientific perspective. Englewood Cliffs, NJ, Prentice Hall, 1988, pp 136-155.
20. Leventhal M et al: Rapid-eye-movement (REM) sleep deprivation: effect on acid mucopolysaccharides in rat brain. Arch Int Physiol Biochim 1975;83:221-232.
21. Shashoua V: The role of extracellular proteins in learning and memory. Am Sci 1985;73:364-370.
22. Drucker-Colin R, Bowersox S, and McGinty D: Sleep and medial reticular unit responses to protein synthesis inhibitors: effects of chloramphenicol and thiamphenicol. Brain Res 1982;252:117-127.
23. Crick F and Mitchison G: The function of dream sleep. Nature 1983;304:111-114.
24. Roffwarg HP, Muzio JN, and Dement WC: Ontogenetic development of the human sleep-dream cycle. Science 1966;152:604-619.
25. Anch AM and Tepas DI: Paradoxical sleep in the rat: comparison of early and late blinding. Psychonomic Sci 1970;19:155-156.
26. Rechtschaffen A et al: The relationship of phasic and tonic periorbital EMG activity to NREM mentation. Sleep Res 1972;1:114.
27. Roffwarg H, Herman J, and Lamstein S: The middle ear muscles: predictability of their phasic activity in REM sleep from dream material. Sleep Res 1975;4:165.
28. Aserinsky E: The maximal capacity for sleep: rapid eye movement density as an index of sleep satiety. Biol Psychiatry 1969;1:147-154.
29. Hobson JA, Goldfrank F, and Snyder F: Respiration and mental activity in sleep. J Psychiatr Res 1965;3:79-90.
30. Wolpert EA: Studies in psychophysiology of dreams. II. An electromyographic study of dreaming. Arch Gen Psychiatry 1960;2:231-241.
31. Dement W and Kleitman N: The relation of eye movements during sleep to dream activity: an objective method of the study of dreaming. J Exp Psychol 1957;53:339-346.
32. Herman JH et al: Evidence for a directional correspondence between eye movements and dream imagery in REM sleep. Sleep 1984;7:52-63.
33. Roffwarg HP et al: Dream imagery: relationship to rapid eye movements of sleep. Arch Gen Psychiatry 1962;7:235-258.
34. Hobson JA and McCarley RW: The brain as a dream state generator: an activation-synthesis hypothesis of the dream process. Am J Psychiatry 1977;134:1335-1348.
35. Bizzi E: Discharge pattern of single geniculate neurons during the rapid eye movements of sleep. J Neurophysiol 1966;29:1087-1095.
36. Evarts EV: Activity of individual cerebral neurons during sleep and arousal. Res Publ Assoc Res Nerv Ment Dis 1967;45:319-337.
37. Pompeiano O: Sensory inhibition during motor activity in sleep. In Yahr MD and Purpura DP: Neurophysiologic basis of normal and abnormal motor activities. New York, Raven Press, 1967, pp 323-375.
38. Volkman F: Vision during voluntary saccadic eye movements. J Opt Soc Am 1962;52:571-578.
39. Hobson JA, Goldfrank F, and Snyder F: Sleep and respiration. J Psychiatr Res 1965;3:79-90.
40. Berger RJ and Walker JM: Oculomotor coordination following REM and non-REM sleep periods. J Exp Psychol 1972;94:216-224.
41. McCarley RW: The biology of dreaming. In Kryger MH, Roth T, and Dement WC: Principles and practice of sleep medicine. Philadelphia, WB Saunders, 1989, pp 173-183.
42. Greene RW, Haas HL, and McCarley RW: A low threshold calcium spike mediates firing pattern alterations in pontine reticular neurons. Science 1986;234:738-740.
43. Gabel S: The right hemisphere in imagery, hypnosis, rapid eye movement sleep and dreaming. J Nerv Ment Dis 1988;176:323-331.
44. Meyer JS, et al: Sleep apnea, narcolepsy and dreaming: regional cerebral hemodynamics. Ann Neurol 1980;7:479-485.
45. Angeleri F, Scarpino O, and Signorino M: Information processing and hemispheric specialization: electrophysiological study during wakefulness, stage two and stage REM sleep. Res Commun Psychol Psychiatry Behav 1984;9:121-138.
46. Murri L et al: Automatic analysis of hemispheric EEG relationships during wakefulness and sleep. Res Commun Psychol Psychiatry Behav 1982;7:109-118
47. Gabel S: Information processing in rapid eye movement sleep: possible neurophysiological, neuropsychological, and clinical correlates. J Nerv Ment Dis 1987;175:193-200.
48. Antrobus J, Erlichman H, and Weiner M: EEG asymmetry during REM and NREM: failure to replicate. Sleep Res 1978;7:24.
49. Violani C, DeGennaro L, and Capogna M: EEG and EOG indices of hemispheric asymmetries during sleep. Res Commun Psychol Psychiatry Behav 1984;9:95-107.
50. Armitage R et al: Asymmetrical auditory probe evoked potentials during REM and NREM sleep. Sleep 1990;13:69-78.
51. Parkes JD: Sleep and its disorders. Philadelphia, WB Saunders, 1985, pp 23-26.
52. Monroe LJ et al: The discriminability of REM and NREM reports. J Pers Soc Psychol 1965;2:456-460.
53. Foulkes D: Dream ontogeny and dream psychophysiology. In Chase M and Weitzman ED (eds): Sleep disorders: basic and clinical research, Advances in Sleep Research, 8. New York, Spectrum, 1983, pp 347-362.
54. Foulkes D: Series of dream formation and recent studies of sleep consciousness. Psychol Bull 1964;62:236-247.
55. Van de Castle R: The psychology of dreaming. New York, General Learning Press, 1971.
56. Gaillard JM: Mental activity during sleep. In Monnier M (ed): Functions of the nervous system, vol 4. New York, Elsevier, 1983.
57. Cartwright RD and Ratzel RW: Effects of dream loss on waking behaviors. Arch Gen Psychiatry 1972; 27:277-280.
58. Weinstein L, Schwartz D, and Ellman SJ: The de-

velopment of scales to measure the experience of self-participation in sleep. Sleep 1988;11:437-447.
59. Kramer M et al: Do dreams have meaning? An empirical inquiry. Am J Psychiatry 1976;133:778-781.
60. Winget C and Kapp FT: The relationship of the manifest content of dreams to duration of childbirth in primipara. Psychosom Med 1972;34:313-320.
61. Gottschalk LA et al: Anxiety levels in dreams: relation to changes in plasma free fatty acids. Science 1966;153:654-657.
62. Levitan H: Traumatic events in the dreams of psychosomatic patients. Psychother Psychosom 1980;33: 226-232.
63. Smith RC: Do dreams reflect a biological state? J Nerv Ment Dis 1987;175:201-207.
64. Cartwright RD: A primer on sleep and dreaming. Reading, Mass, Addison-Wesley, 1978.
65. Breger L: Children's dreams and personality development. In Fisher J and Breger L (eds): The meaning of dreams: recent insights from the laboratory. California Mental Health Symposium No. 3, 1969.
66. Foulkes D: Longitudinal studies of dreams in children. In Masserman J (ed): Science and psychoanalysis, 9. New York, Grune & Stratton, 1971.
67. Ames LB: Sleep and dreams in children. In Harmes E (ed): Problems of sleep and dreams in children. New York, Macmillan, 1964, pp 6-29.
68. Foulkes D: The psychology of sleep. New York, Scribner, 1966.
69. Wollman MC and Antrobus JS: Sleeping and waking thought: effects of external stimulation. Sleep 1986;9:438-448.
70. Cavallero C: Dream sources, associative mechanisms, and temporal dimension. Sleep 1987;10:78-83.
71. Purcell S et al: Dream self-reflectiveness as a learned cognitive skill. Sleep 1986;9:423-437.
72. Burton SA, Harsh JR, and Badia P: Cognitive activity in sleep and responsiveness to external stimuli. Sleep 1988;11:61-68.
73. Hobson JA and McCarley RW: The brain as a dream state generator: an activation-synthesis hypothesis of the dream process. Am J Psychiatry 1977;134:1335-1348.
74. Brylowski A, Levitan L, and LaBerge S: H-reflex suppression and autonomic activation during lucid REM sleep: a case study. Sleep 1989;12:374-378.
75. Schenck CH et al: Chronic behavioral disorders of human REM sleep: a new category of parasomnia. Sleep 1986;9:293-308.

7

Disorders of Initiating and Maintaining Sleep

Sleeplessness is one of the most frequent sleep-related complaints brought to the practitioner, since the entire family is affected by a child who cannot sleep at night. Symptoms of sleep deprivation may be identified in one or all members of the family. It is not unusual for a worn, haggard, frustrated parent to seek help for a child who appears happy, active, alert, and well rested.

Sleeplessness appears to be a final common pathway for a heterogeneous group of disorders that may have many causes. Underlying causes may be chronophysiological, medical, psychological, social-environmental, or a combination of factors. Indeed, considerable overlap exists among underlying conditions. Some children have no difficulty falling asleep but awaken several times during the night. Other children have significant difficulty falling asleep at a prescribed time but, once asleep, sleep throughout the night. Still others suffer from both difficulty settling and nighttime wakings.

The typical connotation of the term *insomnia* does not appear to be applicable to sleepless children. Underlying causes of disorders of initiating and maintaining sleep during childhood appear to be considerably different from those causing insomnia in adults, and different approaches to diagnosis and therapy are required.

Sleep onset and maintenance require appropriate interaction between biological and psychological determinants. When one or more of these factors are disrupted or dysfunctional, sleeplessness results. Disorders of partial arousals from sleep stages and sleep-wake transition disorders (such as sleep walking and night terrors) are discussed in Chapter 10.

Accurate diagnosis is essential for appropriate management of these problems. This chapter focuses on epidemiology, clinical presentation, diagnostic features, differential diagnosis, and management paradigms for disorders of initiating and maintaining sleep in childhood.

GENERAL CONSIDERATIONS

The problem of sleeplessness during childhood does not appear to be solely neurodevelopmental. Instead, sleeplessness reflects a pattern of interaction between physiological and behavioral variables.[1] Interactions between the parent and the child at times of sleep transition are important. Parents display a wide variety of normal responses to their sleeping infant, which change as the infant ages. Under normal circumstances parents frequently respond to a signaling (crying) infant during the first few months of life. With an older infant, parental intervention usually involves occasional checks of the sleeping infant. Interestingly, during the first 8 months of life, when infants are undergoing rapid neurodevelopmental changes and entrainment to appropriate sleep-wake cycles, almost half of infants are already asleep when placed in the crib.[2]

As the infant ages, sleeplessness may contribute to significant parental feelings of anxiety, anger, fear, helplessness, and hopelessness. Parental concerns focus not only on the child's difficulty sleeping, but also on their own sleeplessness. Prolonged night wakings result from an interaction between the child's temperamental predisposition for waking at night and other factors of health, development, and parental management.[3] Concerns of parents may be justified. Recent studies of adults have suggested that short sleep durations are related to increased morbidity.[4] During childhood, lack of sleep significantly affects school performance. In a study of 9,000 children, superior school performance[5] and higher scores on intelligence tests[6] were associated with longer duration of nighttime sleep.

Despite nocturnal awakenings, children less than 5 years of age rarely suffer from significant sleep deprivation. Young infants and toddlers sleep when necessary, at any place or any time. Although parents often are concerned that a child waking at night might be sleep deprived, this is not usually the case. Problems arise when social and educational demands are juxtaposed with sleep demands.[7]

Parents of older children often believe that their sleep time is affected by television viewing in the evening. Weissbluth and co-workers have shown that total sleep time is the same today as it was 60 years ago.[8] Television viewing has had minimal or no effect on day or evening sleep in children 5 years of age or older. Although girls sleep slightly longer than boys at night, there appear to be no sex differences for time spent in daytime sleep or television viewing. A sex difference in total nocturnal sleep time is also seen in adults. Although increasing television viewing did not change total sleep time, it was correlated with consistently lower scores on standardized tests for reading, written expression, and mathematics.[8]

INCIDENCE AND PREVALENCE

Brief wakings at night are normal in children and adults. Most often the individual turns over, immediately falls back to sleep, and does not recall the arousal.[7] Studies of incidence and prevalence of night waking in the pediatric population have been limited because they must rely on subjective parental reports and questionnaires. Despite limitations of this method of investigation, the frequency of sleeplessness during childhood seems high. Bax has shown that approximately 20% of children in the birth to 2-year-old age group have problems with nocturnal wakings. There seems to be a slight decline in 3- to 4-year-old children, but the problem is still common in 4- to 5-year-old children, affecting 10% of this group.[7] Of children exhibiting nocturnal wakings at 12 months of age in Bax's study, 40% still woke at 18 months. Forty percent of children with early sleep problems continued to wake at 2 years (but not necessarily the same 40% as at 18 months). When children waking at 18 months were studied, 54% were still waking at 2 years and 23% were still waking at 3 years. At 5 years, nocturnal waking still occurred although less significantly and less frequently after school entry.

In another study Jenkins, Bax, and Hart reported night waking in 23% of children at 1 year, 24% at 18 months, and 14% at 3 years of age.[9] Richman, Stevenson, and Graham showed that at 3 years of age, 13% of children have problems settling and 14% wake at night.[10]

Inherent difficulties are present in evaluation of data collected by parent reports and questionnaires, since parents notice nighttime wakings only if the child is fussy and requires attention. Periods of quiet wakefulness during normal sleep hours are missed. To overcome this problem, Anders videotaped parent and baby interactions during normal sleep periods.[11] Settling was defined as sleeping without removal from the crib from midnight to 5 AM for at least 4 weeks, and night wakings were defined as an arousal during that time at least once weekly for 4 weeks. A simple waking occurred when the baby woke after being asleep, then returned to sleep without fussing and being removed from the crib. A complex awakening occurred when the baby woke after being asleep, fussed, and was removed from the crib. Sixty percent of 2-month-old infants and 62% of 9-month-old infants were awake when initially placed in their cribs. Seventy percent of males were placed into bed awake, compared with

50% of females. There was also a difference between sexes in the time the infants were placed in bed. Females at 2 and 9 months of age were placed in the crib between 8 and 9 PM and removed from the crib at 7 to 8 AM. Males at 2 months were placed in the crib between 7 and 10 PM and removed from the crib between 6 and 8 AM. Males at 9 months were placed into the crib between 7 and 9 PM and removed at 6 to 8 AM. Average sleep onset latency for the group placed in the crib awake was 27.5 minutes at 2 months and 16.4 minutes at 9 months. Two thirds of the infants who were placed in the crib awake *entered active sleep first*. This correlated well with polysomnographic studies, which showed active (REM) sleep onset during infancy.[12] Half of the awakenings at 2 and 9 months were simple and half were complex. Length of simple wakings was 9 minutes at 2 and 9 months and tended to be more frequent as morning approached. Complex awakenings lasted longer, and the duration changed with age, from 75 minutes at 2 months to 24 minutes at 9 months.[11] At 2 months of age, complex awakenings occurred predominantly between midnight and 6 AM. Females seemed to awaken more regularly between 3 and 6 AM. At 9 months males demonstrated two peaks of complex awakenings. The first peak occurred between 9 PM and midnight. The second peak occurred between 3 and 6 AM. Females remained more regular with a single peak between 3 and 6 AM.

Moore and Ucko reported that 50% of infants who had settled successfully again awakened at night during the second half of the first year of life.[13] Most parents and child health care practitioners can attest to the presence of this second peak of nocturnal wakings. The etiology may be developmentally or physiologically based; however, night wakings during this time may also be secondary to shifts and stresses in the environment.[13]

BEHAVIORAL CHARACTERISTICS, TEMPERAMENT, AND NIGHT WAKING

Zuckerman, Stevenson, and Bailey conducted a longitudinal study of night waking based on interviews with 308 parents.[14] For infants 8 months of age, 10% of mothers reported that their babies woke three or more times per night, 8% reported that the babies took an hour or more to settle after waking, 5% complained that their own sleep was severely disrupted by the child, and 18% reported at least one of these problems. By 3 years of age, 29% of the children enrolled in the study had difficulty settling or staying asleep. Of the children with sleep problems at 8 months of age, 41% still had a problem sleeping at 3 years of age. In comparison, only 26% of children without a sleeping problem at 8 months of age developed a problem by 3 years. In this study, children with persistent sleep problems were more likely to have behavior problems, especially tantrums and behavior management problems, than were children without persistent sleep problems. Children with sleep problems, on the other hand, were not more likely to have fears, anxiety, or other behavior problems measured by the Behavior Screening Questionnaire.

Some evidence suggests a temperamental predisposition to night waking. If this is true, evaluation of the sleepless child requires a broader perspective. In a private pediatric practice, 25% of 60 randomly selected patients suffered from night wakings between 1 and 12 months of age. Night wakings and temperamental characteristics of low sensory threshold correlated significantly.[3]

To determine whether common sleep disturbances in young children, such as night waking and bedtime struggles, tend to persist, whether they are related to environmental stress factors and are accompanied by other behavioral problems, and whether their persistence is related to other factors, Kataria, Swanson, and Trevathan studied 60 children between the ages of 15 and 48 months.[15] Mothers were interviewed at the beginning of the investigation and 3 years later. Children identified as having sleep disorders were compared with those not having sleep disorders. Forty-two percent of children studied had disturbed sleep at the initial interview, and 84% of these children had persistence of the sleep disturbance after 3 years. Persistence of the sleep disorder had a significant relationship with increased frequency of stress factors in the environment. Other generalized behavior difficulties were present in 30% of sleep-disturbed children and 19% of non-sleep-disturbed children, which was statistically not significant. Sleeping with a parent or sibling was noted more frequently in sleep-disturbed children (34%) than in non-sleep-disturbed children (16%). Twenty percent of the mothers at the initial interview and 30% of mothers at 3-year follow-up perceived their child's sleep disturbance as stressful to them and to their family life. They concluded that early identification of the child with sleep disturbance and timely intervention would help both the child and the family.

It is apparent that settling problems, night wakings, or a combination of both seriously disrupts family life and leads to fatigue, irritability, limitation of parents' activities, and on occasion, marital strain.[16] *Night waking is undoubtedly a trigger for child abuse on some occasions, and the symptoms of difficulty settling and night wakings should be taken seriously by the practitioner.*[7] Stress and depression, common in parents with young children, are often made worse by a lack of sleep. Parents who themselves have not slept cannot think rationally about ways of coping with their child's night wakings.

Stress in the home is frequently associated with poor sleeping at night. Marital discord, separation, divorce, financial or professional difficulties, parental affective illness, medical disorders, death, family move, school entry or change, toilet training, and the birth of a new sibling may all contribute to poor sleeping.[1] A cry certainly is a powerful biological signal. It is difficult to ignore, whether the response is positive or negative.

Although night waking and settling problems have medical, biological, and psychosocial underpinnings, some consider these symptoms to be a conditioned reflex.[17] Wilks has stated, "The child wakes, cries, the mother intervenes with loving attention and a drink; the child repeats his crying nightly and each time is quickly rewarded. With such regular reinforcement, the reflex is soon established."[17] This proposition, however, is too simplistic when considering disorders of initiating and maintaining sleep, since the interactions of many variables contribute to the final common pathway of sleeplessness.

In contrast to sleep duration in older children, adolescents, and adults (which appears to be related to mental and physical health status, environmental, and social factors), sleep duration in infancy seems determined primarily by neurological maturation and to some degree by infant temperament. Weissbluth compared infant temperament characteristics with total sleep duration and found that four of five infant temperament characteristics (mood, adaptability, rhythmicity, and approach-withdrawal) that are used to establish temperament diagnoses of "easy" or "difficult" were highly negatively correlated with total sleep duration.[18]

Consistent patterns of behavior can be seen in babies. Some children are definitely quieter and less active than others. Therefore a consideration of the baby's personality may be important in the assessment of the sleep disorder.[3,19] Persistent sleep problems are associated with increased rates of temper tantrums and generally greater difficulty in managing the child's behavior at 3 years of age. This suggests that persistent sleep problems are part of more pervasive behavioral conflicts between parent and child involving limits and boundaries.[14]

Sensory thresholds may also be important in evaluating the child's behavior and sleep problems. Sensory threshold is defined as the level of extrinsic stimulation required to evoke a discernible response.[3] Low sensory threshold may partly explain problems such as teething and sleeplessness. In Cary's study of the distribution of temperament, 76% were easy or intermediate low and 24% were intermediate high or difficult. Among infants who woke at night, 13 of 15 had low sensory thresholds. There are two theoretical mechanisms of how low sensory threshold contributes to night waking. First, a greater response to stimuli during the day makes infants more arousable at night. Second, an infant may be generally more responsive to internal and external stimuli at night.[3]

Great care must be taken, however, in evaluating infant temperament and sleep problems. Oberklaid and co-workers have shown that toddler temperament ratings differ according to sex, age, social class, and cultural contexts. Future temperament norms may need to specify characteristics of the group of children from which they were derived to allow more valid comparisons.[20]

After 3 to 4 months of age a major feature of a child's difficult temperament is the proclivity to cry and fuss in many situations.[21] Infants with excessive crying beyond 3 to 4 months tend also to have irregular sleep or sleep patterns characterized by frequent waking.[22] Furthermore, it appears that in the age range of 3 to 18 months, infants who cry more at any time during the day and night are also more likely to cry during sleep-wake transitions.

CO-SLEEPING

Co-sleeping (sharing a bed with another individual) is common in many cultures. Concerns about suffocation of children and night wakings appear unfounded.[7] Parents are often advised to move the infant to a separate room soon after birth so the child will not need a parent present to fall asleep. Parents are often concerned that separate rooms may result in inattentiveness to the child's needs. Bax reports, however, that parents often become *more* attentive to their child when sleeping environments are separated. A cry from a distant bedroom easily wakes the parent to respond to the child's needs.[7] Loudspeaker systems and intercom units have been marketed to ensure this arousal response from the parent. These techniques appear to be in conflict with the idea that co-sleeping is not detrimental. However, Bax reported that 68% of children with sleep problems experienced co-sleeping, compared with 22% of those without sleep problems.

Prevalence and correlates of sleeping in the parental bed among healthy children between 6 months and 4 years of age were studied by Lozoff, Wolf, and Davis.[23] In this cross section of families in a large U.S. city, co-sleeping was a routine practice in 35% of white and 70% of black families. Co-sleeping in both racial groups was associated with approaches to sleep management at bedtime that emphasized parental involvement and body contact. Co-sleeping children were significantly more likely to fall asleep out of bed and to have adult company and body contact at bedtime. Among white families only, co-sleeping was associated with the older child, lower level of parental education, less professional training, increased family stress, a more ambivalent maternal attitude toward the child, and disruptive sleep problems in the child.

Objective evidence of co-sleeping resulting in sleep disruption has been reported by Monroe.[24] Couples who were good sleepers and habitually slept together were studied polysomnographically when they slept together and apart. When the couple slept apart, more slow-wave sleep and less REM sleep were identified. This seems to indicate a rebound of slow-wave sleep similar to that seen in sleep-deprived subjects. Monroe concluded that sleeping together may be good for marital bliss, but sleeping apart eliminates disturbances of sleep when partners change position. Similar studies have not been performed in children.

Breast feeding may be associated with a concurrent mother-infant adaptation that involves frequent night wakings. However, when a mother stops breast feeding, the rate of sleep problems among breast-fed children 8 months of age is the same as that for children whose mothers never breast fed.[14] Breast feeding and ethnic differences may not be linked to persistent sleep problems because these characteristics may be associated with different childrearing expectations and behaviors.[25] Night waking during infancy is considered a normal occurrence in some cultures, especially when children sleep with their parents.

EVALUATION OF THE SLEEPLESS CHILD

Evaluation of the sleepless child should be approached in the same manner as evaluation of any other clinical problem (Figs. 7–1 and 7–2). Evaluation begins with a comprehensive

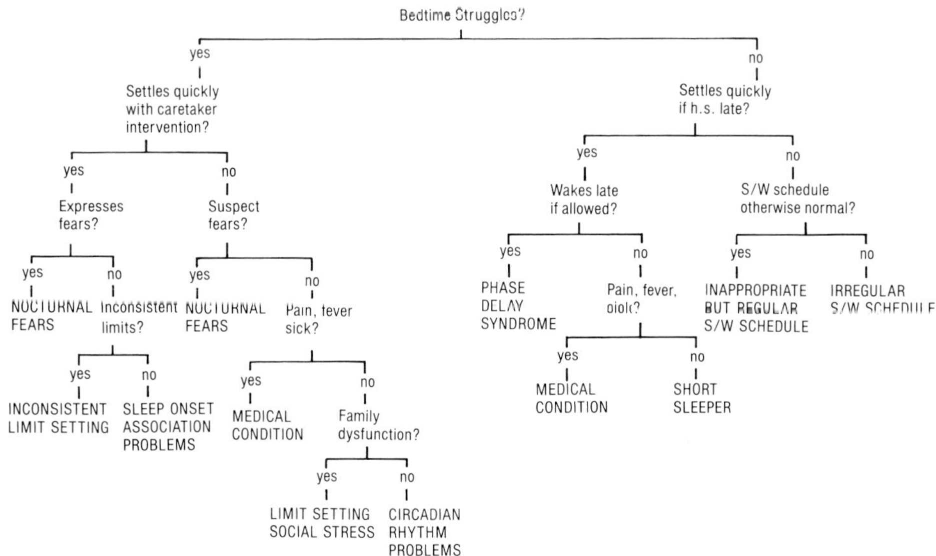

FIGURE 7–1. Evaluation of the sleepless child who does not settle easily at night.

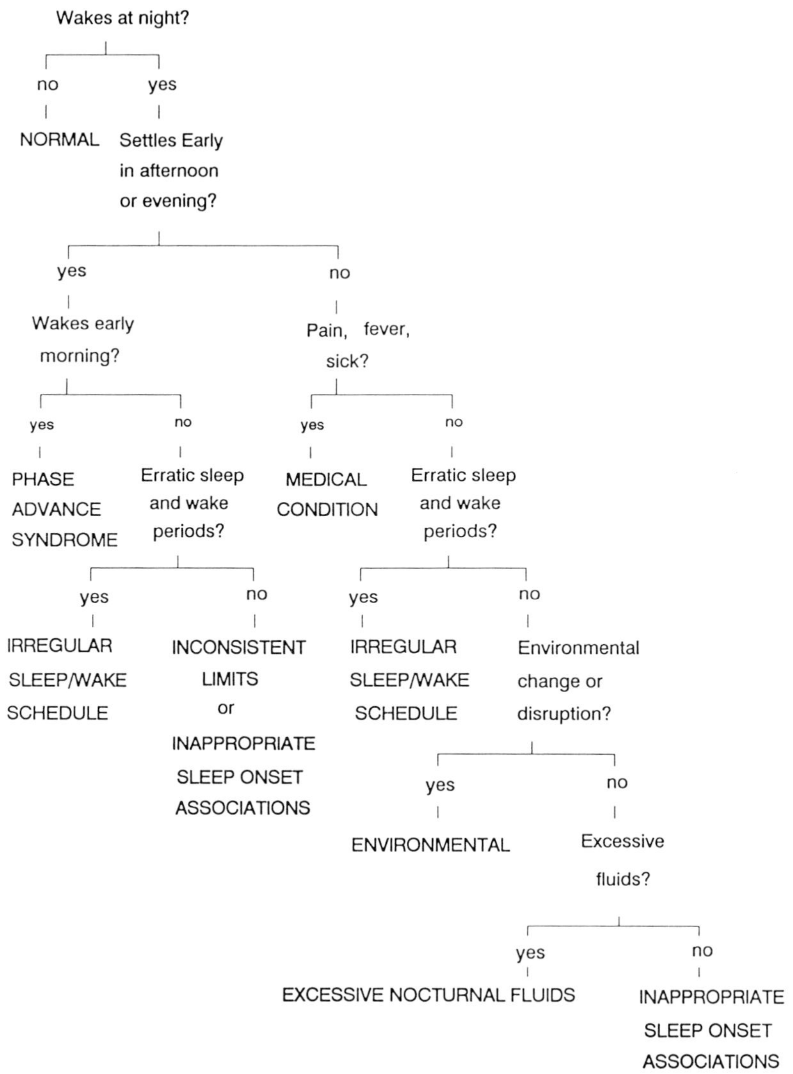

FIGURE 7–2. Evaluation of the sleepless child who initially settles easily at night.

medical, developmental, and behavioral history. Physical examination should be comprehensive, with special attention to developmental landmarks and the central nervous system.[7]

Parents usually seek help for the problem only if the child's sleeplessness has resulted in parental sleeplessness or fear that the child is becoming significantly sleep deprived. Unless the clinician takes the initiative to obtain a *comprehensive sleep history* during the normal course of well child care and health maintenance, many problems will be missed. Persistent night wakings have been frequently ascribed to parental mismanagement of nocturnal arousals. Appropriate attention should be paid to the methods with which the parents have responded to their sleepless child in the past. The following questions may elucidate significant aspects of the patient's history and provide insight into sleep patterns and habits:

1. What is the normal evening bedtime?
2. What specific activities are performed during a period of 2 hours immediately before bedtime?
3. How long does it normally take the child to fall asleep?
4. If it takes the child longer than 30 minutes to fall asleep, what does the child do during the time from lights out to sleep onset? What are the parents' responses to these behaviors?
5. What steps have the parents taken to assist the child in falling asleep?
6. Is the child permitted to fall asleep somewhere other than in his or her own bed and in his or her own bedroom?

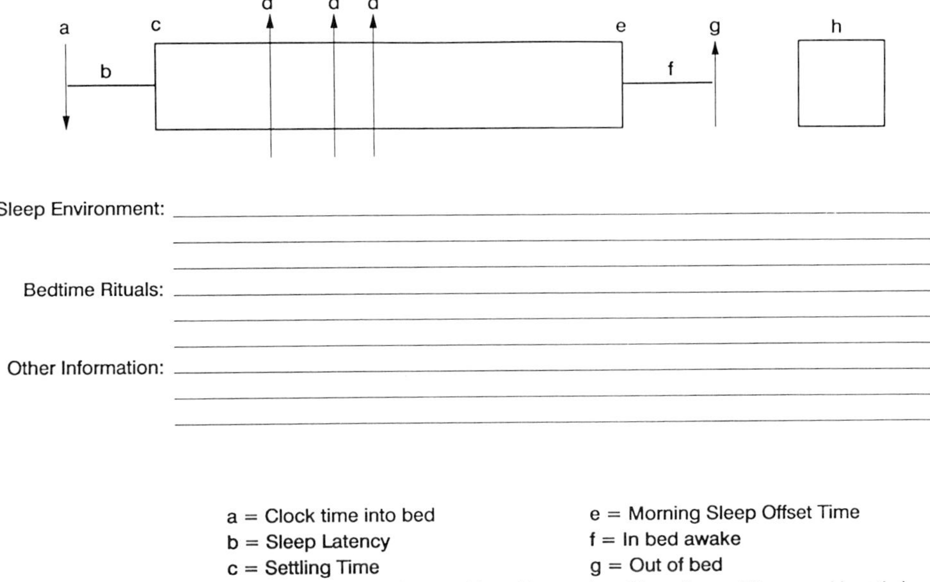

FIGURE 7–3. Recording the sleep history. A comprehensive sleep history includes, but is not limited to, information regarding the sleeping environment (e.g., the bedroom, type of bed, presence of night lights, other occupants of the bedroom); prebedtime rituals; time of lights out on weekdays and weekends; presleep behavior; time of sleep onset on weekdays and weekends; arousals, awakenings, or unusual behaviors during sleep; types of parental intervention during awakenings or unusual behaviors; presence of snoring or other breathing difficulties during sleep; bedwetting; time of morning awakening on weekdays, weekends, and during holidays; time the child gets out of bed in the morning; behavior on awakening; times of maximal alertness (or sleepiness) during the day; presence of excessive daytime sleepiness; and time, length, frequency, and characteristics of daytime naps. Often the information obtained in the sleep history is an approximate perception by the parents and may not describe the sleep-wake pattern in enough detail for accurate evaluation. The sleep history is greatly enhanced by the maintenance of a sleep log for 2 to 4 weeks.

7. Exactly what associations does the child require in order to fall asleep (e.g., stuffed animal, special toy, pacifier, bottle, being held, watching television, night light)?

8. After sleep onset does the child wake? For how long? At what times? How many times per night?

9. If the child wakes at night, what interventions are required for the child to fall back to sleep?

10. Does the child exhibit any unusual behaviors or movements during sleep? Does the child walk in his or her sleep? Bang his or her head? Wake suddenly with a piercing scream? Jerk his or her legs? Grind his or her teeth?

11. Does the child snore? Is the snoring mild, moderate, severe? Does the child snore every night?

12. What time does the child wake in the morning? Does the child wake spontaneously, or is the child awakened by a clock? Parent? Sibling? Is it difficult to wake the child? How does the child feel upon waking? Grumpy? Tired? Happy?

13. At what time during the day is the child most active and alert? Most tired and cranky?

14. Does the child nap during the day? How many times each day? At what times?

15. Does the child exhibit any unusual behaviors during daytime naps?

16. Where does the child nap? Are the same sleep associations present for the child at daytime naps?

Fig. 7–3 depicts a shorthand method practitioners might use for recording sleep patterns and habits.

A sleep diary or sleep log maintained for 2 weeks is of great assistance in analyzing children's sleep problems. The diary provides more objective, longitudinal evidence of sleep patterns and a baseline from which to compare progress and success of treatment regimens. By keeping the sleep diary during the course of treatment, the parents and practitioner have clear evidence of change.

Despite parental concern that their child is being sleep deprived from difficulty in settling or night waking, this is usually not the case. If the child remains active, alert, and playful during normal waking hours, the volume of sleep during the previous 24 hours is probably appropriate.[7] Parental sleep deprivation, on the other hand, is usually real. Treatment of the child's sleep problem generally resolves the parents' sleep problems.

MANAGEMENT OF DISORDERS OF INITIATING AND MAINTAINING SLEEP IN CHILDHOOD

A variety of solutions to sleep onset and maintenance problems have been suggested, and there have been significant contradictory recommendations regarding optimal management. No single approach appears to be universally effective. Recommendations have included attention to nighttime rituals, firm handling, letting the child "cry it out," use of hypnotics and sedatives, general support and sympathy, and a combination of the preceding.[16] Many are appropriate. Some are not. For example, Wilks has described a method for deconditioning night wakings in one night[17]:

> ***The child cries. Father stamps in, flings down the side of the cot, slaps him once. But firmly, flings up the cot side, and stamps out, slamming the door behind him (locking it with older children). The child screams and shouts for hour after hour until, depending on his strength and determination, eventually he subsides in a lather of sweat and exhaustion.***

Obviously, this method of treatment goes against most acceptable methods and may result in numerous difficulties in addition to problems with sleep.

Behavioral methods of treatment have been used successfully in the management of childhood psychological and behavioral problems. However, a behavioral approach may not be appropriate for all problems related to sleeplessness. This approach requires careful analysis of the individual problem, establishment of specific goals of treatment, and then *gradual* steps to their attainment. Emphasis should be placed on removing factors that reinforce the problem and replacing them with appropriate behaviors. Many sleep problems are resolved spontaneously, and time is on the physician's side in the management of many sleep disorders.[7] Simple behavioral procedures may occupy the parents' attention long enough for a spontaneous remission to occur.

Night wakings and settling problems are often interactional, affecting the entire family and not merely the child. Therefore management of the problem should be directed at the family and not only the child. In many circumstances the best method of treatment is habit training (behavior modification) and attention to the principles of sleep hygiene (Table 7–1). If the child fails to respond, some recommend the short-term use of sedation.[3] It is thought that a short course of a hypnotic or sedative may alter the infant's arousal threshold enough to facilitate the learning of a more acceptable sleep pattern. However, this approach is controversial; we and many practitioners think that medication rarely has a place in the management of sleep disorders.

Changes in the sleeping environment may cause dramatic changes in sleep patterns. Children with a persistent problem with sleeplessness may sleep well at a grandparent's home only to have the symptoms return in their own home environment. This is frequently irritating to young parents, who may feel insecure about

TABLE 7–1. Principles of Sleep Hygiene in Childhood

The sleeping environment should be quiet and dark.

Morning wake time should be strictly and consistently enforced. This strengthens circadian cycling.

Bedtime should be strictly enforced.

Room temperature should remain at a comfortable level (<75°). Excessively hot ambient temperatures disturb sleep.

Environmental noise should be kept at a minimum.

Hunger at bedtime should be avoided. However, excessive fluids at bedtime and throughout the night disturbs sleep.

Children should learn to fall asleep alone, without parental intervention.

Vigorous activity should be avoided for an hour or two before bedtime. Baths may be a stimulating activity for some children, and if bedtime struggles are a problem, bath time might be changed to another time during the day.

Food or beverages containing methylxantines (caffeine, theophylline) should be avoided for several hours before bedtime. Common foods and beverages containing these compounds include most colas, chocolate, coffee, and tea.

Some medications contain alcohol or caffeine and may disrupt sleep.

Naps should be developmentally appropriate. However, prolonged and too frequent napping should be avoided.

Modified from Hauri P: Current concepts: the sleep disorders. Kalamazoo, MI, Upjohn Company, 1982, p 22, with permission.

their role.[7] Appropriate support and management of the entire family are essential in this situation.

According to Bax, short-term use of chloral hydrate or promethazine (Phenergan) may be necessary.[7] If so, it is important to start with an adequate dose and wean quickly from the medication. This method appears better than starting with small doses and increasing until a desired effect is achieved. The latter method may result in increasing tolerance to the medication and the need for larger doses.

During any behavioral management regimen, parents must be warned that the child's sleep problem may appear to worsen for a few days at the beginning of treatment. This apparent setback frequently results in abandonment of the treatment protocol if the parents are not adequately warned, supported, and reassured. When improvement occurs, it tends to happen quickly.

Jones and Verduyn reported that 53% of children's sleep problems resolved completely when a behavioral approach was used.[16] Thirty-seven percent more showed partial resolution, and 10% were unchanged at the end of the treatment regimen. Maternal psychiatric history was unrelated to the outcome. The success of sleeping through the night remained unchanged at 6-month follow-up. The problem was less likely to resolve when marital discord was present. Response was best when both parents were persuaded to attend sessions with the physicians. Consistency and persistency are imperative in management, and cooperation between parents during the treatment regimen will result in more rapid and complete resolution of symptoms.

DIFFERENTIAL DIAGNOSIS OF CHILDHOOD DISORDERS OF INITIATING AND MAINTAINING SLEEP

Behavioral Factors Causing Sleeplessness

Disorder of Sleep Onset Associations

As pointed out in Chapter 1, brief nocturnal awakenings are normal, especially during transitions between REM and non-REM sleep. These brief arousals may serve an important survival function. The sleeping environment may be checked and the body repositioned. Bedclothes may be adjusted to the sleeper's comfort. Return to sleep is most often rapid and the short arousal is not remembered. If the sleeping environment has changed, however, returning to sleep may be difficult and the individual may become fully alert.

Sleep onset occurs through complex behavioral and physiological interactions. First, the body must be physiologically ready for sleep, at its appropriate position in the circadian cycle. A series of bedtime rituals follows. A pillow might be fluffed, covers and blankets positioned. A night light, soft music, television, or presence of a bed partner may be required. Without these behavioral rituals, sleep onset may be difficult. In other words, we *learn* to fall asleep in a particular manner and this learned behavior is repeated night after night. When these *sleep onset associations* are absent, falling to sleep may be troublesome.

Children learn to fall asleep in the same manner. Certain conditions must be present to ease the transition. The child may require a particular bedroom, lying in a certain crib or bed, and holding a favorite stuffed animal or special blanket.[1,26] These conditions are usually present all night. Being held and rocked, the presence of television, being read a story, or suckling a pacifier may not be present all night. After a normal arousal, it may be hard for the child to return to sleep, since the child has not learned to fall asleep without these associations. As Ferber persuasively states, "Thus the problem is not one of abnormal wakings but one of difficulty in falling back to sleep. And the difficulty arises because of the child's particular associations with falling asleep."[26]

Disorder of sleep onset associations occurs most commonly in infants and toddlers. The older the children, the more control they have over their environment and the less likely they are to require associations that are not present within their sleep environment during nocturnal arousals. Association problems become less significant after 4 years of age, although they occasionally persist into adolescence.

Clinical Presentation and Diagnosis. The usual complaint is one of prolonged night wakings. Settling may not be of concern to the parents, since associations may be present early in the evening. During the night the child may fuss significantly until removed from the crib or bed, permitted to sleep in the parents' bed, held, or rocked. Daytime sleepiness is unusual, although parents may be significantly sleep deprived from continually responding to their child's nocturnal crying. Time of settling is usually normal. In most cases review of a sleep diary reveals normal sleep onset latency time and frequent, prolonged nocturnal arousals. Total sleep time, the timing of the major sleep period, and morning wake time are usually normal.

Parents often report that the child rapidly returns to sleep if given a bottle. The volume of fluid consumed by the youngster during these nocturnal feedings is usually small. For the breast-fed infant, sleep returns quickly once nursing begins, and the mother perceives nocturnal feedings as different from daytime feedings. These characteristics help differentiate association problems from disorders of excessive nocturnal fluids. Physiological processes controlling the sleep-wake cycle can be assumed to be functioning normally if the child sleeps well while being held or rocked. If there is significant dysfunction of central mechanisms controlling sleep, the child would not sleep well under any circumstances. Physical examination usually produces normal findings. Rapid return to sleep when habitual associations are reestablished helps to differentiate normal from abnormal arousals and the diagnosis of disordered sleep onset associations as the problem.

Treatment. Treatment is straightforward. The child must learn to make the transition from wake to sleep without expecting a parent's participation. Success rates are high if parents are given sufficient support. Relearning usually takes less than 1 week.[26]

The child must learn to fall asleep alone and under conditions that can be easily reestablished after normal nocturnal arousals. Bedtime rituals should not be stimulating, require ongoing activity, or need parental participation. Holding, rocking, nursing, and suckling on a pacifier should be discontinued. The child should be placed in the crib or in bed alone and should learn to fall asleep by himself or herself.

Two basic principles must be followed. The parents must be *consistent* with reestablishing appropriate sleep onset associations and must be *persistent* with the regimen. The following paradigm usually is rapidly successful if the parents are consistent and persistent. For some families, sleepless nights may seem worse for the first day or two of treatment. Therefore the treatment regimen should begin on days when parental sleeplessness will not affect their performance the following day. Although some degree of crying should be expected during the beginning of the treatment phase, it is usually kept to a minimum by *gradually* establishing appropriate sleep onset associations. Letting the child "cry it out" usually maintains crying at its maximum and often results in parental frustration and treatment failure. The following regimen is recommended:

1. The first night
   a. The child should be placed in the crib or bed with only those association objects that will be present during normal nocturnal awakenings.
   b. The room should be dark (although a small night light may be used), quiet, and at a comfortable temperature. A room that is too hot or too cold may inhibit sleep. When the room temperature cannot be controlled, the child should be dressed appropriately for the ambient temperature.
   c. The parent may soothe and comfort the child until the child is lying quietly. Allowing some crying rarely results in psychological trauma to the child and is often more difficult for the parent.
   d. Once the child is quiet in the bed or crib, the parent should leave the room.
   e. If the child begins to cry, the parents should let him or her cry for a short time. The exact time should be developmentally appropriate, but at least 1 to 2 minutes (according to a clock or a stop-watch) should elapse before the parent responds.
   f. The parent may then return to the room to comfort the child, but *the child should not be removed from the crib or bed.* The parent may remain in the room quietly soothing the child until he or she lies back down in the crib or bed and is quiet. When the child is again quiet, the parent should leave the room.
   g. If and when the child begins to cry again, the parent should wait slightly longer before responding (a period of 2 to 5 minutes is usually appropriate) and repeat the previous step.
   h. The above process should be repeated (keeping the wait-response period at 2 to 5 minutes on the first night) until the child is sleeping.
   i. On the first night this process of cry-wait-respond may last for several hours before the child is sleeping. Parents must be warned that this might occur. They must be supported and reassured that the process will succeed if they are persistent and consistent with the regimen. If they give

up and remove the child from the crib or bed on the first or second night of management, a treatment failure is likely. Involving all caretakers in the treatment program is also important so that responsibilities are shared and consistency is ensured.

2. The second night
   a. Treatment on the second night is similar to the first; however, the wait-response period may be lengthened to 2 to 4 minutes at first, and 5 to 10 minutes for the subsequent waiting times. *If the child is beginning to calm at the end of the wait-response time, the parents should wait slightly longer to see whether the child will settle on his or her own.*
   b. Parental interventions should be *supportive*. The child should know that the parent is nearby and *understanding*.
   c. Parents must not exhibit anger or frustration or allow these feelings to escalate as the night progresses.
3. Subsequent nights
   a. Treatment on subsequent nights should parallel the first two nights.
   b. By the third night improvement is usually seen. Nighttime wakings are usually shorter, loud crying may be replaced with mild whimpering, and return to sleep without parental intervention occurs.
   c. Nocturnal arousals may still occur, but crying does not. The child has learned to fall back to sleep on his or her own without parental assistance.

During the course of management, parents should maintain a sleep diary to record progress. This is important for the parents and practitioner so that improvement may be documented. During the course of treatment, follow-up visits should occur weekly. The sleep diaries should be evaluated at each visit. Once the child is falling to sleep on his or her own, he or she will most often continue to sleep well. Occasional disruptions might occur, especially during times when the usual regimen is altered (e.g., vacations, birthdays, holidays). Parental response and management of these intermittent sleep disruptions will determine whether they will persist. If the disruption is managed in a manner consistent with the original regimen, rapid resolution will occur and the child will continue to sleep well.

If the mother is breast feeding the child, nursing may continue while the sleep onset association is being corrected. It is only necessary to dissociate the act of nursing from falling to sleep. Association problems are most likely present if the youngster falls asleep at the breast during nocturnal feedings after nursing for only a few moments. Moving the last feeding of the evening to a time several hours before bedtime will prevent the association of feeding and bedtime. If the child tends to fall asleep at the breast, the mother may discontinue the feeding before the child falls to sleep and place the child in the crib or bed. The same techniques may be used during daytime naps.

Excessive Nocturnal Fluids

Although considered under the rubric of behavioral etiologies, excessive nocturnal fluids may have a physiological basis for causing sleeplessness. In older children and adults, bladder distention typically results in an arousal (see Chapter 12). In children with primary functional sleep enuresis, this arousal appears to be developmentally delayed. Other evidence that bladder distention has a central arousal effect stems from observations that parasomnias (disorders of sleep stages and partial arousals from sleep) appear to be exacerbated by bladder distention.

Clinical Presentation and Diagnosis. Infants fed excessive quantities of fluid during the night typically wake frequently. This problem occurs in both breast-fed and bottle-fed infants. The volume of fluid consumed during the night may range from 8 to 32 ounces, and these youngsters wake from three to eight times per night.[27] Diapers are usually heavily soaked by morning.

During the second half of the first year of life, infants no longer have a physiological need for feeding during the night. Waking to eat may be secondary to one or more of three major factors: (1) the infant may associate feeding with sleep onset and returning to sleep; (2) the infant may have learned to be hungry during the night; or (3) bladder distention may be present and causing the arousal. Children waking and feeding because of inappropriate sleep onset associations typically wake less often than those waking because of excessive nocturnal fluids. Presence of only one or two arousals per night with rapid return to sleep after only a brief period at the bottle, breast, or pacifier suggests that the nipple or parent is more important than the fluid intake. If sleep onset association problems are present, intake of fluid is usually less than 6 ounces per night. More frequent wakings and the consumption of large volumes of fluid (8 to 32 ounces) suggests excessive fluid intake as the problem. Breast feeding more than two times per night and a nursing session lasting longer than 2 to 3 minutes suggests excessive fluid intake. Finally, if the child has learned to eat during the night, frequent nocturnal waking will occur. Habitual nocturnal feedings may distort the circadian hunger rhythm and disrupt the sleep-wake cycle as much as the fluid and food intake.

Treatment. Although nocturnal wakings are typically frequent and severe in patients ingesting excessive nocturnal fluids, treatment is straightforward and not difficult. The aim of therapy is to *discontinue the nocturnal fluids gradually*. For the bottle-fed infant, gradually decreasing the volume of fluid in each nocturnal bottle over the course of 1 to 2 weeks usually results in rapid improvement. Often infants stop waking to be fed when only 1 to 2 ounces is provided. An alternative is to dilute formula gradually with water before weaning from the bottle. In either case, however, an association of sleep onset with sucking must not be established during the treatment phase. If this occurs, the regimen should be modified to include principles discussed in the section on treatment of sleep onset association disorder. Treatment of the breast-fed infant ingesting excessive nocturnal fluids is slightly more difficult. Nursing mothers may experience a milk "let down" on hearing their crying infant. The nursing mother may have to express her milk manually (or use a breast pump) and let the infant's father or other caretaker respond. The mother's milk is diluted with water and the infant is gradually weaned from the bottle in the same manner as for formula-fed infants. Once the infant is sleeping through the night, maternal let down during sleep usually resolves.

Colic

Infantile colic is one of the more common disorders affecting sleep in young infants. Colic affects about one in five infants.[28] The patient is usually less than 4 months of age, and the typical complaint is unconsolable fussiness during the late afternoon or evening. Often symptoms of colic resolve but disordered sleep remains. The problem does not appear to be biologically based, although it may reflect altered chronophysiological factors during development. More likely the sleep problem occurs in response to altered sleep-wake schedules and habitual patterns of parental responsiveness persisting after the colicky period.[1]

Weissbluth has stated that colicky behavior appears to be a reflection of central nervous system development during the first few months of life.[28] Subsequently, some colicky infants develop irregularity of behavior, heightened activity or arousal, and sensitivity to stimuli that cause, directly or indirectly, difficulty maintaining regular, prolonged, and consolidated sleep patterns.[28] Mismanagement of the infant's sleep schedule and habits after the colicky period has passed, a result of early difficulties in handling the infant, is thought to be the most common cause of sleep problems persisting after 4 months of age.

Clinical Presentation and Diagnosis. Patients suffer violent, rhythmical, screaming attacks that are unresponsive to parental intervention and for which no other cause can be found.[29] Wessel and co-workers described colicky infants as those who experience paroxysms of irritability, fussing, or crying totaling more than 3 hours per day, occurring more than 3 days per week, and continuing or recurring for more than 3 weeks.[30]

Age of onset, time of occurrence, and age of resolution of symptoms are characteristic. "Attacks" seldom occur during the first few days of life. Symptoms typically begin during the third (80%) or fourth week of life (100%).[30] An important exception is the premature infant. Three studies have documented the onset of colic in premature infants within 2 weeks of the expected date of birth (70% between the 39th and 44th gestational weeks) regardless of the gestational age at birth.[31-33] Once symptoms begin in the preterm infant, the duration of colic appears to be similar to that of term infants. Thus the age of onset and age of disappearance of colic appear to be time locked to conceptual age. Episodes of colic tend to start between 5 and 8 PM and end at about midnight. By 2 months of age almost half of infants suffering from colic have resolution of symptoms. Symptoms resolve in 90% of all infants with colic by 4 months of age.

Another characteristic feature of colic is relatively uninhibited motor activity. During the crying spells affected infants have been described as hypertonic or neurolabile. This does not occur at other times during the day or night. Physical movements during the colicky spell include tonic stiffening of the entire body with fists tightly clenched, legs flexed rigidly over the abdomen, writhing, twisting, and turning motions, and jerky, uncoordinated movements such as batting or flapping of the arms or kicking of the legs. Facial grimacing suggests severe pain, and affected infants appear unusually sensitive to light.[34]

Daytime sleep periods in colicky infants are extremely irregular and brief. Some infants temporarily discontinue daytime naps during the period of maximal fussiness (approximately 6 weeks of age). Colicky infants, during their evening "attacks," miss periods of quiet sleep.[28] Interestingly, after cessation of daytime and nighttime "spells" the infant invariably falls asleep. This may be secondary to exhaustion or time of day or could represent a period of transient but excessive neurological arousal, excitation, or lack of inhibition that is terminated by naturally occurring periods of quiet sleep or increased inhibition.[28]

A number of studies have evaluated infants' sleep patterns in the postcolicky period.[35-37] Parents of infants who have had colic report shorter total sleep duration at 4 to 5 months of age. A history of colic appears to be significantly associated (ratio of almost 2.5:1) with frequent night wakings when compared with infants who have no history of colic. Duration of night wakings is a problem for some, as is frequency of waking in others.

Some postcolicky infants are exquisitely sensitive to irregularities of their sleep-wake schedules. Disruptions of sleep-wake routines because of illness, holidays, or vacations cause extreme disruptions of settling and night wakings that may last several nights. According to Weissbluth, these prolonged recovery periods might reflect easily disorganized endogenous biological rhythms caused by enduring congenital imbalances in arousal and inhibition of sleep-wake control mechanisms.[28] This suggests that disordered chronophysiological mechanisms may be significant in postcolicky sleep-wake disturbances, and treatment should focus on mechanisms that may functionally "reset" and entrain the endogenous circadian pacemaker.

Treatment. Infants who suffer from frequent night wakings and short sleep periods in the postcolicky period may be successfully treated only if the parents establish and maintain a regular sleep schedule. Most postcolic sleep problems are the result of the parents' failure to establish regular sleep patterns when the colic dissipates at approximately 4 months of age. Therefore treatment should focus on reestablishment of a normal sleep-wake routine. If parents strictly program their child's sleep schedule, regular day and night sleep patterns will reemerge. The most powerful point of entrainment is *morning wake time*. Morning wake times must be fixed and consistent. Nocturnal bedtime and nap times also require strict adherence. *Consistency* and *persistency* are key factors in establishing a successful regimen. A sleep diary recorded for 1 to 2 weeks before instituting therapy and during the course of treatment greatly assists parents in maintaining an appropriate routine and provides accurate feedback for the practitioner regarding success of the regimen during follow-up visits.

Medical Disorders Resulting in Sleeplessness

Cow's Milk Allergy

Allergy to cow's milk protein may result in severe disturbance of sleep during early infancy. Cow's milk allergy is often difficult to differentiate clinically from colic, since both begin at similar ages and are associated with sleeplessness, fussiness, intermittent crying episodes, and short sleep periods.

Clinical Presentation and Diagnosis. Frequent night wakings (five or more times per night) and short total sleep times (often as low as 4½ hours) are the typical sleep complaints.[1,38] Infants with cow's milk allergy cry frequently during the day and are described by their parents as "fussy." Physical findings may be unremarkable, although some infants have anemia and hematochezia. Polysomnographic analysis reveals a significantly disturbed sleep pattern and is useful in determining the absence of other causes for arousal and short total sleep time. Diagnosis is based on a high clinical index of suspicion of atopy. Allergy testing usually reveals elevated immunoglobulin E (IgE) levels, and radioallergosorbent testing (RAST) is often positive for cow's milk protein. Discontinuing cow's milk–based formula and substituting a hydrolyzed milk protein formula resolves the symptoms.

Treatment. Once the diagnosis is established, treatment consists of replacing cow's milk protein with hydrolyzed milk protein formula. Within 2 weeks of dietary modifications, sleep patterns generally normalize. Daytime symptoms decrease or resolve, total sleep time increases to a developmentally normal level, and nocturnal awakenings end. Reintroduction of cow's milk protein formula exacerbates symptoms. At times exacerbations are severe, and clinical judgment should determine whether reintroduction of the responsible protein is prudent. It should be done only in rare circumstances and only under highly controlled conditions.

Otitis Media

Any condition that results in pain, discomfort, or fever may cause sleep disruption and sleeplessness. Otitis media is one of the most common childhood illnesses, and acute middle ear disease rarely goes unrecognized. The cause for the child's sleep complaint is often readily apparent. In contrast, chronic middle ear disease often is present despite a paucity of clinical symptoms. Serous or secretory otitis media associated with persistent middle ear effusions may be asymptomatic except for the disruption of sleep.

Clinical Presentation and Diagnosis. Children with acute suppurative otitis media often have fever, otalgia, appetite changes, and vomiting. Frequent prolonged nocturnal arousals, associated daytime sleepiness, and significant decrease in daytime activity often occur. Physical examination reveals a bulging tympanic membrane with loss of normal landmarks and immobility of the drum on pneumootoscopy or tympanography.

Chronic serous or secretory otitis media is often associated with few symptoms. Hearing may be decreased, but the loss may be clinically inapparent. Complaints of otalgia may be absent. Physical examination may reveal a retracted, immobile tympanic membrane. Evidence of eustachian tube dysfunction is often present, and air-fluid levels may be visualized. Regardless of the absence of clear clinical complaints during the day, sleep may be significantly disrupted.

Treatment. Treatment of the sleep disturbance associated with acute or chronic middle ear disease first focuses on adequate management of the underlying disorder. Appropriate courses of antibiotic therapy for acute suppurative otitis media should resolve the sleep complaints. Treatment of chronic serous or secretory otitis media and persistent middle ear effusion has included tympanocentesis, tympanotomy tube placement, long-term antibiotic therapy, or a combination of antibiotics and short-course steroid treatment. Resolution of the effusion often results in concomitant resolution of nocturnal symptoms. During the course of medical or surgical therapy, attention must be paid to principles of sleep hygiene. Sleep schedules must be regularized, and parents should adhere to strict patterns of age-appropriate sleep-wake timetables.

Neurological Disorders

Neurologically impaired children frequently wake at night and exhibit disordered sleep-wake schedules. This sleep disruption may be due to chronic cerebral irritability; however, sleeplessness and night waking are also reported by parents of children with other significant handicaps. Children with static encephalopathies, noncortical blindness, and deafness may exhibit significant disorders of sleep-wake cycles.

Clinical Presentation and Diagnosis. Sleep problems in children with neurological disorders may be due to various underlying causes. Indeed, a child with obvious neurological impairment may also exhibit symptoms of sleeplessness secondary to any of the nonneurological conditions discussed in this chapter. Therefore assessment of the child's sleep problem must include a comprehensive evaluation without prematurely attributing the sleep disorder to the prominent neurological condition. All factors that may result in sleeplessness should be considered.

The primary neurological diagnosis is often clinically obvious. Characteristics of the sleep problem, however, may be more obscure, and maintenance of a sleep diary is extremely important in evaluating the sleep-wake cycle of the neurologically impaired child. Sufficient data may be collected to differentiate a primarily behavioral cause from one secondary to impairment of neurological mechanisms responsible for controlling sleep-wake cycles, sleep onset, and sleep maintenance. Medications used for management of the principal neurological condition may themselves be responsible for disordered sleep. Nocturnal polysomnography is often helpful in differentiating a central origin of the sleep disorder and assists in detecting nocturnal seizure activity that may not be apparent during the day. Diagnosis of an organic basis for disordered sleep is one of exclusion. Only after comprehensive evaluation of other possible mechanisms has failed to reveal the reason should neurological mechanisms be considered causative.

Treatment. Treatment of sleeplessness in the neurologically impaired child depends on the identified underlying cause. Attention should be first paid to all factors that may influence sleep and the sleep-wake cycle, other than the neurological disorder. If a behavioral or parental management problem is suspected, it may be managed in a manner previously described. It might be necessary, however, to conduct the therapeutic regimen more slowly than it would be conducted in a nonneurologically impaired child. Appropriate attention should be paid to the child's sleep-wake schedule, circadian rhythms, and zeitgebers, especially in children with special sensory disorders such as blindness. Correction of these schedule abnormalities is usually not difficult and rapidly improves sleep patterns and daytime function.

If medication used in treatment of the principal neurological disorder is considered responsible for the sleep problem, attention should be paid to dosage and timing of administration of the drug. As discussed in Chapter 3, windows of time exist in which a particular medication may significantly affect circadian timekeeping mechanisms. Administration within the window significantly shifts circadian rhythms; administration of the same medication and dosage outside of the window results in little change in pacemaker timing. Therefore a shift in the time of administration of prescribed medications may greatly change the child's sleep-wake patterns. Under certain circumstances dosage of the medication may be modified to improve the child's sleep. In other situations, although less commonly, specific medications may have to be discontinued and replaced with an alternative drug for sleep improvement to occur.

When the underlying neurological abnormality is considered the cause of sleeplessness, attention should still be paid to appropriate sleep hygiene. If improvement of sleeplessness occurs with mild medications, such as diphenhydramine, the child usually shows similar improvement without the use of drugs. Hypnotic or sedative medication is occasionally required. Chloral hydrate is often effective for treating sleeplessness in children with neurological or special sensory impairment. If medication is necessary, use of adequate dosages is important. It is more appropriate to begin with a dosage schedule that is significant enough to control the symptoms, rather than beginning with a small dose and slowly increasing it until a response occurs. Medication resistance is less common in neurologically impaired children than in children without neurological disorders. Once medication is instituted, the child's daytime function must be monitored to ensure improvement. Periodic withdrawal of medication is also recommended. Once the symptoms of sleeplessness are controlled, it may be possible to discontinue the medication without exacerbating the symptoms.[39]

Attention Deficit Hyperactivity Disorder

Parents of hyperactive children consider their children to have many more sleep problems than do parents of children without hyperactivity.[40] Most commonly, night wakings and restless sleep are reported. In a study by Salzarulo and Chevalier, parents of children with attention deficit hyperactivity disorder (ADHD) reported sleep onset problems 16.5% of the time and night wakings 39% of the time.[41] The *Diagnostic and Statistical Manual of Mental Disorders*, ed. 3 (DSM III), lists motor restlessness during sleep as one of the defining characteristics of hyperactivity,[42] even though support from sleep studies is ambiguous and controversial results exist.[43,44] Hyperactivity and attention deficits are probably symptoms of a heterogeneous group of disorders with varied causes, manifesting increased daytime activity and disordered sleep. For example, children with obstructive sleep apnea syndrome manifest daytime symptoms virtually indistinguishable from ADHD on clinical grounds alone. Attention span problems may reflect daytime results of sleep deprivation with the appearance of microsleeps. Further investigation is necessary to determine whether dysfunctional sleep is an effect or a cause of ADHD in some children.

Clinical Presentation and Diagnosis. Diagnosis of ADHD may be difficult. These children tend to be fidgety, have difficulty staying on and completing tasks, often disturb other children in school, are easily distracted, often cry easily, and have rapid mood swings. They may exhibit restlessness and increased activity. They are often easily frustrated in efforts and may become destructive. Physical examination often produces normal findings, and the child may not exhibit increased activity during the clinical evaluation. Soft neurological signs may be present in some children; however, the significance of these findings is questionable. Visual tracking may be poor, and speech may be dysfluent. Letter reversals when writing from dictation, dysdiadochokinesia with significant overflow-associated movements, difficulty hopping and skipping, and right-left confusion have also been reported with increased frequency in children with ADHD.[45,46]

Night wakings and restless sleep are characteristic sleep complaints. There does not, however, appear to be a difference in sleep onset latency or total sleep time between children with ADHD and normal children. Enuresis and night sweats have also been reported more frequently in hyperactive children than in control subjects.[40] Differentiating the sleep disruption of ADHD from that of obstructive sleep apnea may be difficult. Parents of virtually all children with obstructive sleep apnea syndrome notice significant snoring. Daytime symptoms of hyperactivity may also alternate with periods of somnolence in children with obstructive sleep apnea syndrome. Traditional nocturnal polysomnography may or may not be helpful. If significant sleep-related airway obstruction is present, the polysomnogram may reveal apneas, hypopneas, oxygen desaturation, and arousals. In many instances, however, results of noninvasive sleep studies are inconclusive. Despite increased respiratory resistive load during sleep, clear-cut apneas and hypopneas may be absent. In these circumstances diagnosis requires more invasive techniques, such as continuous monitoring of intrathoracic pressure through an indwelling esophageal balloon manometer. Noninvasive techniques for continuous monitoring of intrathoracic pressure during sleep are being investigated.

Treatment. Appropriate treatment for ADHD is controversial and beyond the scope of this text. Stimulant medication, counseling, and behavior modification are the most widely accepted methods of therapy. Sleep problems tend to improve along with daytime symptoms, despite the use of stimulants, which often cause sleeplessness in children without ADHD. At the present time, how the medication functions to improve daytime and nighttime symptoms of ADHD is obscure. It is interesting to speculate on the mechanism of this paradoxical effect. First, stimulant medication may provide enough cortical stimulation to cause an alerting response. Children may then be more capable of focusing attention on the task at hand. On the other hand, if microsleeps are present and responsible for attention span deficits and concomitant symptoms, stimulant medication may decrease the frequency or eliminate these microsleeps, resulting in better attention and focus. If microsleeps are frequent and sleep begins to accumulate during daytime hours, nocturnal sleep may be disrupted. Administration of stimulant medication may then eliminate or reduce the frequency of microsleeps. Since daytime sleep accumulation does not take place, nocturnal sleep improves. Although engaging, these explanations are highly speculative and await documentation.

Medications

Virtually any medication may cause sleep disruption. Hypnotics are the most commonly prescribed drugs in the United States. This classification of medication has resulted in more significant exacerbation of sleep problems than cures. Hypnotics and sedatives are often inappropriately used in children. Rarely does the use of hypnotics result in long-term improvement of sleep in children who are otherwise normal. If improvement occurs initially, a behavioral approach and attention to appropriate sleep hygiene most likely would also have resolved the symptoms without the risk of side effects. The most commonly prescribed medications in childhood are antihistamines (which may themselves cause sleeplessness), major sedatives (such as chloral hydrate and phenobarbital, which may themselves cause paradoxical hyperactivity), and short-acting benzodiazepines. These classes of medications may also adversely affect the child's performance the following day.

Relatively innocuous medications prescribed for acute or chronic illness may also be responsible for sleeplessness. Antibiotics, especially liquid preparations, have been associated with disorders of initiating and maintaining sleep.[39] The vehicle and not the antibiotic itself is thought to be responsible for the sleep disruption. Over-the-counter medications, especially combination drugs, may also be implicated. Oral bronchial smooth muscle relaxant medications often cause sleep disruption, although the exact mechanism is unclear.

Clinical Presentation and Diagnosis. A comprehensive medication history should be taken from the parents. Over-the-counter medication must be included, since the vehicle may be responsible for sleep disruption. If the child is taking medications, the dosage and timing of administration are important. The history may suggest onset of the sleep problem concurrent with the institution of medication. Most medications do not result in any typical patterns of sleep disruptions. Nocturnal settling and waking problems may be present. Hypnotics, sedatives, and neuroleptics may cause significant changes in sleep architecture, and nocturnal polysomnography may be useful in the diagnosis. Depending on the medication, total sleep time may be decreased or shifts in sleep-wake scheduling may occur. Maintenance of a sleep diary for 2 weeks may be valuable in accurately documenting the child's typical circadian sleep-wake rhythm.

Treatment. If possible the suspected offending medication should be discontinued. If this is not possible, modification of timing of administration or dosage may be attempted.

Switching to a similar medication or the same medication prepared differently may be successful (e.g., changing from oral bronchodilators to inhaled preparations). At times, merely changing brands of medication resolves the sleep problem.

Chronic Illness

Any chronic condition may contribute to persistent sleep problems. Pain or discomfort from the illness or from treatment regimens may be contributory. Disorders such as migraine cephalalgia, asthma, diabetes mellitus, gastroesophageal reflux, and seizures have all been associated with sleep disturbances. The problem of sleeplessness may be directly caused by the underlying disorder or may be an indirect consequence of therapy, medication, or anxieties.

Clinical Presentation and Diagnosis. The underlying disturbance may be readily apparent or may be obscure. For example, a child whose sleep is disrupted because of pruritus associated with chronic eczematous dermatitis will probably have easily diagnosable signs. On the other hand, a sleepless child waking from pain secondary to esophagitis and chronic gastroesophageal reflux may exhibit few abnormalities. Similarly, chronic serous or secretory otitis media may present few subjective symptoms.

Sorting out which factors related to the illness are precipitating the sleep problems is often difficult. Confusion regarding whether sleep disruption is caused by the primary illness, associated symptoms, side effects of medication or therapy, or the family's or child's response to the illness is frequently present. Diagnosis rests on a comprehensive history and physical examination.

Treatment. Treatment is based on management of the underlying chronic disorder, control of associated symptoms, and appropriate attention to sleep hygiene. If parental or patient anxiety about the chronic illness is suspected, appropriate supportive interventions should be recommended.

Psychosocial Factors Resulting in Sleeplessness

Childhood Affective Disorders

Depression in children is extremely difficult to diagnose because the clinical picture may vary depending on the child's age and developmental level.[47-49] Disrupted sleep has long been noted as part of the symptom complex. Polysomnographic characteristics seen in adult patients with affective disorders are well defined and reproducible. Kane has described a patient with childhood depression who manifested polysomnographic variables different from those of adults, but more similar to adult studies than to normative data for children of the same age.[47] Significant disturbance in sleep continuity was described. Early morning waking, problems settling, and intermittent nocturnal arousals were all present. Sleep efficiency was decreased. A stable but persistently shortened REM latency was also noted. Although the REM latency was at the lower end of normal for the patient's age, it was significantly shorter than the mean value for the patient's age group.

Stress may be associated with sleeplessness in children. Transient disorders of initiating and maintaining sleep may be precipitated by life events, such as the death of a grandparent or parental marital discord. Persistent disorders of sleeplessness in children are often due to parental mismanagement of transient sleeplessness caused by acute stress reactions. Another possibility is that stressful life events do not affect children directly, but rather are mediated by the parents' affect and changes in their responsivity and caretaking, especially during infancy when an infant's sleep-wake organization may be affected by responsive caretaking.[50]

Depression is not just another problem, but a central link between many kinds of problems: those that lead to depression and those that may follow.[51] Psychosocial factors identified as associated with sleep problems may represent a parent's withdrawal of psychological attention.[52] Evidence indicates that parental depressed feelings are associated with children's sleep problems. Maternal depression, rather than other measured psychosocial stresses such as separation experiences, is associated with the development of sleep problems. Long-term sleep continuity problems and the association of persistent sleep problems with parental difficulty in behavior management have been reported.[14]

To determine whether sleep problems commonly seen in pediatric practice are associated with more pervasive disturbances in the child or family, Lozoff, Wolf, and Davis studied two groups of healthy children.[52] Five experiences distinguished children with sleep problems from those without: an accident or illness in the family, unaccustomed absence of the mother during the day, maternal depressed mood(s), sleeping in the parental bed, and maternal attitude of ambivalence toward the child. These findings attest to the importance of sleep problems as an early childhood symptom. Bedtime conflicts and night waking seem to be quantifiable, easily ascertainable behavior patterns that could alert pediatric health professionals to the existence of more pervasive disturbance in the child and family.

NIGHTTIME FEARS

Childhood fears are normal. Most often they are developmentally related and are manifested in a variety of ways. At 2 to 3 years of age, children may exhibit aggression directed toward siblings (sibling rivalry), may fear death or loss of a parent, or may be troubled by separation from parents and emerging socialization. Clinical presentation may vary significantly, and developmentally appropriate fears may be generally obscure. Children may complain of a fear of robbers or monsters. These fears may be manifest as frightening dreams. In general, the reasons for nocturnal fears and nightmares are similar.[1] If these fears are extreme, excessive limit setting by parents requires the child to deal alone with the fears, is usually unsuccessful in resolving the sleep disturbance, and may be detrimental to the child's emotional health.

To determine the origin of the fears that may be manifest as nocturnal fears and sleep disturbances, the physician should evaluate the child during waking hours. Evaluation and intervention by a psychologist or psychiatrist should be considered, especially if the problem has persisted for some time. If fears (and symptoms) have been present for only a short time, parental understanding and firm support may be all that are necessary. Positive reinforcement, progressive relaxation techniques, biofeedback, and techniques of self-control may be attempted. A change in bedtime ritual, in which the parent remains close to the child for support with gradual withdrawal, may be successful in some children. Others may respond well to modifications in the physical sleeping environment.

INADEQUATE LIMIT SETTING

Disordered sleep secondary to inadequate limit setting is most often seen in children during middle childhood and early adolescence. The usual complaint is difficulty settling at night and bedtime struggles. Frequently the child refuses to remain in bed or even in the bedroom. Although the child is physiologically prepared for sleep, the parents give in to the child's protestations easily and are unwilling or unable to enforce nighttime rituals and routines consistently. The child therefore does not remain in bed long enough to fall asleep. The child repetitively gets out of bed and protests, the parents become disturbed, tension escalates, the parents ultimately give in, and the child's behavior is reinforced. Parents may lack knowledge regarding limit setting or be aware that they are not appropriately setting limits for the child. Environmental factors, such as marital discord or sharing a bedroom with a sibling or with parents, may contribute to sleep disruption. Parental lack of recognition of the intensity of the child's fears and the inability to provide supportive firmness in the face of the child's protestations may increase the child's anxiety and exacerbate the problem.

Bedtime struggles by children who are not physiologically ready for sleep because of circadian rhythm disturbance or who suffer from inordinate nighttime fears may appear similar to those of children who do not have appropriate limits set. Clinical differentiation may be difficult, and evaluation of the family, intrafamilial relationships, and adequacy of parenting is necessary.

If inappropriate limit setting is suggested by the clinical assessment, treatment should address the underlying cause. Psychological problems and parental dysfunction should be addressed first. Parents should be counseled in mechanisms to enforce consistency and to provide *supportive* firmness. The parents must implement a regular bedtime ritual, which they must be unwilling to modify, regardless of the child's protestations. Door closure or a gate might be used to keep the child in his or her room. However, door closure must be associated with a supportive parental response, and this may be difficult if significant parental dysfunction is present. Anger, punishment, and escalation of tension must be eliminated. Children over 3 years of age may respond to specific behavior modification techniques and contracting using positive reinforcement for appropriate behavior and compliance with objectives of the regimen. Concepts of *persistency*, *consistency*, and *winning* should be stressed. Parents must decide who will win, the parents or the child. Often the child is more patient and persistent than the parents, who find giving in to the child easier than struggling. By letting the child "win," parents reinforce similar behaviors that are often manifested during waking hours as well.

Chronophysiological Factors Resulting in Sleeplessness

Advanced Sleep Phase Syndrome

Advanced sleep phase syndrome is a less common chronophysiological disorder resulting in sleeplessness. Total sleep time is normal, but sleep occurs at an inappropriate time. When sleep phase is advanced, children retire and settle early and easily. Bedtime struggles are not characteristic, and children may become cranky and disagreeable if kept awake when they are physiologically ready for sleep. Nocturnal wakings and protestations are infrequent or absent. Parental complaints most often center on early morning waking. The child is awake, alert, happy, and playful during early morning hours. Advanced sleep phase syndrome often goes unrecognized because early bedtime and wake time may fit well with parental schedules and cause little social interruption. School attendance and performance are rarely affected, and parents may appreciate the free time afforded them in the evening. Maintenance of a sleep diary greatly assists in diagnosis.

Treatment is straightforward, and a rapid response should be expected. Delaying the sleep phase is significantly easier than advancing the phase, since the master circadian pacemaker, under free-running, unentrained conditions, is spontaneously delayed (usually by 1 hour for each 24-hour period). Bedtime should be gradually delayed by 30 to 60 minutes per night (depending on the child's developmental level). Morning wakes should remain spontaneous and will become delayed reflexively once settling time is delayed. When the desired bedtime and wake time have been achieved, they should be fixed and enforced every night (including weekends and holidays). Again, persistency and consistency are imperative for success of the regimen. A sleep diary should be maintained during the course of treatment to monitor progress objectively.

Delayed Sleep Phase Syndrome

Delayed sleep phase syndrome is a result of a shift of the normal period of sleep to hours later than expected or desired. Characteristics of sleep are normal, but the children sleep at the wrong times. Children are physiologically ready for sleep late in the evening, and the morning spontaneous wake time may occur during the late morning or early afternoon (depending on the degree of shift). Nocturnal wakings do not appear to be a problem. Once asleep, the child tends to stay asleep.

Parental expectations for bedtime may be much earlier than the time the child is biologically ready for sleep, resulting in the typical complaint of sleep onset difficulties and significant bedtime struggles. Because the normal sleep period has shifted to a time later in the day, parents usually report profound difficulties waking the child in the morning. The child's behavior and activity in the morning hours are sluggish. School performance in morning classes (compared with classes that occur in the afternoon) may be poor, and the child may fall to sleep in school, especially at the beginning of the week. On weekends and holidays, when bedtime tends to be later in the evening, there are fewer struggles and the latency from lights out to sleep is shorter. Children suffering from delayed sleep phase syndrome tend to be sleep deprived during the week (because of the early morning wakings) but catch up on the weekends. Delayed sleep phase syndrome may be difficult to differentiate from other disorders with sleep onset difficulties, such as inappropriate and inconsistent limit setting. A comprehensive evaluation and maintenance of a sleep diary for 2 to 3 weeks are of great assistance in evaluating a child for a phase delay.

Small phase shifts in younger children are usually best treated with a controlled phase advance. The regimen should begin when the child does not have important daytime social and developmental responsibilities (i.e., school), since some degree of sleep deprivation occurs during the first few days of management. The regimen is begun by delaying the hour of bedtime for 2 to 3 days to a point at which the child is physiologically ready for sleep and sleep onset latency is relatively normal. Bedtime struggles disappear quickly. At the same time the morning wake-up time should be strictly fixed and maintained, even on weekends and holidays. If developmentally appropriate, naps should be continued, but prolonged naps should be avoided. If the child should not normally nap, daytime sleep should not be permitted, since the child may accumulate sleep during these hours at the expense of nocturnal sleep. Once the child is settling easily, the bedtime should be slowly advanced until the desired bedtime is reached. The degree of advance should be determined by the child's tolerance and response to treatment. However, the total sleep time should remain appropriate for the child's age and development. Parents should be counseled regarding appropriate sleep period times at various ages and should develop realistic expectations for their child. Again, maintenance of a sleep diary greatly assists in the assessment and monitoring of the therapeutic regimen.

Treatment of large sleep phase delays in adolescent patients may involve further delaying the sleep phase around the clock (moving in the direction of a free-running pacemaker) until desired sleep and wake times are reached. This should be accomplished only when the youngster has no other social responsibilities, since for a time he or she will sleep all day and remain awake all night. In addition, a parent may have to stay up with the youngster and phase delay with him or her for the regimen to succeed. This form of treatment may be extremely difficult and inappropriate for younger adolescents and prelatency children.

Exposure to intense light, especially when it occurs during windows of entrainment, may quickly shift the sleep phase to an appropriate time. This form of therapy appears promising in adult patients (although still experimental). Similar trials have not been performed in children with phase shifts.

Regular But Inappropriate Sleep-Wake Schedule

Children may nap too late or too early in the day. Naps may be too frequent or prolonged. Daytime sleep may also be too infrequent for the child's developmental level. Occasionally the complaint is one of inappropriately early bedtime or early morning wakings (which appear similar to a phase advance), but significant daytime sleep also occurs, resulting in appropriate total sleep times. Although any of these symptoms may be present, they tend to be consistent and recur daily. A sleep diary kept for 2 to 3 weeks reveals these regularly recurring but inappropriate times of sleep.

Treatment is directed at normalization of the sleep-wake schedule. Once a regular and appropriate sleep-wake schedule is attained, sleep normalizes.

Irregular Sleep Schedules

Entrainment of circadian rhythms occurs only if appropriate zeitgebers are present and if sleep-wake schedules remain constant. Inappropriate naps and schedules may result in internal desynchrony of other systems as well. In these patients, not only is bedtime disrupted, but also life in general is chaotic and lacks formal structure. Social instability is often present. Meal times tend to be irregular from day to day, and meals may be taken by different family members at different times.

Family dysfunction must be addressed first. With little structure in the lives of all members of the household, there is little chance that structuring sleep for the child will be successful unless the entire ecology of the family is treated. Sleep should be charted regularly, and appropriate schedules for meals and sleep should be established. Appropriate time cues must be provided, and structured wake time and bedtime must be maintained in a consistent and persistent manner.

Other Factors Resulting in Sleeplessness

Childhood Onset Disorders of Initiating and Maintaining Sleep

One form of primary insomnia in adults has its onset before puberty. Some evidence places the presence of this disorder early in infancy.[53] Sleep onset or sleep maintenance complaints may be present. Daytime symptoms of inadequate sleep may occur. This disorder of initiating and maintaining sleep is difficult to differentiate from others, since it may be finally diagnosed only if the sleep complaint persists through puberty and into adulthood. No precipitating cause can be identified. Childhood onset disorders of initiating and maintaining sleep may also constitute a shift in balance of the circadian pacemaker responsible for generation of the sleep-wake rhythm. Patterns of poor sleep are often more difficult to treat than the other forms of insomnia during childhood, and poor sleep tends to continue throughout both poor and good periods of emotional and developmental adaptation. This group is also differentiated from short sleepers by the presence of daytime symptoms of fatigue, irritability, tenseness, mild depression, difficulties in awake attention, and at times daytime sleepiness.

Short Sleeper

Although not typically discussed in the pediatric literature, the short sleeper is presented here because this condition may be genetically or congenitally determined. Short sleeper is the designation for an individual who consistently sleeps substantially less in a single day than the customary amount of sleep for the patient's age and developmental level.[53] Sleep, although short, is normal. There are typically no specific complaints about the quality of sleep, although bedtime struggles or early morning wakings may occur during childhood. Daytime sleepiness, difficulty with daytime behavior, and poor performance are notably absent. No true disorder of initiating or maintaining sleep exists, despite the occasional desire and unsuccessful attempts to sleep longer. Short sleep appears to be at one end of the normal, individual sleep requirement continuum.

As previously mentioned, short sleep has been linked to reduced life expectancy. This relationship probably has its source mainly in short total sleep time patterns resulting from medical or other sleep disorders, not in short sleep itself as represented by the short sleeper.[53]

REFERENCES

1. Ferber R: Sleeplessness in the child. In Kryger MH, Roth T, and Dement WC: Principles and practice of sleep medicine. Philadelphia, WB Saunders, 1989, pp 633-639.
2. Anders TF: Night-waking in infants during the first year of life. Pediatrics 1979;63:860-864.
3. Carey WB: Night waking and temperament in infancy. J Pediatr 1974;84:756-758.
4. Palmer CD, Harrison GA, and Hirons RW: Sleep patterns and life styles in Oxfordshire Village. J Biosoc Sci 1980;12:437.
5. California Assessment Program. Student achievement in California Schools: 1979-1980. Annual report, prepared under the direction of Alexander I. Law, Chief, Office of Program Evaluation and Research, 1980.
6. Hayashi Y: On the sleeping hours of school children of 6 to 20 years. Psychol Abstr 1927;1:439.
7. Bax MCO: Sleep disturbance in the young child. Br Med J 1980;280:1177-1179.
8. Weissbluth M et al: Sleep duration and television viewing. J Pediatr 1981,99:486 488.
9. Jenkins S, Bax MCO, and Hart H: Behaviour problems in preschool children. J Child Psychol Psychiatry 1980;21:5-17.
10. Richman N, Stevenson JE, and Graham PJ: Prevalence of behaviour problems in 3-year-old children: an epidemiological study in a London borough. J Child Psychol Psychiatry 1975;16:277-287.
11. Anders TF: Night-waking in infants during the first year of life. Pediatrics 1979;63:860-864.
12. Metcalf D: The ontogenesis of sleep-awake states from birth to 3 months. Electroencephalogr Clin Neurophysiol 1970;28:421.
13. Moore T and Ucko C: Night waking in early infancy: Part I. Arch Dis Child 1957;32:333.
14. Zuckerman B, Stevenson J, and Bailey V: Sleep problems in early childhood: continuities, predictive factors, and behavioral correlates. Pediatrics 1987;80:664-671.
15. Kataria S, Swanson MS, and Trevathan GE: Persistence of sleep disturbances in preschool children. J Pediatr 1987;110:642-646.
16. Jones DPH and Verduyn CM: Behavioural management of sleep problems. Arch Dis Child 1983;58:442-444.
17. Wilks JM: The sleepless child [letter]. Br Med J 1977;2:704-705.
18. Weissbluth M: Sleep duration and infant temperament. J Pediatr 1981;99:817-819.
19. Thomas A, Chess S, and Birch HG: Temperament and behavior disorders in children. New York, New York University Press, 1968.
20. Oberklaid F et al: Assessment of temperament in the toddler age group. Pediatrics 1990;85:559-566.
21. Lounsbury ML and Bates JE: The cries of infants of differing levels of perceived temperamental difficulties: acoustic properties and effects on listeners. Child Dev 1982;53:677-686.
22. Snow ME, Jacklin CN, and Maccoby EE: Crying episodes and sleep-wakefulness transitions in the first 26 months of life. Infant Behav Dev 1980;3:387-394.
23. Lozoff B, Wolf AW, and Davis NS: Cosleeping in urban families with young children in the United States. Pediatrics 1984;74:171-182.
24. Monroe LJ: Transient changes in EEG sleep patterns of married good sleepers: the effects of altering sleeping arrangement. Psychophysiology 1969;6:330-337.
25. Caudill W and Ploth D: Who sleeps by who. Psychiatry 1964;32:12-43.
26. Ferber R: Solve your child's sleep problems. New York, Simon & Schuster, 1985.
27. Ferber R and Boyle MP: Nocturnal fluid intake: a cause of, not treatment for, sleep disruption in infants and toddlers. Sleep Res 1983;12:243.
28. Weissbluth M: Sleep and the colicky infant. In Guilleminault C (ed): Sleep and its disorders in children. New York, Raven Press, 1987, pp 129-141.
29. Illingworth RS: "Three months" colic. Arch Dis Child 1954;29:167-174.
30. Wessel MA et al: Paroxysmal fussing in infancy, sometimes called "colic." Pediatrics 1954;14:421-434.
31. Pierce P: Delayed onset of "three months" colic in premature infants. Am J Dis Child 1948;75:190-192.
32. Breslow L: A clinical approach to infantile colic: a review of 90 cases. J Pediatr 1957;50:196-206.
33. Meyer JE and Thaler MM: Colic in low birth weight infants. Am J Dis Child 1971;122:25-27.
34. Jorup S: Colonic hyperperistalsis in neurolabile infants: studies in so-called dyspepsia in breast fed infants. Acta Paediatr 1952;85:1-92.
35. Weissbluth M, Christoffel KK, and Davis AT: Treatment of infantile colic with dicyclomine hydrochloride. J Pediatr 1984;104:951-955.
36. Weissbluth M and Liu K: Sleep patterns, attention spans, and infant temperament. J Dev Behav Pediatr 1983;4:34-36.
37. Weissbluth M, Davis AT, and Poncher J: Night waking in 4- to 8-month-old infants. J Pediatr 1984;104:477-480.
38. Kahn A et al: Insomnia and cow's milk allergy in infants. Pediatrics 1985;76:880-884.
39. Ferber R: The sleepless child. In Guilleminault C (ed): Sleep and its disorders in children. New York, Raven Press, 1987, pp 141-163.
40. Kaplan BJ et al: Sleep disturbances in pre-school-aged hyperactive and non-hyperactive children. Pediatrics 1987;80:839-844.
41. Salzarulo P and Chevalier A: Sleep problems in children and their relationship with early disturbances of the waking-sleeping rhythms. Sleep 1983;6:47-51.
42. Diagnostic and statistical manual of mental disorders, ed 3. Washington, DC, American Psychiatric Association, 1980.
43. Greenhill L et al: Sleep architecture and REM sleep measures in pre-pubertal children with attention deficit disorder with hyperactivity. Sleep 1983;6:91-101.
44. Busby K, Firestone P, and Pivik RT: Sleep patterns

in hyperkinetic and normal children. Sleep 1981;4:366-383.
45. Peters JE, Romaine JS, and Dyckman RA: A special neurological examination of children with learning disabilities. Dev Med Child Neurol 1975;17:63-78.
46. Touwen BCL and Prechtl HFR: Neurological examination of the child with minor nervous dysfunction. London, Spastics International Medical Publications, 1970.
47. Kane J et al: EEG sleep in a child with severe depression. Am J Psychiatry 1977;134:813-814.
48. Cytryn L and McKnew D: Proposed classification of childhood depression. Am J Psychiatry 1972;129:149-155.
49. Poznanski E and Frull JP: Childhood depression: clinical characteristics of overtly depressed children. Arch Gen Psychiatry 1970;23:8-15.
50. Sander LW et al: Early mother infant interaction and 24-hour patterns of activity and sleep. J Am Acad Child Psychiatry 1970;9:103-123.
51. Brown GW and Harris T: Social origins of depression. London, Tavistock, 1978.
52. Loxoff B, Wolf AW, and Davis NS: Sleep problems seen in pediatric practice. Pediatrics 1985;75:477-483.
53. Association of Sleep Disorders Centers: Diagnostic classification of sleep and arousal disorders. Prepared by the Sleep Disorders Classification Committee, H.P. Roffwarg, Chairman, Sleep 1979;2:1-137.

8

Disorders of Excessive Somnolence

In contrast to the sleepless child, the abnormally sleepy child often goes undetected for a long time. One major factor in delays in seeking medical attention is uncertainty about what constitutes normal total sleep times.[1] Although normative data are available for age-related weight, height, head circumference, and laboratory values, observations of normal amounts of sleep and wakefulness and sleep stages in children are still sparse and fragmented. Little information is available regarding what constitutes normal daytime alertness (and sleepiness) during early childhood. Sleep-wake schedules are usually well established by 6 months of age. Daytime napping is common until 3 to 4 years of age. However, the acceptable interval of napping depends largely on social and cultural factors. What is normal for one child may be considered abnormal for another.

The sleepy child has been ignored for too long by both parents and health care professionals. Sleepy children generally do not bother parents. Identification is difficult because behaviors associated with sleepiness may be attributed to a variety of other factors. Underlying disorders inducing sleepiness and its resultant behaviors therefore go undetected. Excessively sleepy children are most often recognized only after they begin school, have trouble participating in regular classroom activities, and manifest impaired learning.[2] Indeed, symptoms are often first recognized by teachers or other school personnel, who pressure parents into obtaining an evaluation because of repeated naps during class hours. Delays in seeking medical attention after recognition of the problem have been reported to range from 7 months to 7 years, with an average of 28 months.[1]

Daytime sleepiness and hypersomnia may be caused by a variety of disorders, some of which are narcolepsy, obstructive sleep apnea, idiopathic central nervous system (CNS) hypersomnia, neurological disorders, seizure disorders, and environmental, toxic, and medical problems (Fig. 8–1). No comprehensive study of the incidence and prevalence of these disorders in children has been published. As Guilleminault has stated, "Daytime sleepiness may be just one of many problems these children have, and the sleep disorder may go untreated, which can have important consequences."[2]

Sleepiness in both children and adults can be mild, with subtle signs and symptoms, or can be severe and brutal. Symptoms may range from brief lapses in concentration, decreased motivation, easy distractibility, frustration, and aggressiveness to more overt signs of somnolence such as slow speech, bland facial expression, droopy eyelids, and increased effort in movements.

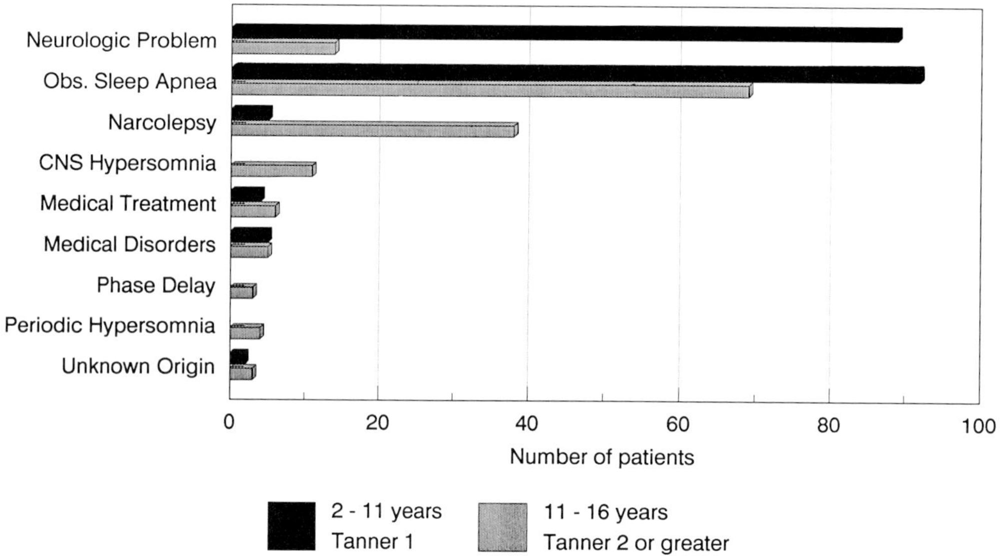

FIGURE 8–1. Distribution of diagnoses when excessive daytime sleepiness is the presenting complaint. (Modified from Guilleminault C: Disorders of excessive daytime sleepiness. In Guilleminault C [ed]: Sleep and its disorders in children. New York, Raven Press, 1987, pp 178-179, with permission.)

Despite objective signs of sleepiness, the way a child feels or appears may be misleading. The degree of sleepiness is related to a number of factors, including circadian influences; time since the last sleep period; previous quantity, quality, and continuity of sleep; and level of CNS stimulation at a given time. *Physiological sleep tendency* refers to the degree to which an individual's CNS is compatible with sleep.[3] The degree of CNS stimulation interacts with this physiological state to determine the degree of subjective sleepiness. *Manifest sleep tendency* is the degree to which sleepiness is experienced or is evident in behavior. Different individuals with the same physiological sleep tendency may manifest different levels of sleepiness and have different symptoms.

A report of sleepiness is not necessarily the same as high physiological sleep tendency. Frequently lethargy, malaise, muscular exhaustion, or fatigue is described as sleepiness. Clearly, being tired and being sleepy are not the same. Given soporific conditions, sleepy patients manifest their sleepiness; patients who are tired but have a low physiological sleep tendency do not. In general, daytime sleepiness should be considered excessive if subjective symptoms or signs *interfere with normal waking function, social responsibilities, or quality of life.*

Terms used to describe sleepiness are difficult to define and are often misleading. *Narcolepsy* is a "disorder associated with excessive daytime sleep, sleep attacks and cataplexy, hypnogogic hallucinations, and/or sleep paralysis."[4] Although sleep is disrupted in the narcolepsy syndrome, total sleep time at night is not usually prolonged. The term narcolepsy has been used to describe short sleep attacks during the day, as well as the syndrome itself. *Hypersomnia* differs from narcolepsy and is more difficult to define. Sleep periods occur during daytime hours, and nocturnal sleep is often prolonged. Hypersomnia generally refers to a disorder associated with significantly prolonged total sleep time over a 24-hour period, and not necessarily sleep attacks at inappropriate times. *Subwakefulness* syndromes also occur. This term refers to a reduction in normal levels of alertness during periods of wake, and not short or long daytime sleep periods. Narcolepsy and hypersomnia are sometimes, but not always, accompanied by subwakefulness.[4] In all instances, differentiating daytime sleepiness from less specific symptoms of tiredness and excessive fatigue is important.

Drowsiness in adults has simple electroencephalographic (EEG) correlates consisting of a decrease, intermittency, and dropout of alpha activity followed by a relatively low-voltage, mixed-frequency pattern and later by vertex waves (analogous to the EEG pattern seen in Stage 1 sleep).[5] Whether these simple EEG correlates of drowsiness are applicable to children, however, is controversial.[6]

Symptoms of sleepiness and drowsiness in children are often confusing. They may overlap and be mistaken for signs and symptoms of other conditions that do not, on the surface, appear to be linked with sleepiness. For example, Weinberg and Brumback[7] have described a *primary disorder of vigilance* in which vigilance is considered to be the state of being watchful, awake, and alert. When vigilance is lost, difficulty sustaining attention occurs. Manifestations of motor restlessness (fidgeting and moving about), yawning and stretching, talkativeness, or a combination of symptoms follows. Motor restlessness has been ascribed to attempts to improve alertness when sitting or standing still or when involved in tasks requiring continuous mental performance. When prevented from being active, the person stares off, daydreams, exhibits minor hyperactivity, loses attention to current activities, avoids or loses interest in structured repetitive activities, and possibly falls asleep. These symptoms are remarkably similar to those of other described syndromes, such as attention deficit–hyperactivity disorder (ADHD). Easy distractibility, difficulty concentrating on schoolwork or other tasks requiring sustained attention, shifting frequently from one activity to another, fidgeting, moving about excessively during sleep, and being always "on the go" are characteristics of ADHD.[8] No clear data have delineated the relationship of objective sleepiness with this symptom complex. Children with obstructive sleep apnea syndrome also suffer from learning problems, morning headaches, nocturnal enuresis, hyperactivity, aggressiveness, attention span problems, and excessive daytime sleepiness.[9,10] Further investigation into the cause of hyperactivity, attention span problems, and learning disabilities will require close attention to the possibility of primary sleep-wake disorders as a significant contributor.

Kahn and co-workers[11] have shown that school achievement difficulties are encountered significantly more often among preadolescent children who are considered poor sleepers than among children without sleep problems. Their preliminary study suggested that pediatric practitioners should *look more closely for the presence of chronic sleep problems in apparently normal preadolescents*.

INCIDENCE AND PREVALENCE

Few studies have adequately assessed the incidence of excessive daytime sleepiness, and still fewer have addressed this symptom during childhood. The exact incidence and prevalence remain unknown. Indeed, obtaining adequate data is difficult for several reasons. First, most epidemiological data regarding sleep-wake problems in childhood have relied on subjective parental reports. Because of the problem of identifying exact symptoms in children, significant underreporting occurs. Second, daytime sleepiness and hypersomnia are not synonymous. Daytime sleepiness may in fact be due to problems of circadian rhythms (e.g., sleep phase delay syndrome) or other abnormalities that result in insufficient sleep at night and sleepiness during the day.

Surveys of adult populations that have focused on hypersomnia or excessive sleep suggest an incidence of 4.2% to 4.4%.[12,13] Lavie, in a study of excessive daytime sleepiness (EDS) in industrial workers in Israel, found that 4.9% of the study population complained of this problem and 7.8% reported falling asleep regularly during at least two of six passive activities.[14] Polysomnographic studies on a subsample of this population suggested that the majority of individuals complaining of EDS had sleep-related breathing disorders. Another survey of more than 2,500 unselected hospitalized patients found that 3.4% of the sample reported EDS when it was defined as more than 8 hours of sleep in each 24-hour period, or more than one nap per day.[15] All patients reporting EDS in the study underwent polysomnographic investigation. Approximately one third had physiological evidence of EDS, the majority because of sleep-related breathing disorders. Data from other questionnaire surveys or those reported from sleep laboratories show the prevalence of EDS to range from 0.3% to 4%.[16-18]

The preceding data indicate that EDS is less common than insomnia. However, looking at subjects with sleep-wake disorders, Coleman found that hypersomnia was a more common complaint than insomnia in a sample population of 8,000 patients.[19] Nonetheless, a conservative estimate would be that 1% to 4% of the adult population has EDS serious enough to affect their health or quality of life. Similar estimates for children are not available.

EVALUATION OF EXCESSIVE DAYTIME SOMNOLENCE

Of prime importance in evaluating EDS is a determination of whether the child's symptoms might be related to excessive sleepiness. This is often more demanding than it sounds. Extreme degrees of sleepiness are obvious, but milder degrees are harder to detect on clinical evaluation.

Discriminating normal from abnormal total sleep requirements is sometimes difficult. If the usual total sleep time in a 24-hour period is 2 hours greater than the average for the child's age, this is cause for concern. However, this does not always mean the child is pathologically sleepy. A child who sleeps up to 2 hours longer than the average total 24-hour sleep time, but is active and alert during the day, most likely is normal but has a long sleep requirement.[20] Daytime napping decreases significantly after the age of 3 years. By 5 years of age the need for daytime naps is uncommon. Therefore, habitual napping by children during middle childhood is another clue that EDS may be present.

Unlike disorders of initiating and maintaining sleep, EDS is less commonly related to behavioral and psychosocial factors than to biological factors. Evaluation of a child with excessive sleepiness should begin with a comprehensive history and physical examination (Fig. 8–2). Historical information regarding the child's normal sleep-wake pattern should include the following:

1. The child's normal, habitual bedtime and wake time.
2. The time it takes the child to fall asleep. A truly sleepy child falls asleep quickly. Prolonged sleep onset latency at night suggests that the daytime problem is not due to hypersomnolence but may be caused by a circadian rhythm problem or insufficient sleep.
3. Total sleep time. It should be compared with the mean sleep time for the child's age. Nocturnal sleep patterns should be well documented; a sleep diary maintained for 2 weeks provides more objective information re-

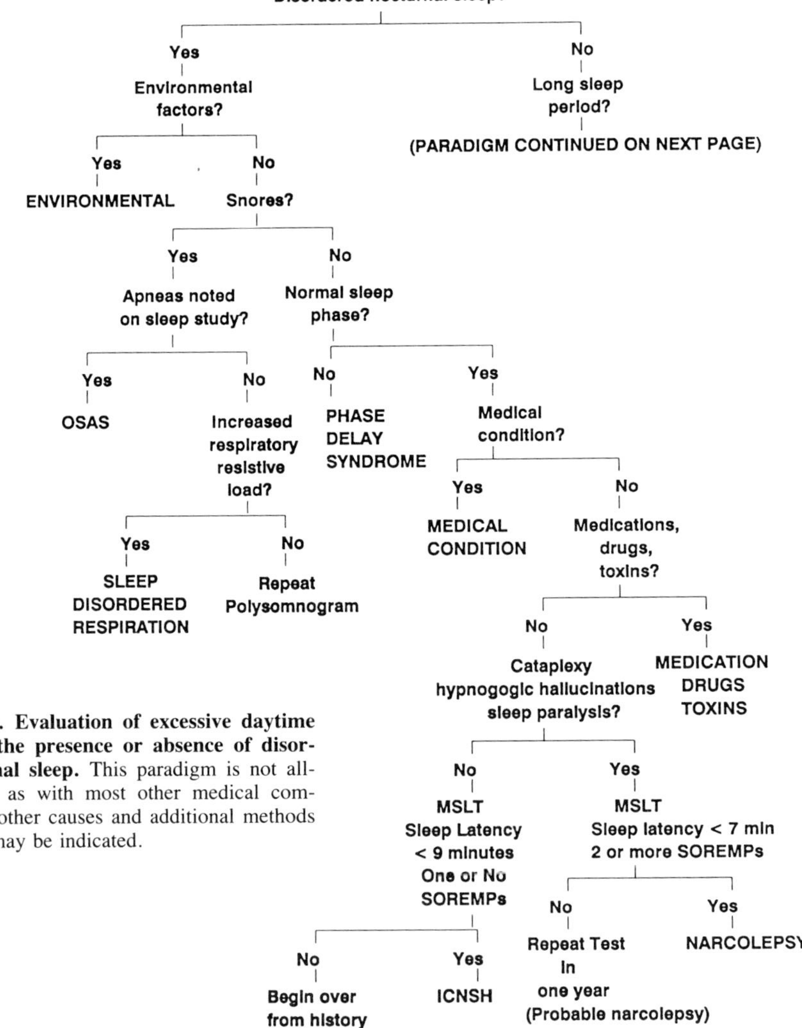

FIGURE 8–2. Evaluation of excessive daytime sleepiness in the presence or absence of disordered nocturnal sleep. This paradigm is not all-inclusive, and as with most other medical complaints, many other causes and additional methods of evaluation may be indicated.

garding the child's sleep-wake pattern (Fig. 8–3).

4. Presence of sleep disruptions, interruptions, snoring, or unusual behaviors during sleep. These may indicate a lack of continuity or deprivation of various sleep stages.

5. Daytime behavior and degree of alertness. Symptoms of EDS include overactivity, attention span problems, aggressiveness with other children, daydreaming, learning problems, sleep attacks, or frequent napping. The focus should be on the length, frequency, and time of day of naps and the activities interrupted by naps. The child's behavior and subjective feeling on waking from naps should also be recorded.

Polysomnographic studies are often necessary to assess a patient with possible EDS. Polysomnography can provide information regarding progression and volume of sleep stages, disruptions of architecture by frequent arousals, presence of sleep-disordered respiration, and EEG abnormalities that may suggest seizures or other intracranial disorders. Since it is often difficult to determine whether a child is sleepy just by the way the child looks or acts, the Multiple Sleep Latency Test (MSLT) may be required to objectively assess the degree of sleepiness and to evaluate the patient for sleep-onset rapid eye movement periods (SOREMPs).

Multiple Sleep Latency Test[21-23]

The MSLT was developed at Stanford University to provide objective information about the degree of daytime sleepiness and the presence of abnormal SOREMPs. SOREMPs are REM sleep episodes that occur less than 15 minutes after sleep onset. The MSLT is interpreted as an operationally defined measure of sleepiness or alertness. The more prolonged the latency to sleep onset, the more alert the individual; conversely, the shorter the delay to sleep onset, the sleepier the individual.[24]

MSLT scores vary and may be related to the amount of sleep obtained on one or several nights preceding the testing, degree of maturation of the subject, age of the subject, continuity of the previous sleep periods, time of day, and presence of drugs or medications. An average sleep onset latency time of less than 5 minutes is associated with decrements in performance and unintentional sleep episodes. One night of polysomnography conducted the night before the MSLT is required. A prior polysomnogram provides information about any disorders that may disrupt sleep continuity or alter the test results. A sleep diary kept for 1 to 2 weeks before the MSLT is also helpful, since MSLT results may be influenced by sleep habits up to 7 nights before testing. Careful consideration of drug ingestion and medication sched-

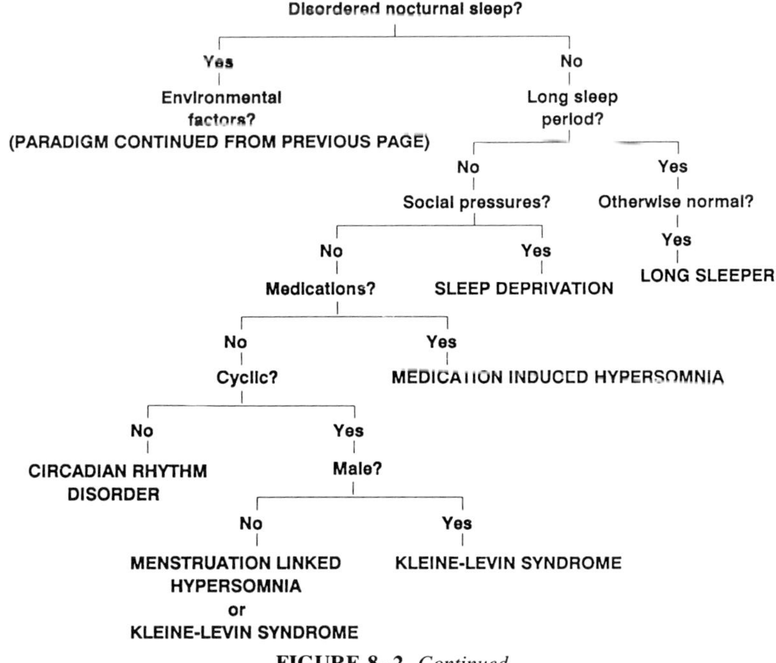

FIGURE 8–2. *Continued*

CENTER FOR CHILDHOOD SLEEP DISORDERS STUDIES

Day	6	7	8	9	10	11	Midnight	1	2	3	4	5	6	7	8	9	10	11	Noon	1	2	3	4	5	Comments

Child's Name: __________

Parent's Name __________

Child's Age: _____ Birth Date: ________

Phone: ( ) ________

Directions:

1. Draw an arrow down (↓) when your child gets into bed.
2. Shade in the boxes ▒ when your child is sleeping.
3. Leave the boxes blank when your child is awake, even if in bed.
4. Draw an arrow up (↑) when you child gets out of bed.
5. NOTE: Each line of boxes represents parts of TWO days!

Example:

Day	6	7	8	9	10	11	Midnight	1	2	3	4	5	6	7	8	9	10	11	Noon	1	2	3	4	5	Comments

FIGURE 8–3. Sleep log. (Modified from Ferber R: Solve your child's sleep problems. New York, Simon & Schuster, 1985, p 105, with permission.)

uling is important in interpreting the results. A urine drug screen before testing may be helpful, especially if the veracity of the history is questionable.

Five test nap periods are attempted at 2-hour intervals, beginning 1½ to 3 hours after the morning wake time. For validity of testing it is important to prevent the patient from sleeping between test naps. Sleep may accumulate and artifactually prolong sleep onset latencies. When testing begins, the patient, wearing street clothes, is placed in a quiet, temperature-controlled room. The lights are turned out, and the patient is instructed to lie quietly (to reduce tossing and turning), to close his or her eyes (to keep the patient from looking about the room), and to try to sleep (or not to resist falling asleep). The same instructions are given immediately before each nap. Nap periods are ended after 20 minutes (if sleep does not occur), after three consecutive 30-second epochs of Stage 1 sleep, or after one 30-second epoch of another sleep stage. If the presence of SOREMPs is an issue, the nap is ended 15 minutes after the first epoch of sleep.

The sleep onset latency is defined as the time from lights out to when sleep occupies greater than 50% of any 30-second epoch. REM latency is measured from the onset of sleep to the onset of the first epoch of REM sleep. For each nap the sleep onset latency and REM latency (if any REM is present) are measured. Averages are calculated for all naps across the day's testing. The preceding night's polysomnographic summary is included in the report.

If the mean sleep onset latency is less than 5 minutes, pathological sleepiness is present. An average sleep onset latency of this magnitude is typically associated with impaired performance and uncontrollable sleep attacks. In adults a mean sleep onset latency of 10 to 20 minutes is considered normal. Latencies between 5 and 10 minutes are diagnostic gray areas. Short sleep onset latencies are extremely rare in children, and these criteria may not hold true during middle childhood. Normal children in this age group rarely fall asleep during testing, and those who do achieve sleep have latencies greater than 15 minutes. Indeed, patients during middle childhood are normally very alert—probably the most alert of any age group.

Presence of two SOREMPs in a five-nap study is characteristic of narcolepsy. SOREMPs are rare in normal individuals. They are occasionally recorded in patients with sleep apnea syndrome or significant sleep deprivation. For these patients SOREMPs reflect a chronic pattern of disturbed or fragmented sleep. However, two or more SOREMPs may indicate the coexistence of narcolepsy and sleep apnea syndrome.

Patterns of daytime alertness and the degree of daytime sleepiness appear to depend on age. A high level of alertness seen in middle childhood gives way to augmentation of daytime sleepiness during pubertal development, even in the presence of a constant total sleep time.[24] At the Stanford Sleep Camp, Carskadon and coworkers have scrupulously described changes that occur during puberty.[25] Their data suggest that older adolescents do not have less need for sleep than younger adolescents. Children across all Tanner stages averaged slightly more than 9 hours of sleep when given the opportunity to remain in bed for 10 hours. The volume of REM sleep remained constant across all maturational levels. Slow-wave sleep decreased significantly in a linear fashion across maturational groups, with an almost 35% decline from Tanner Stage 1 to Tanner Stage 5. In a parallel manner, daytime alertness, as measured by the MSLT, declined at midpuberty (Tanner Stage 3) and remained at the reduced level, *even though total sleep time remained constant*. Carskadon and associates concluded that the need for sleep does not decline during adolescence but may in fact increase.

As described in Chapter 2, adolescents tend to spend less time in bed as they grow older. Carskadon and Dement have dramatically shown that older adolescents (college students) were very sleepy all day long. In comparison, younger adolescents were very alert during the day.[24] Sleep loss from restricted time in bed had significant consequences the next day. MSLT scores reached their minimal values immediately after the night of sleep loss and remained low until recovery sleep was permitted. Unlike adults, adolescents did not recover to baseline MSLT scores until after a second recovery night of sleep. Further assessment of the consequences of the night of restricted sleep revealed significant performance deficits on a number of tasks after sleep restriction, and performance decrements were clearly related to the occurrence of sleep episodes during the tasks.

Not all adolescents are significantly sensitive to sleep restriction, although all are affected to some degree. Most respond moderately and can perform simple, brief tasks adequately after restricted sleep. Some adolescents, however, are affected to a point at which pathological sleepiness occurs and recovery is not fully established after a full night's sleep. Since recovery is delayed, the degree of alertness or sleepiness and performance does not depend entirely on the immediately preceding night's sleep. As Carskadon and Dement point out[24]:

> ***A percentage of normal adolescents have a significant disturbance of waking function as a result of the pubertal increase in daytime sleepiness, the restriction of nocturnal sleep to meet societal expectations or obligations, and the additive impact of chronic sleep restriction. The susceptibility to each of these factors is variable. Additionally suggested, the percentage of impaired adolescents rises as the structure enforcing bedtimes is reduced, e.g., when an adolescent goes away to school or when parents exert less control over sleeping hours at home.***

Their experimental studies in the sleep laboratory have shown a clear relationship between excessive sleepiness and performance on tasks involving attention, memory, and motor and cognitive skills. The impairment of performance usually does not become significant until episodes of sleep intrude during the tasks, especially when the tasks are long, dull, and repetitive.

Several normative studies of sleep in preadolescent children have been published,[26-29] and Carskadon and Dement have performed studies on patients during middle childhood similar to those performed on adolescent patients.[22] The most notable feature of the MSLT data was that subjects in middle childhood rarely fell asleep. *Sleep was seen within the 20-minute test period on fewer than one fourth of the tests*. In those tests in which sleep was noted, the children never fell asleep in less than 15 minutes. These data appear to document the extreme level of alertness of children during this developmental period. Children during middle childhood who exhibit significant sleep tendency on the MSLT most likely are excessively sleepy during the daytime, regardless of daytime symptoms.

CLINICAL DISORDERS OF EXCESSIVE SOMNOLENCE

Narcolepsy

Narcolepsy is a serious, lifelong, disabling disorder characterized by a tetrad of symptoms including EDS, cataplexy, hypnogogic hallucinations, and sleep paralysis.[30] Most commonly a single symptom or a combination of symptoms appears in the second decade of life, during puberty or postpubertal adolescence.[31] Narcolepsy is rarely diagnosed in prepubertal children, although symptoms can be recognized in some children during middle childhood.

The exact prevalence of narcolepsy in the general population is unknown but is estimated to range from 0.04% to 0.09%.[32] Investigations in California have found the prevalence to be 0.067% in Los Angeles and 0.05% in San Francisco.[33] According to the American Narcolepsy Association (ANA), narcolepsy frequently goes undiagnosed; therefore these data may be significantly underestimated.[34] Significant delays often occur between the onset of symptoms and the time of diagnosis. The ANA reports that the average delay is approximately 15 years!

Clinical Presentation. Symptoms most commonly begin during puberty and postpubertal development.[31] The most common symptom is EDS. If, however, cataplexy (a more striking symptom) is present, parents seek medical attention more quickly. The classic tetrad of EDS, cataplexy, hypnogogic hallucinations, and sleep paralysis may be absent, although varying manifestations occur. Patients may have a single symptom or a combination, with any degree of intensity and severity. Auxiliary symptoms of automatic behaviors and disrupted nocturnal sleep often occur.

Daytime sleepiness and sleep attacks are the most characteristic symptoms of narcolepsy. Affected patients may not feel their sleepiness, and therefore uncontrollable sleep episodes occur during periods of sedentary, monotonous, or sporific activity. Sleep attacks occur without warning. Occasionally sleepiness can be detected and resisted, but the onset of sleep cannot be delayed indefinitely.

Narcoleptic naps are typically *short and refreshing* and are followed by 1 to several hours of refractory alertness. Naps that last longer than 60 minutes may include slow-wave sleep and may result in confusion and disorientation on awakening (sleep drunkenness). Adolescent patients may complain of difficulty in waking after a night's sleep. Disorientation, abusive behavior, aggressiveness, and confusion may occur.

Cataplexy is a sudden, reversible decrease in voluntary muscle tone. Extraocular muscles and the diaphragm are usually spared. This decrease in muscle tone may be generalized or localized. A cataplectic attack is usually precipitated by emotions (e.g., laughter, fear, anger). Cataplexy may be complete or partial. When it is complete, patients may fall to the ground or slump. If it is partial, they may experience brief periods of head rocking or tilting. Chronic cephalalgia and neck pain may occur. During these brief attacks patients may complain of a sudden *draining* feeling. Consciousness is maintained during an attack.

Sleep paralysis usually occurs as the patient is falling alseep or on waking. Patients report a subjective feeling of inability to move, open their eyes, or talk. Breathing may feel shallow and difficult. These episodes are often frightening. Patients report that they can hear people taking to them during the episode but they cannot move or respond. Sleep paralysis may be aborted in some patients by rapidly moving the eyes back and forth or by being touched or shaken by another person.

Hypnogogic hallucinations are auditory or visual hallucinations that occur at the onset or ending of the sleep period and may occur during daytime sleep as well. Hallucinations are often frightening and involve the sleep environment. Hearing noises that resemble footsteps or breaking glass is common. Less often the hallucinations involve some environment other than the bedroom.

Disturbed nocturnal sleep is frequently reported by narcoleptic patients. Night sleep is often unstable and is interrupted by repeated awakenings and frightening dreams.[35]

Constant drowsiness may occur. Repetitive microsleeps have been demonstrated during periods of extreme drowsiness. A microsleep usually lasts 1 to 10 seconds, and continuous monitoring of the EEG reveals a replacement of low-voltage alpha activity (characteristic of relaxed wakefulness) with relatively low-voltage, mixed-frequency activity (characteristic of Stage 1 sleep). As sleep is resisted, microsleep periods increase in frequency, occurring in clusters that may result in automatic behavior and memory lapses.[36] Automatisms usually involve activities that do not require extensive skill. Lapses are more frequent during late afternoon and evening hours and rarely occur in the morning.[31] Microsleeps and automatisms can result in poor school performance and may be mistaken for learning disabilities or behavior disorders.

Diagnosis. The diagnosis of narcolepsy is based on a high index of suspicion, comprehensive historical information, and a complete physical examination. A history of EDS and cataplexy is nearly pathognomonic of narcolepsy. Since sleepiness, rather than cataplexy, is usually the initial symptom, the clinical diagnosis may be difficult. Diagnosis may be confirmed, however, with nocturnal polysomnography, MSLT, and ruling out other causes for excessive somnolence. The presence of pathological sleepiness and two or more SOREMPs on a five-nap MSLT is characteristic of narcolepsy, although not specifically diagnostic.

The differential diagnosis can be extensive. Conditions that should be considered include obstructive sleep apnea syndrome, sleep deprivation, dyssomnias, drugs and medications, CNS insult or trauma, seizure disorders, psychological and psychiatric conditions, myotonic dystrophy, idiopathic CNS hypersomnia, tumors, metabolic disorders, Kleine-Levin syndrome, and menstruation-linked hypersomnia.[4] Many of these disorders may be differentiated on historical and clinical grounds alone. Others require additional laboratory evaluations such as EEG, radiography, and electromyography.

Clearly narcolepsy should be considered in the evaluation of children and adolescents with EDS, disrupted nocturnal sleep, unusual behavior in the morning, or poor school performance. Symptoms of narcolepsy may be similar to those of substance abuse and should be considered in the evaluation of an adolescent who is suspected of using drugs, yet denies drug misuse.

A strong association between narcolepsy and the histocompatibility antigen complex HLA-DR2 has been described. Honda and co-workers discovered that almost all narcoleptic patients in Japan were HLA-DR2 positive.[37,38] This finding has been confirmed by studies in England, France, and Canada.[39,40] Studies in the United States have shown a slightly smaller correlation.[41] Nonetheless, the link between this histocompatibility complex and narcolepsy is strong and provides the basis for future research into the etiology and transmission of this disorder.

Treatment. Treatment initially focuses on behavioral management and life-style modification. Major goals of treatment are the control of excessive sleepiness and the elimination of cataplexy. Close attention to sleep hygiene and regularly scheduled naps may significantly improve EDS in some patients. If the initial approach is insufficient to control the symptoms, EDS and sleep attacks should be treated with analeptic medications, such as methylphenidate, pemoline sodium, or amphetamines. Cataplexy sometimes decreases in frequency (although is usually not eliminated) when sleepiness is controlled. Tricyclic medication, such as protriptyline, amitriptyline, or imipramine, is usually effective.[42] Abrupt discontinuation of CNS stimulants may result in extreme sleepiness and significant depression. Rapid withdrawal from tricyclic compounds may dramatically increase cataplectic symptoms, and therefore withdrawal should be gradual.

Sleep Apnea–Hypersomnia Syndrome

In its complete presentation, sleep apnea–hypersomnia syndrome includes symptoms of loud snoring during sleep, enuresis, morning headaches, EDS, decrease in school performance, behavioral changes during daytime hours, gain or loss of weight, and if protracted, cardiovascular abnormalities. Adenoidal hypertrophy and chronic nasopharyngeal obstruction have been reported as possible causes of pulmonary hypertension and cor pulmonale.[43-46] Childhood sleep apnea differs significantly from apnea of infancy and apnea of prematurity.

Clinical Presentation. Childhood sleep apnea syndrome is a fairly common course of EDS in children. After narcolepsy, it was the second most frequent cause of EDS in patients at a large sleep disorders center.[47] It results from respiratory abnormalities that occur only during sleep. Loud snoring interrupted by numerous respiratory pauses is the hallmark of this nocturnal breathing abnormality. Apneic episodes are frequently associated with hypoxemia, hypercapnia, and mild acidosis. Although children with sleep apnea do not reveal the alveolar hypoventilation typically seen in the Pickwickian syndrome, the secondary daytime sleepiness and cardiovascular complications are similar. Pulmonary function test findings are most often normal in patients with sleep apnea.

The cause of EDS in children with sleep apnea is related to significant lack of continuity of nocturnal sleep. Apneic episodes associated with secondary oxygen desaturation profoundly disrupt sleep. Partial awakenings occur at the end of each apnea, and normal sleep architecture is disrupted. Total sleep time may appear abnormally prolonged. Most often, Stage 1 and 2 sleep increases and slow-wave sleep progressively disappears. REM sleep is also affected, and the total REM volume may be markedly reduced. Early in the course of the disorder a compensatory rebound of slow-wave sleep may take place, with a resultant increase in Stage 3 and 4 volume. This may be a protective mechanism against the repetitive disruptions induced by respiratory events or a rebound from prior sleep continuity deprivation. As the disorder progresses, slow-wave sleep and normal sleep architecture are obliterated. Apneas of 10 seconds or longer, occurring at a frequency of at least five per hour (apnea index of 5), are considered abnormal in adults. Children may become affected at indices somewhat less than those of adults, and classic obstructive apneas may not be appreciated polysomnographically. Increased respiratory resistive load without clearly defined apneas may disrupt sleep continuity and architecture sufficiently to cause daytime symptoms.

EDS in the sleep apnea syndrome is similar to that in narcolepsy. Microsleep episodes intrude during the waking state, become frequent, and have a similar impact on behavior and learning.[47]

When obstructive sleep apnea is suspected clinically, polysomnography and comprehensive evaluation of the upper airway are recommended. Sleep apnea has been associated with micrognathia, Pierre-Robin syndrome, Arnold-Chiari syndrome, bilateral high cervical cordotomy, Pickwickian syndrome, and chronic upper airway obstruction resulting from hypertrophied tonsils and adenoids (the most common underlying cause of obstructive sleep apnea during childhood).[43,44] Therefore patients with documented obstructive sleep apnea should be evaluated for possible neurological abnormalities and malformations of the neck and mandible. Allergic reactions that result in partial obstruction of the pharyngolaryngeal junction should also be considered.

Treatment. Once the obstruction is identified, management must focus on appropriate treatment of any abnormality of the pharynx, neck, or mandible. Treatment of a local obstruction (e.g., tonsillectomy and adenoidectomy) may be all that is necessary. In adults palliative treatment with nasal continuous positive airway pressure (CPAP) and weight loss are usually recommended. Nasal CPAP has also been successfully used in children and may be used as a temporizing measure while the cause of the airway obstruction is being sought. The minimum pressure required to eliminate the apnea and regularize sleep architecture is prescribed. Pressure is titrated under controlled conditions in the sleep laboratory while the patient is monitored polysomnographically during the normal sleep period.

Although extremes are self-evident, how much persistent respiratory irregularity can be considered normal during sleep in childhood is unknown. Whether children with sleep apnea will develop sleep apnea–hypersomnia syndrome as adults is also unknown.

Idiopathic Central Nervous System Hypersomnia

Some patients with severe daytime sleepiness have none of the auxiliary symptoms characteristic of narcolepsy (cataplexy, sleep paralysis, hypnogogic hallucinations).[48] Idiopathic central nervous system hypersomnia (ICNSH) is a disorder characterized by EDS and occurs in adolescents and young adults. It has been referred to in the literature under various names: *essential narcolepsy, independent narcolepsy, NREM sleep narcolepsy, functional hypersomnia,* and *harmonious hypersomnia.*

ICNSH is often difficult to differentiate from narcolepsy syndrome when associated symptoms are absent, since ICNSH is also characterized by a persistent pathological sleep tendency.[49] The two syndromes have many similarities, including age of onset, nonremission of symptoms over the life span, and a heredofamilial tendency.[50] The disabling effect of this condition varies among individuals but is frequently as great as or greater than that seen in narcolepsy.

Several factors may be responsible for the isolated daytime somnolence occurring in ICNSH. Three subgroups of patients have been described by Guilleminault and co-workers at Stanford University.[32] Hypersomnia in the first group of patients is clearly related to infection, most commonly with Epstein-Barr virus or *Mycoplasma pneumoniae*. Hypersomnia may also be caused by Guillain-Barré syndrome. Patients usually complain of fatigue, excessive tiredness, and prolonged nocturnal sleep despite resolution of their primary infection. Patients with hypersomnia secondary to communicating hydrocephalus or to closed head trauma must be clearly distinguished from patients with ICNSH. A second subgroup consists of patients with no significant medical history but with a strong family history of hypersomnolence. Onset of symptoms most commonly occurs at the end of puberty, and associated symptoms of migrainous cephalalgia, syncope, mild to moderate orthostatic hypotension, and peripheral vascular complaints are present. The last subgroup consists of teenagers who have isolated daytime sleepiness without any identifiable medical etiology. Diagnosis of ICNSH should probaby be reserved for these patients in whom specific causes for sleepiness cannot be found.

Clinical Presentation. ICNSH should be suspected when the patient has EDS in the absence of cataplexy, sleep paralysis, and hypnogogic hallucinations and in the absence of significant snoring associated with sleep apnea–hypersomnia syndrome. The age at onset of symptoms varies but is frequently between 15 and 30 years.[50] ICNSH develops progressively over several weeks or months, and once established, symptoms persist with little change. Patients usually have long periods of daytime sleepiness that significantly disturbs function and performance. Daytime somnolence leads to naps that are *frequently lengthy and unrefreshing*.[32] Although recurrent daytime sleepiness occurs, sleep attacks as seen in narcolepsy are uncommon.[51] Daytime sleep episodes are less discrete than in narcolepsy, and the need to sleep can be resisted somewhat.[48] When daytime sleep does occur, patients wake feeling lethargic, in contrast to the brief refreshed state that often follows a sleep attack in narcolepsy.

Nighttime sleep in ICNSH seems to be relatively normal,[52] although patients have a longer total sleep time, fewer awakenings, and fewer episodes of wake after sleep onset than do narcoleptics.[53-55] Slow-wave sleep may be reduced, and volume of Stage 2 sleep may be increased.[3]

Patients with ICNSH may sleep for excessive periods at night and may be difficult to awaken in the morning. In addition, sleep drunkenness after nighttime sleep or daytime naps may be reported.[32,56] Aggressiveness may occur on awakening, and patients may be verbally and physically abusive during this state. The unrefreshing quality of napping and the sleep drunkenness associated with awakenings lead patients to fight sleepiness as long as they can.[50]

During periods of resisted drowsiness, short microsleeps occur, resulting in automatic behavior.[57] As the patient continues to resist sleep, microsleeps become more frequent and intrude more repetitively into the waking state. These episodes are characterized by a "blank stare," and patients may subsequently act in an unplanned and often inappropriate way.

Diagnosis. Diagnosis is based on a high index of suspicion and the absence of other causes for excessive daytime somnolence. The patient should be evaluated for the presence of intracranial disease or injury, seizure disorder, past infections, trauma, and medications or drugs.

Nocturnal polysomnography is relatively normal, although total sleep time may be unusually long. Sleep onset latency on the MSLT is abnormally short, with a mean of less than 7 minutes. *SOREMPs are notably absent*.[58,59] Microsleeps may be seen before actual sleep onset, indicating more impairment in waking function than the mean sleep onset latency suggests.[3]

Treatment. Because the etiology is unknown, treatment is difficult and directed at the symptoms. Many different medications have been tested, including CNS stimulants, tricyclic antidepressants, monoamine oxidase inhibitors, clonidine, L-dopa, bromocriptine, amantadine, and 5-hydroxytryptophan.[50] None has successfully controlled the hypersomnia. Only the CNS stimulants have brought partial, although intermittent, resolution. Pemoline is usually inadequate. Methylphenidate has been the most commonly used treatment, though the results have been disappointing. Large doses may be required, but therapeutic protocols should strive to maintain the patient on a schedule that prevents side effects. A daily dose of 60 mg of methylphenidate (or 40 mg of dextroamphetamine) in divided doses should not be exceeded. Tolerance to CNS stimulants is common. Behavioral management and sleep hygiene have been attempted and are recommended, but they seem to have little effect. These interventions only prevent abrupt exacerbation of sleepiness that is temporarily seen with transient sleep deprivation or abrupt time shifts.[50]

Hypersomnolence Associated with Medical or Toxic Conditions

Increased sleep and excessive somnolence are symptoms well known to practitioners who treat children for acute and chronic illnesses. Any illness may cause the child to feel fatigued and, to some extent, hypersomnolent. Excessive sleepiness, however, should not persist for a significant time after the acute illness has resolved. Many medical, toxic, and environmental conditions are associated with disorders of excessive somnolence as a primary cause. In addition, excessive somnolence may be a consequence of nocturnal sleep disruption secondary to the underlying condition.

There is little published data regarding the objective measurements of physiological sleep tendency in various illnesses. Nonetheless, neurological dysfunction, nutritional deficiencies, endocrine and metabolic conditions, hypercapnia, anemia, hepatic inflammation and failure, CNS tumors (especially those that impinge on the third ventricle and those located in the posterior hypothalamus), intracranial hemorrhage, toxic encephalopathies, and increased intracranial pressure may all be associated with hypersomnolence.[60] Hypersomnia may also occur 6 to 18 months after head trauma.[61] Daytime somnolence is a common, and sometimes the only, symptom of progressive hydrocephalus in both children and adults. Medications and intoxications may also be associated with hypersomnolent states and should be considered in any child with unexplained sleepiness.

Clinical Presentation. Presenting signs and symptoms may vary significantly and depend on the underlying cause. A comprehensive history and physical examination may yield significant information pointing to the etiology. True daytime sleepiness must be differentiated from lethargy, fatigue, and malaise, as well as from signs of disordered consciousness such as stupor, coma, and catatonia.[62]

Diagnosis and Treatment. Severe forms of EDS and hypersomnia are usually associated with physiological and medical abnormalities. Many of the possible underlying disorders are treatable. Differentiation must be made between true sleepiness and fatigue. Sleepiness caused by medical, toxic, and environmental factors must also be distinguished from other causes, particularly those that are psychological, from persistent disturbances of the sleep-wake cycle, and from self-induced sleep deprivation.

Great strides in the methods of diagnosis of excessive sleepiness have been made in the past decade. Thorough evaluation in a sleep disorders center often yields dramatic insights into the patient's condition.[63] A comprehensive medical evaluation is necessary and should be based on the presenting signs and symptoms. Urine drug screening and toxicological assessment are essential in the evaluation.

Sleep Deprivation, Insufficient Sleep, and Circadian Rhythm Abnormalities

Sleep deprivation, insufficient sleep, and circadian rhythm abnormalities are considered together, since the primary cause of sleepiness is insufficient sleep, rather than pathological sleep states or other medical conditions. Circadian rhythm disturbances are considered in greater detail in Chapter 9.

The most common cause of EDS is *insufficient sleep*.[64] Life-styles and responsibilities that lead to insufficient time in bed result in somnolence during the day. Insufficient sleep is defined as an earnest complaint of daytime sleepiness and associated waking symptoms presented by an individual who gives evidence of persistently failing to obtain sufficient daily sleep to support wakefulness.[60] The individual is voluntarily, but often unwittingly, chronically sleep deprived. This, along with the normal increase in daytime sleepiness that occurs during puberty, may result in significantly decreased daytime alertness and performance deficits. Although the cause of sleepiness should be self-evident, in many instances the symptoms cause a person to seek professional assistance without realizing that restricted sleep is the underlying cause. Children with daytime sleepiness caused by restricted nocturnal sleep tend to sleep considerably more on weekends than on schooldays.

Diagnosis. A clear and detailed history of past and current sleep patterns in relation to the volume of sleep normally obtained, the amount desired, and the amount possible to achieve may suggest sleep restriction as the primary cause. The disparity between the amount of sleep needed and the amount actually obtained is usually substantial and unappreciated by the patient or parents. A sleep diary maintained for 2 to 3 weeks usually reveals a decrease in total sleep time. A therapeutic trial of longer sleep that alleviates daytime symptoms confirms the diagnosis.

Depending on the chronicity of sleep loss, secondary daytime symptoms may develop. Irritability, difficulty concentrating, reduced vigilance, distractibility, reduced motivation, depression, fatigue, motor restlessness, incoordination, malaise, loss of appetite, gastrointestinal disturbances, and muscle pains may occur.[60]

Patients are most often healthy. Polysomnography may reveal relatively efficient sleep and a prolonged total sleep time. The patient falls asleep and remains asleep normally. Sleep architecture is normal, although a rebound increase in slow-wave sleep and REM sleep volume may be noted (depending on the number of consecutive nights of study). Children may not show a rebound on the first night after deprivation, and several nights may be required to document the increase.

Treatment. Treatment is focused on reestablishing an appropriate sleep-wake schedule. Educating the parents and patient regarding suitable total sleep time and the effects of sleep loss on daytime functioning and performance is essential. Modification of daytime routines and social responsibilities may also be necessary. Allowing more time for homework and shifting play to different times during the day may be helpful. *Parents who perform shift work must pay close attention to the sleep-wake patterns of their children, in addition to their own.* Children who are kept up late in the evening or are awakened by a parent who works unusual hours may experience significant disruption of their sleep continuity and develop symptoms during the daytime.

Congenital Long Sleeper

Long sleepers are individuals who regularly sleep significantly more in each 24-hour period than the conventional volume for their age group.[60] They usually have no complaints about the quality of sleep, excessive daytime sleepiness, or changes in daytime behavior or performance. No true disorder of excessive somnolence exists unless the patient restricts sleep because of societal pressures and responsibilities. Sleep restriction is especially likely during adolescence. Because of pressures and demands, long sleepers may develop daytime symptoms characteristic of insufficient sleep. The patients usually have no problem with time distortion or ability to be accurate about the quality of sleep.

Diagnosis. Essential to the recognition of a long sleeper is documenting a consistent pattern of long sleep. A sleep diary maintained for 2 to 3 weeks should reveal sleep volume at least 2 hours longer than the average total sleep time for the patient's age group, without reversion to shorter sleep duration on schooldays. The sleep period may range from 9 to 14 hours per night. Differentiating simple long sleep from other pathological conditions that may begin during adolescence is often difficult. Accurate diagnosis is made chiefly by excluding specific diagnostic features associated with other causes of excessive sleepiness and is also based on a lack of complaints concerning behavior and performance during the waking state. Polysomnography reveals normal architecture and absolute amounts of slow-wave sleep, but REM sleep and Stage 2 sleep are at slightly higher levels than normal for the patient's age. Pathological conditions resulting in hypersomnolence often have an acute onset and rarely reveal the stable sleep duration of the long sleeper.

Periodic Hypersomnias

Kleine-Levin Syndrome

Kleine-Levin syndrome is an unusual disorder occuring predominantly in males. Symptoms usually begin in middle or late puberty.[66] The main clinical features are episodic hypersomnia and overeating. Overeating appears to be compulsive and not due to pathological hunger. Billiard has estimated a male/female ratio of 4:3 to 4:1.[67] The age at onset in males is classically between 13 and 18 years, but onset as early as 10 years of age has been reported. Symptoms usually appear spontaneously. Beginning and ending of an "attack" are variable and may be rapid or gradual. Periods of hypersomnolence and overeating last from a few days to several weeks with an average of 5 to 7 days and recur monthly to yearly.[4] Intervals between episodes usually vary in a patient, and during these intervals the patient's physical and mental health is completely normal. The syndrome does not appear to be related to seizure activity or other neurological disorders.

During episodes the patient is characteristically tired, sleeps for prolonged periods (up to 20 hours), and appears lethargic, irritable, and apathetic. Other inappropriate and sometimes bizarre behavior occurs, with changes in awareness, speech, mood, cognition, and sexual function.[68] No convincing evidence of metabolic or endocrine abnormalities has been identified. Laboratory findings are usually normal both during and between attacks. The EEG between attacks is usually normal. A variety of inconsistent EEG changes have been reported during sleep attacks.[69,70] These have included early onset REM periods, decrease in slow-wave sleep and REM sleep, frequent interruption of REM sleep by Stage 2 NREM and alpha activity, and severe sleepiness documented by MSLT during an attack. The sleepiness is as severe as that in narcolepsy and obstructive sleep apnea.

Treatment. Many therapeutic regimens have been attempted.[71-73] Amphetamines have been claimed to reduce the frequency and severity of attacks but are not prophylactic. Phenmetrazine and amphetamine both improved the condition of a woman described by Roth[72] but did not shorten the duration of the attack. Psychotherapy, electroconvulsive therapy, and neuroleptics appear to be unsuccessful. Lithium carbonate abolished attacks in one patient described by Ogura and co-workers[73]; when the medication was withdrawn, the attacks recurred.

Menstruation-Linked Periodic Hypersomnia

More common than the Kleine-Levin syndrome, but still rare, is menstruation-linked periodic hypersomnia. This unusual cause of periodic hypersomnia begins within months before or during the first 2 years after menarche.[74] The overeating and bizarre behavior seen in the Kleine-Levin syndrome are absent. Recurrent episodes of extreme sleepiness last for 6 to 10 days and usually end when menses occurs. Symptoms frequently disappear when the patient reaches the third decade of life or subsequent to pregnancy. In the few examples described in the literature, sleep patterns have been relatively or entirely normal, although unusual EEG features have been described in two subjects who had epileptiform discharges during the hypersomnolent periods.[75] More typical is a pattern of prolonged nocturnal sleep with diffuse EEG abnormalities at the time of waking during attacks but normal patterns during the interparoxysmal period.[74]

Treatment. Hypersomnia usually ceases when ovulation is inhibited by birth control pills.[74,76] Symptoms often reappear if the medication is discontinued. Billiard thought that progesterone triggered the hypersomniac episodes, and the beneficial effect of estrogen in the case described by Billiard was attributed to its inhibitory effect on progesterone secretion. If contraceptive medications with low drug content are used initially, stronger dosages may have to be prescribed after several years to maintain complete control.[32]

REFERENCES

1. Guilleminault C and Anders TF: Pathophysiology of sleep disorders. II. Sleep disorders in children. In Schulman I (ed): Advances in pediatrics, vol 22. Chicago, Year Book, 1976, pp 151-174.
2. Guilleminault C: Disorders of excessive daytime sleepiness. In Guilleminault C (ed): Sleep and its disorders in children. New York, Raven Press, 1987, pp 177-179.
3. Anch AM et al: Sleep: a scientific perspective. Englewood Cliffs, NJ, Prentice Hall, 1988, pp 196-218.
4. Parkes JD: Sleep and its disorders. London, WB Saunders, 1985, pp 267-334.
5. Santamaria J and Chiappa KH: The EEG of drowsiness. New York, Demos, 1987.
6. Egg-Olofsson O: The development of the electroencephalogram in normal adolescents from the age of 16 through 21 years. Neuropaediatrie 1976;3:11-45.
7. Weinberg WA and Brumback RA: Primary disorder of vigilance: a novel explanation of inattentiveness, daydreaming, boredom, restlessness, and sleepiness. J Pediatr 1990;116:720-725.
8. American Psychiatric Association: Diagnostic and statistical manual of mental disorders, ed 3. Washington, DC, American Psychiatric Association, 1981, pp 43-44.
9. Guilleminault C: Sleep apnea in 8 children. Pediatrics 1976;58:28-31.
10. Guilleminault C and Winkle R: A review of 50 children with OSAS. Lung 1981;159:275-287.
11. Kahn A et al: Sleep problems in healthy preadolescents. Pediatrics 1989;84:542-546.
12. Lavie P et al: Prevalence of sleep complaints in Israel. Sleep Res 1979;8:198.
13. Bixler EO et al: Prevalence of sleep disorders in the Los Angeles metropolitan area. Am J Psychiatry 1979;136:1257-1262.
14. Lavie P: Sleep habits and sleep disturbances in industrial workers in Israel: main findings and some characteristics of workers complaining of excessive daytime sleepiness. Sleep 1981;4:147-158.
15. Smirne S et al: Prevalence of sleep disorders in an unselected inpatient population. In Guilleminault C and Lugaresi E (eds): Sleep/wake disorders: natural history, epidemiology and long-term evolution. New York, Raven Press, 1983, pp 61-71.
16. Bixler EO et al: Incidence of sleep disorders in medical practice: a physician survey. Sleep Res 1976;5:160.
17. Coleman RM et al: Sleep-wake disorders in a family practice clinic. Sleep Res 1980;9:192.
18. Karacan I et al: Prevalence of sleep disturbances in a primarily urban Florida county. Soc Sci Med 1976;10:239-244.
19. Coleman RM: Diagnosis, treatment and follow-up of about 8000 sleep/wake disorder patients. In Guilleminault C and Lugaresi E (eds): Sleep/wake disorders: natural history, epidemiology and long-term evolution. New York, Raven Press, 1983, pp 87-97.
20. Ferber R: Solve your child's sleep problems. New York, Simon & Schuster, 1985, pp 214-232.
21. Carskadon MA et al: Guidelines for the multiple sleep latency test (MSLT): a standard measure of sleepiness. Sleep 1986;9:519-524.
22. Carskadon MA and Dement WC: The Multiple Sleep Latency Test: what does it measure? Sleep 1982;5:S67-S72.
23. Carskadon MA and Dement WC: Sleep tendency: an objective measure of sleep loss. Sleep Res 1977;6:200.
24. Carskadon MA and Dement WC: Sleepiness in the normal adolescent. In Guilleminault C (ed): Sleep and its disorders in children. New York, Raven Press, 1987, pp 53-66.
25. Carskadon MA et al: Pubertal changes in daytime sleepiness. Sleep 1980;2:453-460.
26. Feinberg I: Changes in sleep cycle patterns with age. J Psychiatr Res 1974;10:283-306.
27. Coble PA et al: EEG sleep of normal healthy children. I. Findings using standard measurement methods. Sleep 1984;7:289-303.
28. Ross JJ et al: Sleep patterns in preadolescent children: an EEG-EOG study. Pediatrics 1968;42:324-335.
29. Williams RL, Karacan I, and Hursch CJ: Electroencephalography (EEG) of human sleep: clinical applications. New York, Wiley, 1974.
30. Yoss RE and Daly DD: Criteria for the diagnosis of the narcoleptic syndrome. Mayo Clin Proc 1957;32:320-328.
31. Dement WC: Narcolepsy—not as rare as we believed! Med Times 1979;107:51-55.
32. Guilleminault C: Narcolepsy and its differential diagnosis. In Guilleminault C (ed): Sleep and its disorders in children. New York, Raven Press, 1987, pp 181-193.
33. Dement WC et al: The prevalence of narcolepsy, Part II [abstract]. Sleep 1973;2:147.
34. Baird WP: Narcolepsy: a non-medical presentation. American Narcolepsy Association, San Carlos, Calif, 1987.
35. Billiard M: Narcolepsy: clinical features and aetiology. Ann Clin Res 1985;17:220-226.
36. Guilleminault C et al: Altered states of consciousness

in disorders of daytime sleepiness. J Neurol Sci 1975;26:377-393.

37. Honda Y et al: Discrimination of narcoleptic patients by using genetic markers and HLA [abstract]. Sleep 1983;12:254.
38. Honda Y et al: A genetic study of narcolepsy and excessive daytime sleepiness in 308 families with a narcolepsy or hypersomnia proband. In Guilleminault C and Lugaresi E (eds): Sleep/wake disorders: natural history, epidemiology, and long-term evaluation. New York, Raven Press, 1983, pp 187-199.
39. Langdon N et al: Genetic markers in narcolepsy. Lancet 1984;2:1178-1180.
40. Billiard M and Seignalet J: Extraordinary association between HLA-DR2 and narcolepsy. Lancet 1985;1:226-227.
41. Guilleminault C and Grumet C: HLA-DR2 and narcolepsy: not all narcoleptic cataplectic patients are DR2. Hum Immunol 1986;17:1-2.
42. Guilleminault C: Narcolepsy syndrome. In Kryger MH, Roth T, and Dement W (eds): Principles and practice of sleep medicine. Philadelphia, WB Saunders, 1989, pp 338-346.
43. Levy A et al: Hypertrophied adenoids causing pulmonary hypertension and severe congestive heart failure. N Engl J Med 1967;277:501.
44. Luke M et al: Chronic naso-pharyngeal obstruction as a cause of cardiomegaly, cor pulmonale and pulmonary edema. Pediatrics 1966;37:762.
45. Cox MA et al: Reversible pulmonary hypertension in a child with respiratory obstruction and cor pulmonale. J Pediatr 1965;67:192.
46. Djalilian M et al: Hypoventilation secondary to chronic upper airway obstruction in childhood. Mayo Clin Proc 1975;50:11.
47. Guilleminault C: Obstructive sleep apnea syndrome in children. In Guilleminault C (ed): Sleep and its disorders in children. New York, Raven Press, 1987, pp 213-224.
48. Mendelson WB: Human sleep: research and clinical care. New York, Plenum, 1987, pp 221-245.
49. Guilleminault C and Faull KF: Sleepiness in nonnarcoleptic, non–sleep apneic EDS patients: the idiopathic CNS hypersomnolence. Sleep 1982;5:S175-S181.
50. Guilleminault C: Idiopathic central nervous system hypersomnia. In Kryger MH, Roth T, and Dement WC: Principles and practice of sleep medicine. Philadelphia, WB Saunders, 1989, pp 347-350.
51. Guilleminault C, Carskadon M, and Dement WC: On the treatment of rapid eye movement narcolepsy. Arch Neurol 1974;30:90-93.
52. Passouant P et al: Etude polygraphique des narcolepsies au cours du nychemere. Rev Neurol (Paris) 1968;118:431-441.
53. Montplasir J and Godbout R: Nocturnal sleep of narcoleptic patients. Sleep 1986;9:159-161.
54. Rechtschaffen A and Roth B: Nocturnal sleep of hypersomniacs. Activ Nerv [Suppl] 1969;11:229-233.
55. Baker TL et al: Comparative polysomnographic study of narcolepsy and idiopathic central nervous system hypersomnia. Sleep 1986;9:232-242.
56. Roth B, Nevsimalova S, and Rechtschaffen A: Hypersomnia with "sleep drunkenness." Arch Gen Psychiatry 1972;26:456-462.
57. Guilleminault C, Phillips R, and Dement WC: A syndrome of hypersomnia with automatic behavior. Electroencephalogr Clin Neurophysiol 1975;38:403-413.
58. Hishikawa Y and Kaneko Z: Electroencephalographic study on narcolepsy. Electroencephalogr Clin Neurophysiol 1965;18:249-259.
59. Roth B, Bruhova S, and Lehovsky M: REM sleep and NREM sleep in narcolepsy and hypersomnia. Electroencephalogr Clin Neurophysiol 1969;26:176-182.
60. Association of Sleep Disorders Centers: Diagnostic classification of sleep and arousal disorders. Prepared by the Sleep Disorders Classification Committee, H.P. Roffwarg, Chairman, Sleep 1979;2:1-137.
61. Zarcone V: Narcolepsy. N Engl J Med 1973;288:1156-1166.
62. Mendelson WB, Gillin JC, and Wyatt RJ: Human sleep and its disorders. New York, Plenum, 1977.
63. Hauri P: The sleep disorders. Kalamazoo, Mich, Upjohn, 1982, pp 52-62.
64. Roehrs T et al: Excessive daytime sleepiness associated with insufficient sleep. Sleep 1983;6:319-325.
65. Zorick F et al: Patterns of sleepiness in various disorders of excessive daytime somnolence. Sleep 1982;5:S165-S174.
66. Critchley M: Periodic hypersomnia and megaphagia in adolescent males. Brain 1962;85:627-656.
67. Billiard M: The Kleine-Levin syndrome. In Koella WP (ed): Sleep 1980. Basel, S Karger, 1981, pp 124-127.
68. Earle BV: Periodic hypersomnia and megaphagia (the Kleine-Levin syndrome). Psychiatr Q 1965;39:79-83.
69. Wilkus RJ and Chiles JA: Electrophysiological changes during episodes of the Kleine-Levin syndrome. J Neurol Neurosurg Psychiatry 1975;38:1225-1231.
70. Reynolds CF et al: Multiple sleep latency test findings in Kleine-Levin syndrome. J Nerv Ment Dis 1984;172:41-44.
71. Gallinck A: The Kleine-Levin syndrome: Hypersomnia, bulimia and abnormal mental states. World Neurol 1962;3:235-241.
72. Roth B: Narcolepsy and Hypersomnia. Basel, S Karger, 1980, pp 261-262.
73. Ogura C et al: Treatment of periodic somnolence with lithium carbonate. Arch Neurol 1976;33:143-153.
74. Billiard M, Guilleminault C, and Dement W: A menstruation-linked periodic hypersomnia: Kleine-Levin syndrome or new clinical entity? Neurology 1975;25:436-443.
75. Elian M and Bornstein B: The Kleine-Levin syndrome with intermittent abnormality in the EEG. Electroencephalogr Clin Neurophysiol 1969;27:601-604.
76. Sachs C, Persson HE, and Hagenfeldt K: Menstruation-linked periodic hypersomnia: a case study with successful treatment. Neurology 1982;32:1376-1379.

9

Sleep-Wake Schedule Disorders

Circadian physiology (see Chapter 3) and several disorders of the sleep-wake schedule have been presented in the context of the sleepless child (see Chapter 7). Indeed, sleep-wake schedule disorders are characterized by extreme variability in presentation: some exhibiting difficulty initiating or maintaining sleep, others manifesting excessive somnolence, and still others showing symptoms of both.

Every physiological function exhibits rhythmical variability across a 24-hour period; the most obvious is the sleep-wake cycle. Sleep-wake schedule disorders are therefore a group of clinical syndromes characterized by a *misalignment between a person's sleep-wake behavior and the individual's (or society's) phase matrix* in which they are contained.[1] The cause may be exogenous or endogenous. Usually the ability to initiate or maintain sleep or wakefulness is normal. The only abnormality clearly identified is in the *rhythm* of sleep and wake when compared with physiological function (or the phase of expected functioning).

Young infants normally exhibit an ultradian rhythm of sleep and wake of about 3 to 4 hours and alternating sleep cycles with a period of about 50 minutes.[2-4] Periodicity of sleep stage cycling increases gradually throughout infancy and childhood until the adult level of 90 minutes is reached.[5]

Even early in infancy there is evidence that the rest-activity cycle is controlled by an endogenous circadian pacemaker.[6] Circadian regulation of sleep begins to appear between 6 and 12 weeks of age. During this time the most functional time cue (zeitgeber) appears to be the feeding schedule.[7-9] Without external time cues, human infants appear to free run at a rate of approximately 25 hours, similar to that of the healthy adult.[7,9] Clearly the circadian clock is functional in infancy and is exogenously influenced as much as it is in adults (though the zeitgebers may be different).

Maturation of the sleep-wake schedule develops through direct interaction between the infant and caretaker.[10] Development of stable cycling of behaviors depends on the parent(s) responding to cues given by the infant and reciprocal interactional responses from the infant to recurrently reproducible and predictable cues provided by the parent(s) and environment. If the cues remain stable and cycle appropriately, entrainment to a 24-hour period occurs. If these interactional events are disordered because of parental failure to recognize the cues, respond appropriately, or provide stable and consistent input to establish routines, proper entrainment may fail and a disorder of the sleep-wake schedule may result.

Like any other physiological system, the circadian system may malfunction. Consequent symptoms may be obvious or subtle. Since each physiological process follows a rhythmical pattern, disrupting normal phase relationships can compromise function.[11] However, whether such disruptions are associated with serious disease is not certain.[12,13] When the phase relationship of the sleep-wake cycle becomes misaligned, symptoms may appear. All other processes and rhythms must realign themselves on the new phase. Although the stimulus for change in chronobiological schedule begins immediately on the new schedule, actual realignment may take several weeks or months, depending on the physiological parameter.[1] This inertia in movement of phase relationships occurs in many other processes as well as in the neurophysiological mechanisms related to the sleep and wake states. After an acute sleep-wake cycle shift, waking may be superimposed on brain function preferenced toward sleep. The position replaced by attempts to sleep maintains its physiological relationship to the awake state.[1]

Changes in the circadian cycle have profound clinical significance. Almost all physiological parameters used in medical diagnosis exhibit circadian rhythmicity,[12] and internal variables wax and wane throughout the day. Consequently, physiological measurements and laboratory studies must be interpreted in the context of the circadian phase in which they were obtained. Some fluctuations are small, but others are large. For example, a theophylline level measured in an asthmatic patient in the emergency room at 3 AM may seem low because of circadian change in the metabolism of the drug and not because of poor compliance with the therapeutic regimen.

The human body may be more susceptible to insult at certain phases of the circadian cycle.[14-16] For example, circadian changes in airway resistance are normally of such low amplitude that they have no noticeable effect on ventilation. Some patients with ventilatory failure secondary to asthma, however, have been shown to have a greatly exaggerated rhythm of bronchoconstriction.[17] Maximum airway constriction and respiratory arrests in these patients are noted during early morning hours. Efficacy and toxicity of medications have also shown circadian rhythmicity.[14] The rhythms of many physiological components appear to change the effectiveness of medicinal therapy because of the waxing and waning of drug metabolism and tissue susceptibility. The toxicity and effectiveness of medications may have circadian rhythms that are separately timed.[18] Attention must be paid to the timing of administration of medications to minimize toxic effects and maximize the efficacy of therapeutic regimens.

Disorders of the sleep-wake schedule may have a multitude of causes associated with the timing of the sleep-wake cycle. Disorders may be transient, appearing and resolving in less than 3 weeks, or may be persistent, lasting longer than 3 weeks. Neurological mechanisms responsible for these shifts are typically intact but cannot be turned on or off at will,[19] since a strong circadian rhythm underlies related neural activity.

Individuals with disorders of the sleep-wake schedule usually do not complain of sleep-wake schedule problems.[19] Typical symptoms center on an inability to initiate or maintain sleep, excessive daytime sleepiness, or both. Despite these complaints, most patients have no physiological abnormality in the initiation or maintenance of sleep or wakefulness.[1] Abnormalities exist only in the rhythm of the occurrence of the sleep and wake states with respect to the phase of internal rhythms or the phase of the person's expected state of functioning. Indeed, any sleep complaint is possible (including parasomnias such as sleep walking and sleep terrors). Evaluating a sleepless child, a sleepy child, or a child with a parasomnia requires a detailed understanding of the child's 24-hour schedule. Comprehensive histories must include longitudinal patterns rather than the typical or average. Knowledge of the sleep-wake pattern on schooldays, weekends, and holidays improves understanding of the disorder. Consistency and day-to-day variability in pattern should also be assessed.[20] Maintaining a log or diary of sleep and wake habits is important in obtaining an accurate description of the problem; however, continuing the diary during the course of treatment is one of the most powerful and useful tools of successful management.[21-23] It provides the practitioner and parents with objective evidence that change is occurring. The sleep diary may, in fact, be therapeutic by itself.[24] Without a continuous record of sleep-wake patterns, the history may be confusing and inaccurate diagnosis may result.

SLEEP PHASE RELATION DISORDERS

The range of entrainment of circadian rhythms in humans is limited.[11] The typical period is about 25 ± 2 hours but may be even narrower. Entrainment to a 24-hour period occurs because of time cues from the environment. Clearly, however, the circadian pacemaker reveals varying degrees of responsiveness depending on the circadian time of day.[25-27] For example, in experimental animals a light pulse falling early in the sleep phase can cause a phase delay of the circadian system, the same light pulse falling late in the sleep phase can cause a phase advance, and a light pulse falling during the middle of the wake phase may have no effect at all.[11] Therefore the timing of appearance of the zeitgeber is of paramount importance in bridging the gap between the intrinsic period of the pacemaker and the 24-hour day. Not only is timing of the stimulus important, but also intensity of the stimulus may determine the degree of shift. Light and meals appear to be strong zeitgebers for humans, and the most powerful window of entrainment appears to be the morning wake-up time.

Once the windows of susceptibility for delaying and advancing the sleep phase are determined, a *phase response curve* can be constructed. The phase response curve (Fig. 9–1) is the key to understanding a wide range of sleep-wake disorders and the limits within which the human can adapt to imposed light-dark cycles.[11] The typical range of entrainment for the human circadian system is 23½ to 26½ hours. This easily accommodates the 24-hour imposition of the light-dark cycle. In any one light-dark cycle, this range permits a phase advance of approximately 30 minutes, while a phase delay can be up to 2½ hours. Several days are needed for resynchronization to occur if the environmental shift is larger than the maximum achievable according to the phase response curve.

Individual variations in the range of entrainment may be considerable. The concept of "morning larks" and "night owls" is based on diversity of the position of the sleep-wake cycle with respect to the light-dark cycle. Existence of night owls and morning larks has been well documented in the literature.[28,29] Morning larks go to bed early in the evening, wake easily (and early) in the morning, and are most alert during morning hours. In contrast, the night owl goes to bed late in the evening, functions best at night, and sleeps late into the morning (or early afternoon) if permitted. When social responsibilities require the owl to wake early, functioning is difficult. Many children can be classified as owls or larks.[10] During childhood the lark tends to fall asleep early in any setting, despite the presence of environmental stimulation. These children wake early in the morning, are alert and active, and resist sleeping to a later time. Sleep-wake schedules of these children are not prone to significant disruption, and generally few complaints are heard, except that the child wakes too early in the morning. In contrast, the

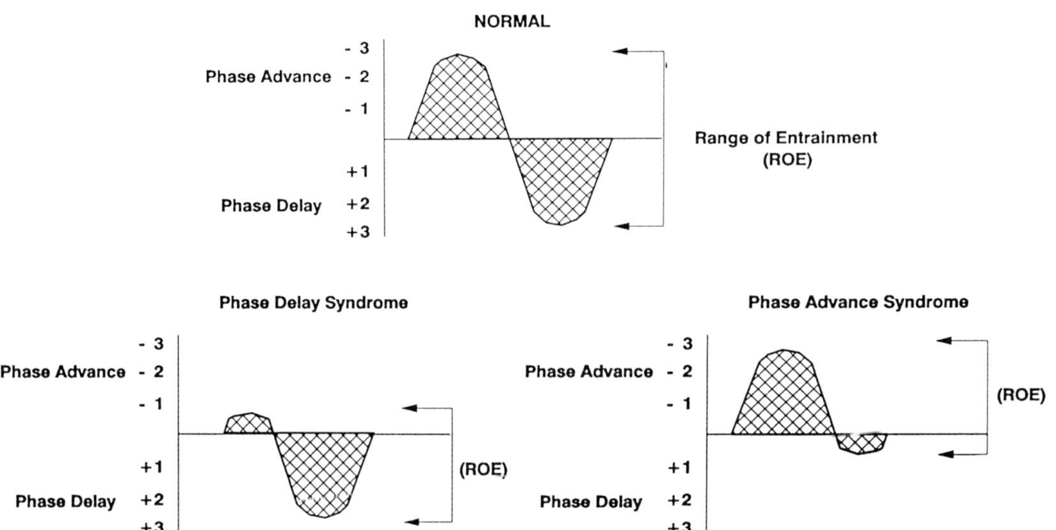

FIGURE 9–1. Phase response curves. Phase delay syndrome is represented by a limited ability to phase advance. In contrast, phase advance syndrome is represented by a limited ability to phase delay. (Adapted from information appearing in *NEJM*. Moore-Ede MC, Czeisler CA, and Richardson GS: Circadian timekeeping in health and disease. I. Basic properties of circadian pacemakers. N Engl J Med 1983; 309:469-475, with permission.)

childhood owl often has difficulty in settling at night, may resist bedtimes, and requires highly stable and consistent bedtime rituals to maintain a constant schedule.[10] The owl's sleep-wake schedule can be easily disrupted by social events or minor illnesses. In both cases, if parental interaction and the presence of other zeitgebers support the shift in sleep phase to earlier or later periods, chronic sleep phase shifts may result (Fig. 9–2).

Transient Disorders

Jet Lag Syndrome

Jet lag, which has been well described in adults, also occurs in children. Because of the limited range of entrainment and difficulty of shifting physiological parameters in a direction opposite to the direction of the endogenous circadian clock, west-to-east travel of two or more time zones (1-hour required phase *advance* for each time zone) is difficult. A longer adaptation phase is usually necessary. East-to-west travel of two or more time zones (1-hour required phase *delay* for each time zone) is usually easier and requires less adaptation time. This difference in adaptation based on direction of travel is caused by the underlying 25-hour period of the free-running pacemaker. East-to-west travel requires a shift in the same direction as the inherent drift of the pacemaker, whereas west-to-east travel requires a phase change opposite to the inherent pacemaker's preference. Once a child is entrained to the new time schedule, a shift back to the original time zone may be difficult. Depending on the number of time zones traversed and the direction of travel, reentrainment to the original sleep-wake schedule may take from 1 to 3 days in the case of east-to-west travel, or up to 3 weeks when traveling from west-to-east. In some cases reentrainment fails completely, resulting in a persistent phase shift.

The degree of symptoms depends on the degree of shift. Typical complaints include excessive daytime sleepiness and difficulty falling to sleep at night. Early morning waking may occur. The best method for readjusting the sleep phase to the new time zone involves stringent adherence to new time cues so that sleep occurs at the appropriate time. Timing of sleep onset and awakening should be in concordance with those of the new location. Meals should also be taken at the appropriate new times. Exposure to sunlight in the new time zone suppresses melatonin secretion and assists in shifting the sleep phase.

Shift Work

Other transient disturbances in the sleep phase, such as shift work, are not typically discussed in the context of childhood sleep disorders. However, parental shift work may have a significant effect on a child's sleep, resulting in sleep fragmentation, disruption of continuity, and ultimately performance decrements during daytime hours. Frequently with good intentions, parents delay their child's sleep phase so they can spend time with the child before or after

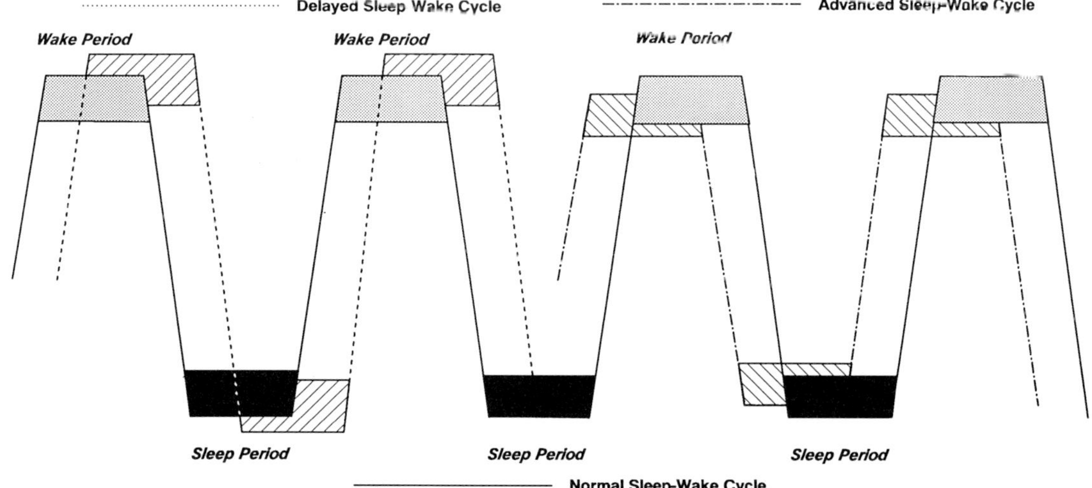

FIGURE 9–2. Phase relation disorders. The physiological sleep period is later in the 24-hour cycle when the sleep phase is delayed, and earlier when the sleep phase is advanced. (Modified from Anch AM et al: Sleep: a scientific perspective. Englewood Cliffs, NJ: Prentice Hall, 1988, p 223, with permission. © 1988 Prentice Hall.)

work. The child's sleep environment may also be disturbed while the parent is preparing for work or sleep. Finally, a child's sleep phase may be shortened or fragmented because of the need to prepare for day care (or night care) so that a work schedule can be met. Although parents' sleep disruption may be transient and regularize on days off, weekends, and vacations (or during rotations to more traditional hours), disturbances in the child's sleep-wake cycle may persist.

Persistent Disorders

Sleep Phase Delay Syndrome

Sleep phase delay syndrome (SPDS) is common and occurs at all ages.[23,30-33] The etiology is typically multifactorial, but one of the most important underlying mechanisms involves the near 25-hour period of the endogenous circadian pacemaker.[10] SPDS is thought to be due to movement of the sleep phase in the direction of the endogenous rhythm and may be the result of failure of normal entrainment mechanisms.[34-36] The result is a stable but delayed relationship to the normal day-night time cues. The SPDS has been theorized to result from a narrow range of entrainment that may be equal to or greater than the normal 24-hour period.[23] This could be the result of a low response in the *advance* portion of the phase response curve or an unusually long endogenous cycle.[21,37]

Occasional late bedtimes followed by recovery morning sleep is enough to shift some children's sleep phase.[10] Holidays on which the child is allowed to stay up, illness delaying sleep onset, bedtime struggles or fights with parents or siblings, and travel may lead to later bedtimes. The child delays regular sleep and morning wake times, resulting in a phase delay.

Clinical Presentation. SPDS is characterized by difficulty falling to sleep at night and difficulty waking in the morning when the child has socially imposed responsibilities (such as school). Sleep is normal if the attempt to sleep is delayed significantly and the child can sleep as long as he or she wishes.

Initial complaints usually center on *bedtime struggles,* difficulty waking in the morning, poor functioning during morning hours, school tardiness, and falling to sleep in morning classes. Children with SPDS are often described as most alert and active in the evening, often coincident with the parentally imposed bedtime. However, the child's physiological sleep phase occurs some time *after* the regularly scheduled bedtime. Physiological sleep offset time is also delayed. The child remains awake for long periods at night (in bed or continually getting out of bed), is awakened for school substantially earlier than the physiological wake time, and suffers sleep deprivation during the first portion of the school week. On weekends bedtime typically occurs later and the child is usually permitted to sleep longer in an attempt to "catch up on sleep." Unfortunately, these recovery days allow the circadian shift to continue and support the phase delay, rather than resolving the underlying problem. If later waking time is not permitted on weekends or vacations, sleep loss may be recovered by daytime naps and the phase delay may persist.

Infants and toddlers may also have significant phase shifts.[10] Total sleep time may be normal. Often a sleep phase delay does not pose a problem for parents of these younger children, and rarely are problems brought to the attention of the practitioner. Extra time spent with the child in the evening may be a positive factor for the entire family, and parents may appreciate sleeping later in the morning. Difficulties arise when social responsibilities of the parent or child change, requiring earlier morning waking for work, day care, or school. Complaints then center on difficulty waking the child in the morning, significant crankiness, and performance or behavior problems during morning hours.

Bedtime struggles are the most common reason for parents to seek medical attention. Sleep at night is generally not interrupted by wakings: children sleep normally throughout the night. Sleep offset is difficult. The child may be excessively sleepy during the day, may nap well in a day care setting, or may fall asleep in school. The sleepy child may, on the other hand, be restless, overactive, irritable, cranky, or manifest other behavior problems such as aggressiveness. Nightime fears may also develop.

Diagnosis is based on the history and physical examination, maintenance of a sleep diary, and sometimes polysomnography. A sleep diary maintained for 2 to 3 weeks greatly assists in diagnosis and management. Polysomnography reveals normal sleep. If the study is done on a recovery night, findings may include an increase in slow-wave sleep, a decrease (or an increase) in rapid eye movement (REM) sleep, and a short sleep onset latency. Absence of abnormalities on the polysomnogram and in the physical examination, a characteristic history, and a sleep diary compatible with a phase shift confirm the diagnosis.

Treatment. Once the diagnosis is made, treatment is straightforward. For the child or young adolescent with a phase delay of 3 hours or less, a slowly progressive phase advance (against the direction of the endogenous pacemaker) may be attempted (Fig. 9–3). Resolution may take one to several weeks. Treatment is usually conducted in five stages, several of which overlap:

STAGE 1. The child should be allowed to fall asleep and wake at times consistent with his or her endogenous sleep phase for 1 or 2 days. Sleep onset may be rather late in the evening, and sleep offset may be late into morning hours. Usually the child falls to sleep easily at this late time, bedtime struggles disappear, and the child wakes without difficulty in the morning.

STAGE 2. On day 3, parents begin to advance the *wake time* by approximately 15 to 30 minutes, keeping the bedtime constant at the endogenous sleep onset time established on the previous 2 days. Sleep offset should be advanced for several days without any change in bedtime.

STAGE 3. When wake time has advanced approximately 45 to 60 minutes, parents begin to advance the bedtime slowly by a period of 15 to 30 minutes.

STAGE 4. When the desired morning wake time is reached, it should be firmly and consistently fixed (on schooldays, weekends, holidays, vacations, etc.).

STAGE 5. Bedtime should be advanced slowly until the desired time is reached and then firmly fixed. The total sleep time should be normal.

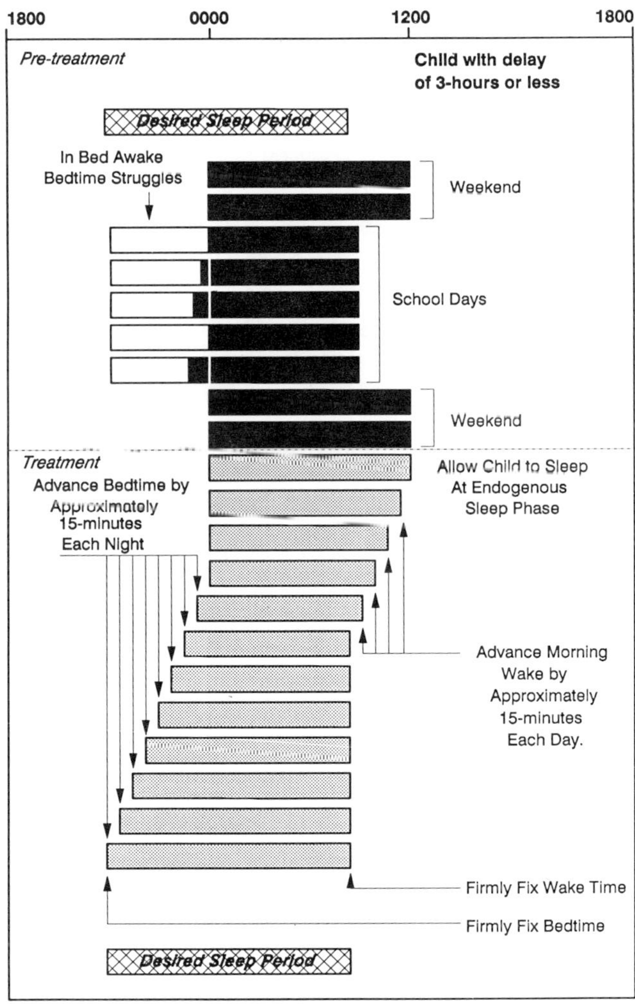

FIGURE 9–3. Paradigm of treatment of a child with a sleep phase delay syndrome by slowly advancing the sleep phase. This regimen is most appropriate for children and adolescents with phase delays of 3 hours or less.

It is not physiologically possible to increase total sleep time to a volume greater than what is developmentally appropriate. Unreasonable expectations by parents to increase total sleep time should be discouraged.

For a short period during treatment, total sleep time is less than is developmentally appropriate and the child is somewhat sleep deprived. Parents should be forewarned of this period of deprivation for two reasons. First, the child's performance and behavior may change and treatment should be scheduled when the child has no significant social responsibilities. Second, during the period of deprivation the child may attempt to nap in the morning, afternoon, or evening. These naps must not be allowed, since sleep recovery may be sufficient to continue the phase delay and interfere with the treatment regimen. Parents need to be supported during treatment, and frequent follow-up visits may be warranted for parent education and reassurance.

For an older adolescent with a phase delay of more than 4 hours, a controlled "around-the-clock" phase delay may be attempted (Fig. 9–4). Chronotherapy of this type must be performed during a time when the patient and parent have no other social responsibilities, since in one period the patient will be sleeping all day and awake all night. Treatment consists of delaying bedtime by approximately 2 hours each night while permitting the patient to sleep as

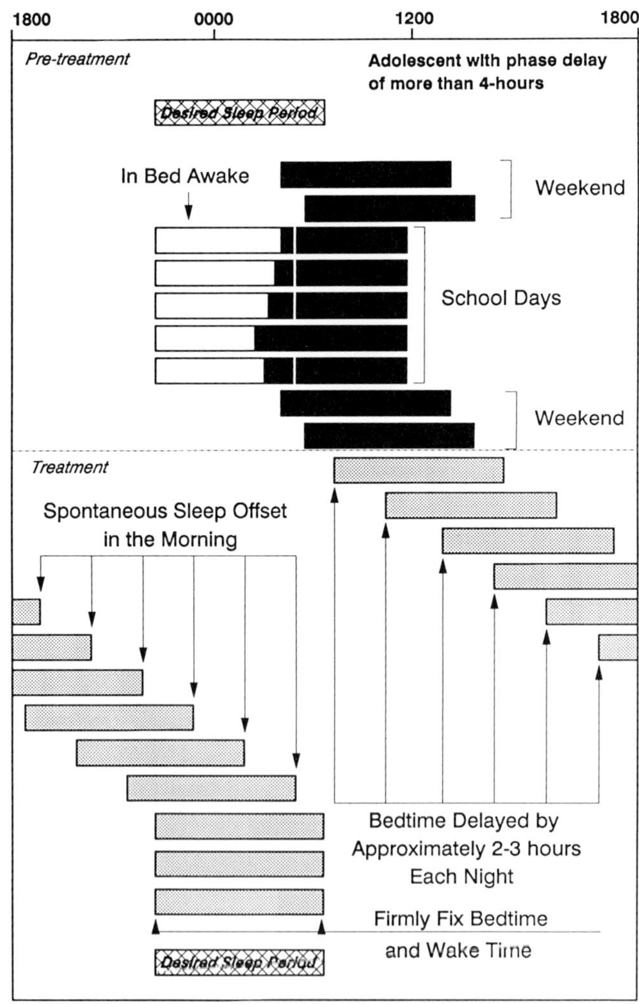

FIGURE 9–4. Paradigm of treatment of an adolescent with a sleep phase delay syndrome by progressive sleep phase delay. This regimen is seldom appropriate for children and young adolescents. It may be indicated for older adolescents with phase delays of more than 4 hours. (Modified from information appearing in *NEJM*. Moore-Ede MC, Czeisler CA, and Richardson GS: Circadian timekeeping in health and disease. II. Clinical implications of circadian rhythmicity. N Engl J Med 1983; 309:530-536, with permission.)

late as he or she wants. Once the progressive sleep onset phase delay begins, spontaneous sleep offset will be delayed by about the same amount each day. Progressive 2-hour delays should continue until the desired sleep phase is reached. When this occurs, morning wake-up time should be firmly fixed and remain consistent on schooldays, weekends, holidays, and vacations. Bedtime should also be firmly fixed. This form of chronotherapy is usually not indicated for younger adolescents and children.

A word about light and phototherapy is warranted. Bright light is a potent entraining zeitgeber and may itself shift phases. Exposing the youngster to a brightly lit environment for several hours after waking in the morning may significantly assist in advancing the sleep phase to more desired times.

Motivated Sleep Phase Delay Syndrome

Motivated sleep phase delay syndrome is most often seen in adolescents. Symptoms are similar to SPDS, with significant sleep onset insomnia, difficulty in awakening in the morning (with or without excessive daytime sleepiness), and prolonged sleep on weekends. In contrast to SPDS, sleep during weekends, holidays, and vacations tends to be normal; sleep and wake occur at appropriate times. The phase delay may be significant and may persist for long periods. Since secondary gains from the complaint are considerable, the patient usually prefers the problem to persist (reminiscent of Munchausen's syndrome). Multiple attempts to correct the sleep phase characteristically fail or are resisted. If chronotherapy with a continued phase delay is attempted, patients often complain that they cannot stay awake according to the prescribed regimen. If school permits a late start, the insomnia worsens and the sleep phase is further delayed. According to Ferber,[38] adolescents with motivated phase delay syndrome exhibit a "reverse vacation effect" and phase advance during this time, wake appropriately at socially important times, are unhappy that the condition is treatable, and often undermine therapeutic efforts. Polysomnography reveals normal sleep, and the patient typically *wakes easily in the laboratory when the study is completed,* even if sleep has been insufficient.

Short-term prognosis is usually poor. Treatment efforts may include family and individual counseling, increasing the youngster's responsibility in managing the problem and day-to-day activities, home tutors, residential school, and residential therapy. Chronotherapy may be attempted but is usually unsuccessful. Use of medication is controversial, but may be helpful, especially if significant depression is present.

Sleep Phase Advance Syndrome[1,11,19,34,39-41]

Sleep phase advance syndrome (SPAS) is uncommon during childhood. It occurs more often in very young children and tends to resolve when evening and nighttime activities (television, homework, peer interaction, and family) entrain a normal sleep phase.

Clinical Presentation. Presenting signs and symptoms are opposite of those seen in SPDS. Typical complaints center on early morning wakings. The problem may come to the attention of the practitioner because parents are being awakened early in the morning by their child who is ready to begin the day. Early evening sleepiness is apparent, and the child falls to sleep several hours earlier than desired. A child who is forced to remain awake may show crankiness, irritability, overactivity, and behavior problems. A thorough review of the child's complete daily schedule usually reveals that the *entire structure of the day is advanced.* Meals and nap times are earlier than the norms for the child's age. Diagnosis is based on the presence of a normal physical examination, historical and sleep diary evidence of early evening sleep onset and early morning awakening (2 or more hours earlier than desired), and evidence of otherwise normal sleep. As with SPDS, sleep is normal in quantity and quality but occurs at unacceptable times.

Treatment. Waking can be delayed only if the entire sleep phase is delayed, and gradual phase delay is most often helpful. Parents should begin a progressive and consistent 30-minute to 1-hour delay of bedtime while allowing spontaneous awakening in the morning (Fig. 9–5). The progressive delay is continued until the desired bedtime and wake time are reached. During treatment it is also important to delay meal times and nap times and to firmly fix these new time relations once the desired schedule is reached. Again, exposure to a bright light environment late in the day (around the endogenous sleep onset time) may assist in delaying the sleep phase. Parents should be warned that total sleep time cannot be extended. As the child grows older, nighttime activities are usually sufficiently stimulating to support the new sleep-wake schedule.

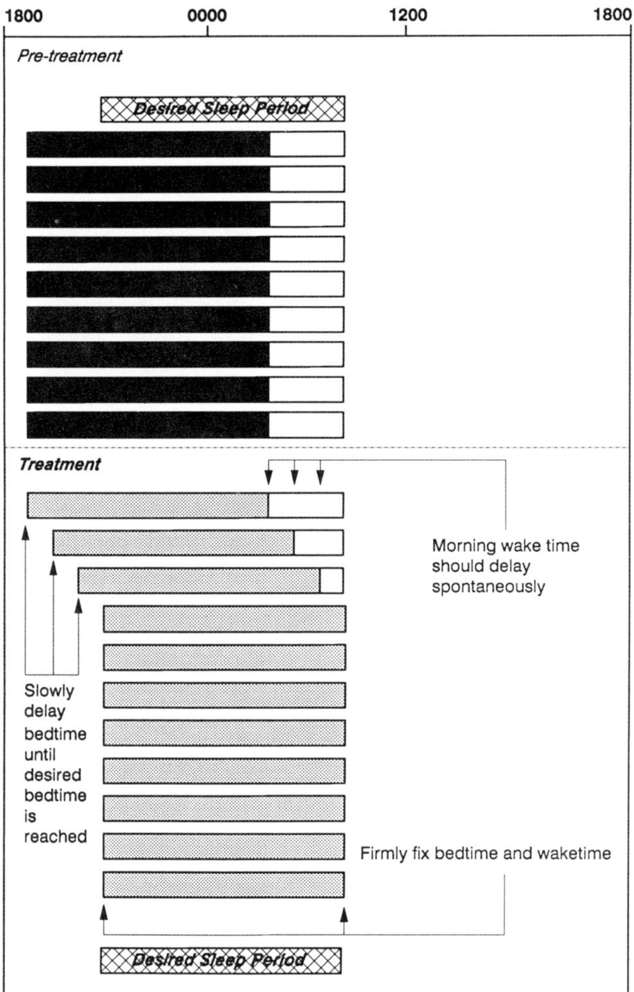

FIGURE 9–5. Paradigm of treatment of a child with a sleep phase advance syndrome by slowly delaying the sleep phase.

Frequently Changing Sleep-Wake Patterns; Irregular Sleep-Wake Patterns[1,10,19,34]

Frequently changing sleep-wake patterns are generally characterized separately from irregular sleep-wake patterns in the adult literature. Little phenomenological distinction is made except for the voluntary component of the former and the apparent involuntary component of the latter. Regardless of this difference, manifestations are similar.

Proper functioning of circadian systems requires entrainment, and entrainment demands resetting the biological clock (and all physiological rhythms) on a daily basis. For entrainment to be successful, zeitgebers, such as light, dark, bedtime, wake time, meals, and patterns of social interaction, must be consistent and predictable. When regular signals are absent, the child may sleep irregularly at night. Little structure may be present in the home. Meal times may vary significantly, and individual members of the household may eat at different times. Naps may occur at different times during the day and are rarely consistent. Bedtimes and wake times fluctuate.

Although it should seem obvious that a child has developed an irregular sleep-wake schedule, this is often overlooked. Irregular sleep-wake pattern is defined as disorganized and variable sleep and waking behavior that disrupts an expected sleep-wake pattern (Fig. 9–6). It is associated with frequent daytime naps at irregular times and excessive bed rest. Sleep periods are not of appropriate volume. Structure of day and night becomes disorganized and extremely variable, and a key feature is the loss of a clear sleep-wake rhythm. Sleep is broken into several

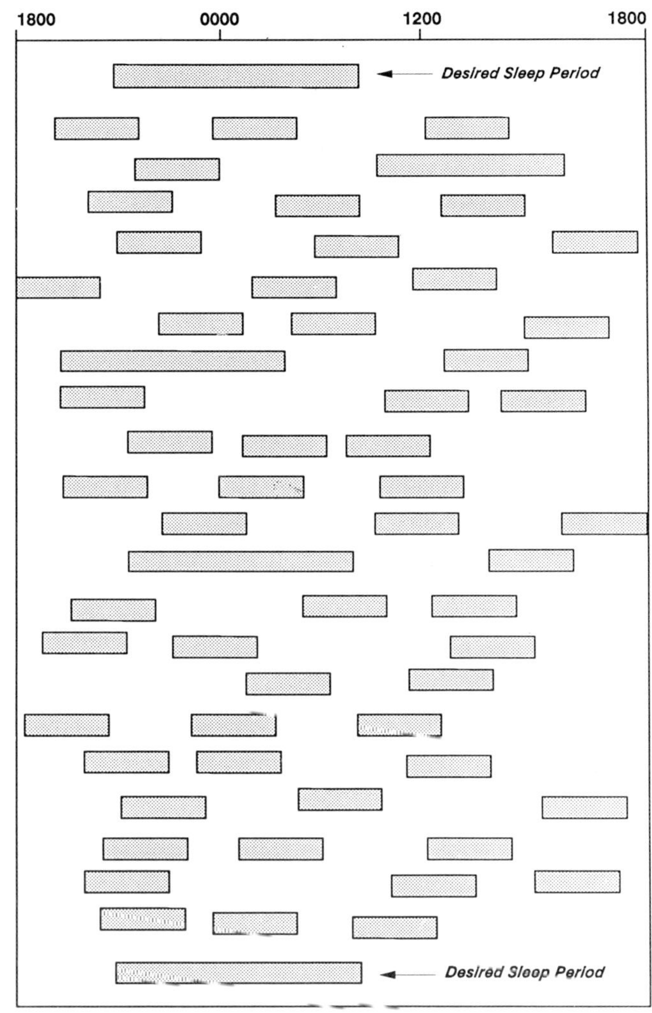

FIGURE 9–6. Schematic representation of an irregular sleep-wake schedule.

short blocks. This condition may begin as a disorder of initiating or maintaining sleep, although sleep diaries reveal that the total 24-hour sleep time is normal for the patient's age. In addition to disruption of the sleep-wake cycle, endocrine, temperature, and other circadian function curves lose their expected circadian waxing and waning. Theoretically an irregular sleep-wake pattern might also result from endogenous causes such as pacemaker failure. Although destruction of the pacemaker in animals results in an irregular and disorganized pattern of behavior, little evidence supports this hypothesis in humans.

Clinical Presentation. The initial complaint may be an inability to fall asleep at the desired bedtime or to remain asleep for an adequate time. Often parents report that their child "never sleeps." Prolonged early nighttime wakings occur, especially after early bedtimes. Under these circumstances the early sleep period actually functions as a late nap. Complaints vary and may include bedtime difficulties, prolonged nighttime wakings, early morning wakings, difficulty waking, or excessive daytime sleepiness.

Varying degrees of internal desynchronization of all physiological systems occur. Some degree of cognitive impairment and sleepiness characterizes the awake intervals. Lassitude, weakness, and somatic symptoms may occur because of loss of fluctuation of most physiological functions. Children are unlikely to feel well or function optimally during daytime hours. Schoolwork may deteriorate, and behavior problems are common. Diagnosis is based on a comprehensive evaluation of the child's and family's daily living patterns. Since family dysfunction is common, compliance with maintenance of sleep diaries may be difficult. If a sleep diary can be maintained, however, it shows the characteristic irregularity of the sleep-wake schedule.

Treatment. Treatment depends on identification of the underlying cause of the irregular schedule. If lack of education or cultural variation is a major etiological factor, treatment consists of following principles of sleep hygiene, emphasizing regular sleep hours, and providing a firm schedule for meals, school, work, and other activities. Inflexible scheduling breaks the cycle of mutually reinforcing naps and disturbed nighttime sleep. Sleep-wake, meal, and activity patterns should be charted during the course of treatment. If family dysfunction is at the root of the problem, solving the sleep problem is more difficult. Psychosocial and stress factors must be managed concomitantly with the sleep complaint, since elements may be interdependent. Family therapy, individual therapy, and parenting education may all be indicated.

Entrainment Failure: Non-24-Hour Sleep-Wake Syndrome[1,10,19,34,42,43]

The non-24-hour sleep-wake syndrome appears to result from a lack of entrainment to a 24-hour period (Fig. 9–7). This may be due to primary pacemaker failure or an inability of the pacemaker to appropriately receive or respond to exogenous time cues. The result is an inability to phase advance each day. Blindness (whether congenital or acquired) appears to increase susceptibility to this syndrome, since the absence of light as a zeitgeber prevents entrainment of endogenous rhythms. The approximate 25-hour

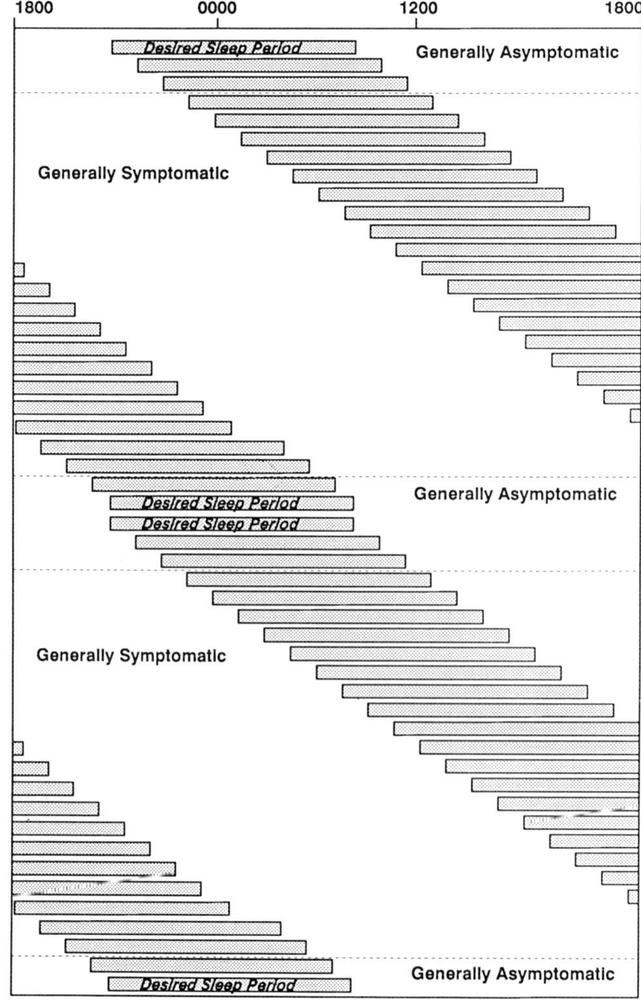

FIGURE 9–7. Schematic representation of a non-24-hour sleep-wake syndrome. The sleep phase seems to free run at its endogenous, unentrained period. This is similar to the pattern seen in the absence of zeitgebers.

period seen in the free-running state is exhibited. Children who have other severe central nervous system damage with retardation, those who have more localized hypothalamic dysfunction, and those who take medication that affects circadian pacing may manifest this syndrome.

Studies in blind subjects have shown that persons with no light perception can be divided into three groups with respect to circadian rhythms: (1) those with normal, stable entrainment and appropriate phase relationships to the 24-hour day; (2) those with a normal, stable period by an abnormal phase relation to the 24-hour day; and (3) those with a period longer than 24 hours whose rhythm does not appear to entrain to the 24-hour day. Because of the disparity in entrainment between the three groups, other, nonretinal entrainment mechanisms must synchronize the circadian system. These include, but are not limited to, social contacts, meals, and behavioral scheduling.

Clinical Presentation. The initial complaint is usually difficulty getting to sleep at night, coupled with inability to remain awake during the day. The patient typically falls to sleep later and later each night. Bedtime struggles appear. Because social responsibilities such as school necessitate a regimented wake-up time, sleep restriction occurs and results in excessive daytime sleepiness, school performance decrements, and behavioral difficulties.

Because of the regularly progressive delay in the circadian rhythm, the sleep period eventually "works its way around the clock" and arrives at a relatively normal phase relationship (although it does not remain in phase for long). The result is a periodic alternation in symptoms. Every few weeks the child's sleep improves greatly as the endogenous rhythm temporarily synchronizes with the environment. A careful sleep-wake diary is required for diagnosis.

Treatment. Entrainment is possible for some patients. The strongest environmental cues possible must be provided to achieve entrainment. Bedtimes and wake times must be consistent and methodically regular. Meal times should be regularly scheduled and firmly fixed. This is especially true of the morning meal. Behavioral cues that fix the time of day (e.g., timing of showers, phone calls, travel to school or day care, and play) should be provided. A consistently structured schedule provides the nonretinal entrainment mechanisms that are most likely to synchronize sleep, wake, and other activities to society's 24-hour day.

REFERENCES

1. Association of Sleep Disorders Centers: Diagnostic classification of sleep and arousal disorders. Prepared by the Sleep Disorders Classification Committee, H.P. Roffwarg, Chairman, Sleep 1979;2:1-137.
2. Lenard HG: Sleep studies in infancy. Acta Paediatr Scand 1970;59:572-581.
3. Stern E et al: Sleep cycle characteristics in infants. Pediatrics 1969;43:65-70.
4. Stern E, Parmelee AH, and Harris MA: Sleep state periodicity in prematures and young infants. Dev Psychobiol 1973;6:357-365.
5. Williams RL, Karacan I, and Hursch CJ: Electroencephalography (EEG) of human sleep: clinical applications. New York, Wiley, 1974.
6. Anders TF: State and rhythmic processes. Am J Child Psychiatry 1978;17:401-420.
7. Kleitman N: Sleep and wakefulness. Chicago, University of Chicago Press, 1939.
8. Kleitman N and Engelmann TG: Sleep characteristics of infants. J Appl Physiol 1953;6:269-282.
9. Ferber R and Boyle MP: Persistence of a free-running sleep-wake rhythm in a one year old girl. Sleep Res 1983;12:364.
10. Ferber R: Circadian schedule disturbances. In Guilleminault C (ed): Sleep and its disorders in children. New York, Raven Press, 1987, pp 165-175.
11. Moore-Ede MC, Czeisler CA, and Richardson GS: Circadian timekeeping in health and disease. I. Basic properties of circadian pacemakers. N Engl J Med 1983;309:469-476.
12. Conroy RTWL and Mills JN: Human circadian rhythms. London, Churchill, 1970.
13. Moore-Ede MC: Hypothermia: a timing disorder of circadian thermoregulatory rhythms? In Pozos RS (ed): The nature and treatment of hypothermia. Minneapolis, University of Minnesota Press, 1983, pp 69-80.
14. Moore-Ede MC, Czeisler CA, and Richardson GS: Circadian timekeeping in health and disease. II. Clinical implications of circadian rhythmicity. N Engl J Med 1983;309:530-536.
15. Halberg F et al: Susceptibility rhythm to *E. coli* endotoxin and bioassay. Proc Soc Exp Biol Med 1960;103:142-144.
16. McGovern JP, Smolensky MH, and Reinberg A (eds): Chronobiology in allergy and immunology. Springfield, Ill, Charles C Thomas, 1977.
17. Hetzel MR and Clark TJH: Clinical importance of circadian factors in severe asthma. In Reinberg A and Halberg F (eds): Chronopharmacology. New York, Pergamon Press, 1979, pp 213-221.
18. Scheving LE et al: Survival and cure of leukemic mice after circadian optimization with treatment of cyclophosphamide and 1-beta-D arabinofuranosylcytosine. Cancer Res 1977;37:3648-3655.
19. Anch AM et al: Sleep: a scientific perspective. Englewood Cliffs, NJ, Prentice Hall, 1988, p 321.
20. Ferber RA: Assessment procedures for diagnosis of sleep disorders in children. In Noshbitz JD (ed): Basic handbook of child psychiatry, vol 5. New York, Basic Books, 1986.
21. Czeisler CA et al: Chronotherapy: resetting the circadian clocks of patients with delayed sleep phase insomnia. Sleep 1981;4:1-21.
22. Kokkoris CP et al: Long-term ambulatory temperature monitoring in a subject with a hypernychthemeral sleep-wake cycle disturbance. Sleep 1978;1:177-190.

23. Weitzman ED et al: Delayed sleep phase syndrome: a chronobiological disorder with sleep onset insomnia. Arch Gen Psychiatry 1981;38:737-746.
24. Largo RH and Hunziker UA: A developmental approach to the management of children with sleep disturbances in the first three years of life. Eur J Pediatr 1984;142:170-173.
25. DeCoursey PJ: Daily light sensitivity rhythm in a rodent. Science 1960;131:33-35.
26. Pittendrigh CS: Circadian rhythms and the circadian organization of living systems. Cold Spring Harbor Symp Quant Biol 1960;25:159-182.
27. Hastings JW and Sweeney BM: A persistent diurnal rhythm of luminescence in *Gonyaulax polyedra*. Biol Bull 1958;115:440-458.
28. Horne JA and Ostberg O: A self-assessment questionnaire to determine morningness-eveningness in human circadian rhythms. Int J Chronobiol 1976;4:97-109.
29. Horne JA and Ostberg O: Individual differences in human circadian rhythms. Biol Psychol 1979;5:179-190.
30. Dement WC, Guilleminault C, and Zarcone V: The pathologies of sleep: a case series approach. In Tower DB (ed): The nervous system. New York, Raven Press, 1975, pp 501-518.
31. Ferber R, Boyle MP, and Belfer M: Initial experience of a pediatric sleep disorders clinic. Sleep Res 1981;10:194.
32. Ferber R and Boyle MP: Phase shift dyssomnia in early childhood. Sleep Res 1983;12:242.
33. Ferber R and Boyle MP: Six year experience of a pediatric sleep disorders center. Sleep Res 1986;15:120.
34. Mendelson WB: Human sleep: research and clinical care. New York, Plenum, 1987, pp 295-314.
35. Ferber R and Boyle MP: Delayed sleep phase syndrome versus motivated sleep phase delay in adolescents. Sleep Res 1983;12:239.
36. Thorpy M: Delayed sleep syndrome of adolescence. In Pediatric sleep disorders. Mercy Hospital and Medical Center, San Diego, Oct 4, 1985.
37. Czeisler CA et al: Entrainment of human circadian rhythms by light-dark cyles: a reassessment. Photochem Photobiol 1981;34:239-247.
38. Ferber R: Motivated sleep phase delay in adolescence. Presented at the annual meeting of the Association of Professional Sleep Societies, Minneapolis, July 1, 1990.
39. Moldofsky H, Musisi S, and Phillipson EA: Treatment of a case of advanced sleep phase syndrome by phase advance chronotherapy. Sleep 1986;9:61-65.
40. Wher TA et al: Phase advance of the circadian sleep-wake cycle as an antidepressant. Science 1979; 206:710-713.
41. Kupfer DJ et al: The application of EEG sleep for the differential diagnosis of affective disorders. Am J Psychiatry 1978;135:64-74.
42. Miles LEM, Raynal DM, and Wilson MA: Blind man living in normal society has circadian rhythms of 24.9 hours. Science 1977;198:421-423.
43. Martens H et al: Sleep/wake distribution in blind subjects with and without sleep complaints [abstract]. Presented at the annual meeting of the Association of Professional Sleep Societies, Minneapolis, June 27–July 1, 1990, p 93.

10

Parasomnias

Parasomnias are classified as dysfunctions associated with sleep, sleep stages, or partial arousals from sleep.[1-3] They are a group of disorders with strikingly dissimilar presentations but share many clinical and physiological characteristics. Many parasomnias present *clear and dramatic* symptoms (e.g., sleep walking, head banging, bruxism). Manifestations appear early in childhood and are often considered by parents and practitioners as normal, benign behavioral features. As the child ages, benign characteristics become exaggerated. Steady, gradual transformation of normal phenomena into "pathological" symptoms suggests that parasomnias may be a deviation from normal psychophysiological development or result from central nervous system immaturity. However, few pathophysiological abnormalities can be identified, despite the severe and explosive features. Resistance to therapeutic interventions and spontaneous remissions as the child ages are common to many parasomnias. Treatment regimens often result in only transient resolution of symptoms. Exacerbation of features occurs, or one characteristic may be substituted for another. Therapeutic failures and increase in intensity are typically followed by spontaneous remission, usually at the time of puberty.

Longitudinal observations have shown that many parasomnias follow a course that comprises several phases (Fig. 10–1). A stage of *undifferentiation* occurs between infancy and 2 years of age. Sleep-wake cycles may shift or become reversed; children may confuse day with night. At this age striking symptoms characteristic of many parasomnias are absent and manifestations may be confused with infantile colic, behavioral problems, or sleep phase or schedule problems. After 2 years of age symptoms gradually change and coalesce during a *crystallization phase*. Characteristic symptoms appear. Parasomnic episodes may be infrequent or mild, and many are considered minor deviations from normal developmental phenomena. During crystallization a variety of symptoms may occur at different times. A *monosymptomatic phase* follows. A single, striking symptom becomes dominant. Agitated sleep walking, violent head banging, or night terrors may occur and are frightening to the observer. Symptoms may range from single episodes to nightly events that persist for a protracted period. The patient appears well and developmentally normal while awake, only to express bizarre and sometimes violent behaviors during sleep. The monosymptomatic phase may persist for years, undergo a phase of *spontaneous remission* or *decompensate* to a more severe symptom, or lead to multiple parasomnic symptoms.

ETIOLOGY

The cause of parasomnias is unknown. They may be due to a developmental dysfunction, immaturity of the central nervous system, or

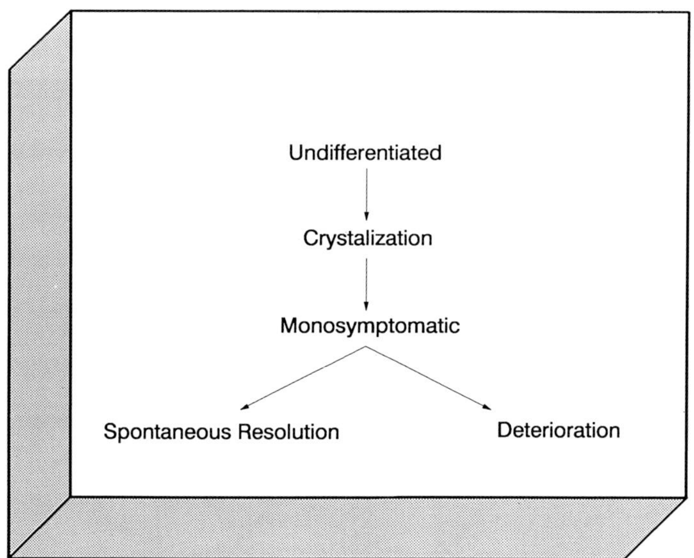

FIGURE 10–1. Ontogenetic stages of parasomnias.

dysfunction of distant organ systems. Any theoretical basis of the genesis of parasomnias, however, must address their common features as listed in Table 10–1. In this context the entire group of parasomnias may be considered clinical and physiological syndromes, specific in manifestation and compensatory in mechanisms. Compensation as an internal physiological principie unites parasomnias into a special class of syndromes with a certain hierarchy. This *set hypothesis* proposes that the organism "sets up" parasomnias as biological tools to serve specific adaptive functions. These functions might include compensation for existing dysfunction to maintain or to change sleep stages, to avoid impending danger (real or imagined), to achieve a higher level of functioning, or to avoid emotional or physical tension.

The International Classification of Sleep Disorders[2] organizes the parasomnias into four major categories: arousal disorders, sleep-wake transition disorders, parasomnias usually associated with rapid eye movement (REM) sleep, and other parasomnias (Table 10–2). This classification is congruent with the proposed set hypothesis in that each parasomnia may be considered a compensatory symptom of a primary underlying dysfunction and manifestations.

EVALUATION OF A CHILD WITH A PARASOMNIA

As with all other disorders of sleep and wakefulness, evaluation begins with a comprehensive history and physical examination. Special attention must paid to a detailed description of the events, including (but not limited to) the following factors:

1. Usual time of occurrence
2. *Exact* behaviors, movements, or symptoms manifested
3. Whether intervention efforts by the caretaker exacerbate the symptoms
4. Displacement of the child from the bed
5. Occurrence of symptoms during the immediate presleep period or during sleep
6. Occurrence of symptoms on waking from sleep or during daytime naps
7. Recall or amnesia concerning the events
8. Occurrence of symptoms during daytime wakefulness
9. Presence of stereotypical movements or rhythmical behaviors during the episode
10. Presence of multiple symptoms

Basic neurodevelopmental landmarks must be carefully assessed for the presence of daytime or waking behavioral or developmental abnormalities. Typical sleep-wake schedules, habits, and patterns should be clearly delineated. Morning wake time, evening bedtime, bedtime rituals, and nap time rituals should be described. The presence of excessive daytime sleepiness, snoring, or restlessness during sleep should be ascertained. The parents should be asked whether the child has a concurrent medical illness or is taking any medications or drugs.

A complete physical examination must be performed. Emphasis should be placed on a comprehensive neurological and developmental evaluation. The existence of developmental delays or symptoms suggestive of neurological disorders might indicate an organic basis for the

TABLE 10–1. Common Features of Parasomnias

Clear and dramatic symptoms
Age related
No gross medical disorder
No gross polysomnographic abnormalities
Therapeutic resistance
Spontaneous resolution

patient's symptoms. Evidence of other medical disorders should be noted, and they should be assessed as possible contributing factors.

Laboratory evaluations should be guided by the signs and symptoms. A urine drug screen may be helpful if the practitioner suspects that symptoms may be side effects of medication. Polysomnography with continuous video monitoring is mandatory. A minimum of eight channels of electroencephalographic (EEG) recording is recommended. An expanded EEG montage assists in differentiating a parasomnia from sleep-related seizures and might pinpoint a focal disorder. The video recording of the sleeping patient clearly demonstrates manifestations of the parasomnia (if they occur during the study) and chronicles stereotypical movements. The study should begin no later than 10 PM to avoid an artificially short sleep onset latency and should end no earlier than 6 AM to avoid missing the last rapid eye movement (REM) period. It is important to permit the patient to wake spontaneously so that a realistic, natural recording may be achieved. Having the patient drink fluids and avoid urination before settling is often helpful, since bladder distention may precipitate some parasomnias.

When patients with nocturnal enuresis are evaluated in the laboratory, uroflowmetry may be added to the montage in order to record the beginning and end of the void during sleep. Special emphasis is placed on analyzing the amplitude of delta waves, REM density, and transitional (or unscorable) stages. These unscorable stages are clinically meaningful, although many sleep laboratories do not concentrate on this area. The need for all-night EEG recordings, routine EEG, and radiographic studies depends on the presenting situation, nighttime manifestations, and clinical symptoms.

SLEEP-WAKE TRANSITION DISORDERS

Sleep-wake transition disorders are parasomnias that occur mainly during transitions from wakefulness to sleep, from sleep to wakefulness, or from one sleep stage to another. All generally occur in otherwise healthy children and are regarded as manifestations of altered physiology. All can occur in frequent episodes, and symptoms can vary from mild movements during sleep to violent, alarming behavior. All have the potential to result in discomfort, pain, anxiety, embarrassment, and disturbance of sleep.

Rhythmical Movement Disorders (Stereotyped Parasomnias)[4-13]

Although the phenomenon of stereotypical movements has been recognized for a long time, little is known of the cause. Stereotyped parasomnias are characterized by repetitive, meaningless movements or behaviors. Large muscle groups are typically involved, and the patient manifests rhythmical, repetitive movements

TABLE 10–2. International Classification of Parasomnias

Arousal Disorders
Confusional arousals
Somnambulism
Pavor nocturnus (sleep terrors)
Sleep-Wake Transition Disorders
Rhythmic movement disorders
Sleep starts
Somniloquy (sleep talking)
Nocturnal leg cramps
Parasomnias Usually Associated with REM Sleep
Nightmares
Sleep paralysis
Sleep-related priapism
Sleep-related sinus arrest
REM sleep behavior disorder
Other Parasomnias
Bruxism
Enuresis
Abnormal swallowing syndrome
Paroxysmal nocturnal dystonia
Unexplained nocturnal death syndrome
Primary snoring
Infant sleep apnea
Congenital central hypoventilation syndrome
Sudden infant death syndrome
Benign neonatal myoclonus

From Diagnostic Classification Steering Committee, Thorpy MJ, Chairman: International classification of sleep disorders: diagnostic and coding manual. Rochester, Minn, American Sleep Disorders Association, 1990, p 16, with permission.

such as *body rocking, head banging, head rolling,* and *body shuttling*. The movements typically are associated with the transition from wakefulness to sleep, are sustained into light sleep, and occur after arousal from sleep. Children are usually developmentally, behaviorally, and medically normal. Movements may be alarming in appearance, and parents often become concerned for the child's physical and mental well-being.

Stereotyped movements occur in normal infants and children. Lack of rhythmical activity during infancy has been associated with developmental delays. When stereotypical movements during wakefulness persist into older childhood and adolescence, a psychogenic component may be present. Stereotypical movements may be a form of attention getting or a mechanism of self-stimulation or self-soothing. They may also be purely functional. In normal children stereotypy seems to be *primary* and serves a developmental function, whereas in children with pathological development (e.g., autism or schizophrenia), stereotypy may be a result of several abnormal factors and is therefore *secondary*.

In normal infants rhythmical movements seem to occur during transitional stages of motor development. It has been theorized that, as a biological state, stereotypy is an attempt at transition or maintenance of various states of vigilance. Standard rotational testing indicates that children who manifest rhythmical stereotypical parasomnias have vestibular asymmetry. Stereotypical movements occur commonly at times of transition to different levels of vigilance, characteristically during the transition from wakefulness to sleep, but also during transitions from one sleep stage to another. During sleep, rhythmical movements seem to cease when the polygraphic EEG tracing shows synchronous delta frequency patterns. Rhythmical body movements have also been shown to correlate with vegetative functions and with EEG synchrony. It seems logical therefore that the vestibular system may play a significant role. Rhythmical movements of the body and head might exogenously stimulate the central vestibular system and mediate state changes that may be dysfunctional or immature. The importance of this hypothesis lies in the development of a rational approach to treatment. As yet, however, evidence is indirect and circumstantial. Further investigation is required to elucidate the function of the vestibular system in rhythmical movement disorders.

Stereotypical rhythmical movements can be observed in two thirds of normal children by 9 months of age. In the normal population the incidence of head banging ranges from 3% to 6.5%, body rocking takes place in 19.1% to 21%, and head rolling occurs in 6.3%. By 18 months of age the prevalence decreases to less than 50% and by 4 years of age to approximately 8%. The consistent decrease and spontaneous resolution of symptoms as the child matures support a developmental origin of the disorder. Rhythmical body movements are 3½ to 4 times more common in males than females. They do not seem to be significantly correlated with birth order or socioeconomic status. A familial pattern has been occasionally reported.

Symptoms most often appear by 1 year of age. Body rocking (shuttling) begins earliest, at about 6 months of age, and is characterized by rocking of the entire body while the child is supported on hands and knees (Fig. 10–2). This symptom may progress to the more violent head banging (jactatio capitis nocturna) at about 9 months of age. Head banging is characterized by forceful movement of the head in an anterior-posterior direction as shown in Figure 10–3. The head may be vigorously thrust against the mattress, against the headboard of the bed, or against the child's hands.

The average age at onset of head rolling is 10 months. The child moves the head (and occasionally the entire body) laterally from a supine position as shown in Figure 10–4. This is in contrast to head banging, in which the head is moved anteriorly-posteriorly from a prone position.

When symptoms begin, the rhythmical movements may appear normal and are not particularly troublesome. Movements may remain mild and resolve spontaneously or may progress to highly vigorous activity, shaking the crib or bed, producing loud noise, and arousing other family members. Indeed, symptoms can be violent and alarming.

Although the movements are turbulent, physical injury is rare. Cutaneous ecchymosis, callous formation, subdural hematoma, and retinal petechiae have been reported. Rhythmical movements usually decrease in intensity and often resolve spontaneously between 2 and 4 years of age; however, they may transform into another parasomnic symptom. Rarely, symptoms persist into adolescence and adulthood.

Diagnosis of rhythmical movement disorders is based on identification of characteristic symptoms in the absence of other medical or psy-

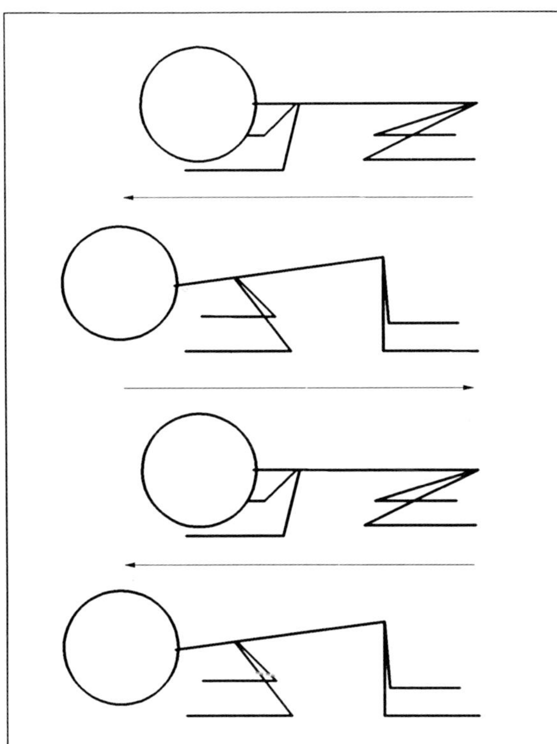

FIGURE 10–2. Schematic representation of body rocking (shuttling).

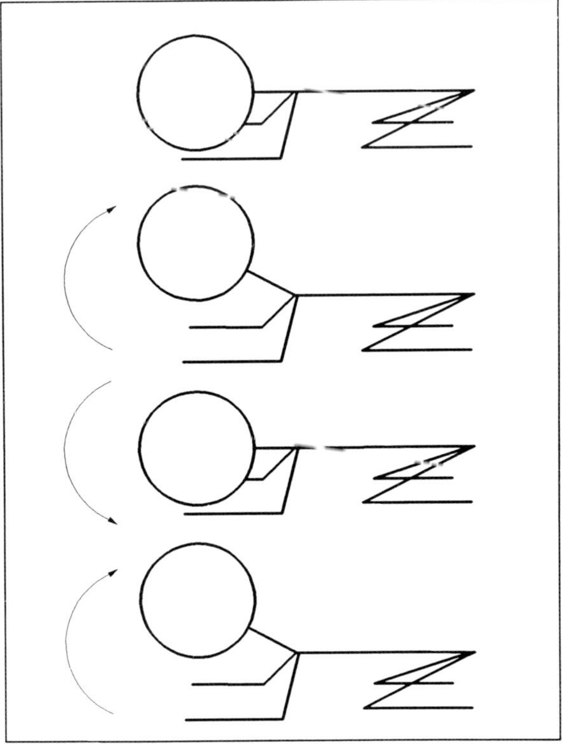

FIGURE 10–3. Schematic representation of head banging (jactatio capitis nocturna).

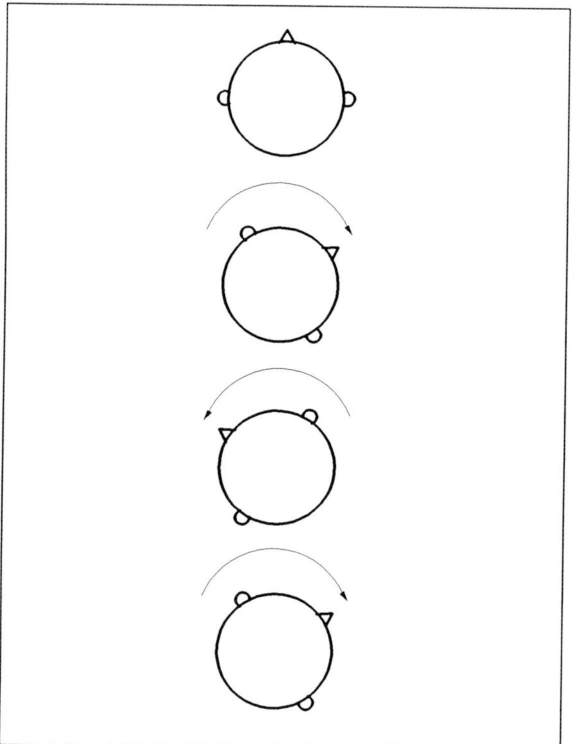

FIGURE 10–4. Schematic representation of head rolling.

chiatric disorders that may have similar symptoms. Polysomnography demonstrates typical rhythmical movements during the immediate presleep period and early in Stage 1 non-REM (NREM) sleep. Occasionally activity is noted during slow-wave sleep, but it is rare during REM sleep. No focal, paroxysmal, or epileptiform EEG activity is associated with the stereotypical activity, but a full-montage EEG may be necessary to rule out epilepsy. Sleep architecture, stage progression, and stage volumes are typically normal.

Hypnic Myoclonia (Sleep Starts)[14-18]

Also termed hypnogogic jerks, hypnic myoclonia is a sleep-wake transition disorder characterized by a sudden, single, brief muscular contraction of the legs. Occasionally patients also have contraction of the arms, head, and other postural muscles. Hypnic myoclonia typically occurs during the transition from wake to Stage 1 sleep. At times visual or sensory hallucinations or the subjective feeling of falling may occur. Sleep starts occur in most individuals at one time or another and are not considered pathological unless they are frequent and result in sleep onset insomnia. Hypnic myoclonia may occur at any age and may frighten the parents, especially if the child cries out. Injury from the massive movement is rare, but foot injuries from kicking a bedpost or crib rail may occur.

Hypnic jerks have been reported to occur in 60% to 70% of normal individuals and are considered a common component of the wake-to-sleep transition. They occur with equal frequency in males and females, and there does not seem to be a familial predisposition.

Clinically, there is a complaint of a single, massive contraction of the legs (and sometimes the arms and head) during the transition to sleep. Occasionally the contraction is unilateral and asymmetrical. A sharp cry may occur at the time of the contraction. This massive jerking movement and cry may be alarming to observers and may or may not wake the child. Sleep starts are benign and do not indicate disease or dysfunction. Affected children are developmentally normal. Polysomnography is rarely indicated; when it is performed, hypnic myoclonia is noted as the appearance of brief, high-amplitude muscle potentials during the transition from wake to Stage 1 sleep at the beginning of the sleep period. A brief arousal or full awakening may follow.

Sleep starts may be differentiated from myoclonic epilepsy by the absence of concomitant abnormal EEG discharges and clinical symptoms of myoclonus during wakefulness (as well as during other stages of sleep). Periodic limb movements (such as "periodic leg movements of sleep" and "restless leg syndrome") are brief small twitches of the lower leg muscles, lasting considerably longer than sleep starts, exhibiting a clear periodicity, and occurring during all stages of NREM sleep. Benign neonatal sleep myoclonus is a marked, fine twitching of the fingers, toes, and face during sleep in newborn infants.

Somniloquy (Sleep Talking)[1,19-21]

Somniloquy is common during childhood, is often amusing, and should be of little concern to parents. Sleep talking is a normal variant of the sleep process. Although the exact incidence is unknown, this parasomnia appears to be common. Severe outbursts and loud talking or utterances are rare but occasionally may be significant enough to disturb the sleep of parents and other family members. Clinically significant somniloquy is more common during periods of stress and febrile illnesses. The child may speak in long sentences, but most often the utterances are brief. Episodes are not associated with pathological states. Somniloquy may be precipitated by talking to the sleeping child, but the child rarely remembers the conversation. Sleep talking may be associated or concurrent with other parasomnias such as night terrors, confusional arousals, and sleep walking.

Diagnosis is based on identification of typical manifestations of coherent speech, incoherent mumbling, or utterances during the sleep period. The patient is unaware of the talking episode. The course of somniloquy is usually self-limited, but symptoms may persist for years or be transformed into other parasomnias.

Polysomnography reveals that somniloquy can occur in any stage of sleep. The polysomnogram can be helpful in recognizing sleep talking that occurs secondary to obstructive sleep apnea or a REM sleep behavior disorder.

Nocturnal Leg Cramps[22-24]

Leg pains associated with sleep are common during middle childhood and are often (perhaps inappropriately) considered analogous to growing pains. Patients have a perception of muscular tightness or aching of the lower leg, foot, or thigh. The pains may be isolated phenomena or related to other medical conditions such as diabetes mellitus, abnormalities in calcium metabolism, neuromuscular disorders, or electrolyte disturbances. The leg pains may wake the child from sleep and result in a sleep maintenance insomnia or complaints of excessive daytime sleepiness. Few complications are noted, however, and no marked psychological or social dysfunctions are identified.

Definitive data on leg pains in children are unavailable. Nocturnal leg cramps occur in about 16% of healthy adults and tend to become more frequent with age. Females are more often affected than males, although this distribution has not been shown to occur during childhood. Some familial patterns have been observed.

Patients generally complain of painful sensations, usually localized to the lower leg and foot, but pain may also occur in other major muscle groups of the leg. Discomfort may result in nocturnal arousals or may occur during the transition from sleep to wake at the end of the sleep period. Often the leg pains are diminished by rubbing, massage, or local application of heat. Diagnosis of benign nocturnal leg cramps requires the elimination of other possible causes for the clinical manifestations (e.g., metabolic abnormalities, endocrinopathies, seizure disorders, dystonia).

Polysomnography may reveal brief, *nonperiodic* bursts of muscle activity, often in the gastrocnemius muscle (although other muscle groups may reveal similar activity). Apnea is, by definition, absent. Other parasomnias may be present but usually do not account for the painful symptoms. Diagnosis is based on the presence of characteristic symptoms and the absence of other disorders that may account for the clinical manifestations.

AROUSAL DISORDERS: PARASOMNIAS ASSOCIATED WITH SLOW-WAVE SLEEP

Arousal disorders are thought to be due to impaired or "partial" arousal from slow-wave sleep. A hierarchical model may exist, since a continuum of manifestations of each of these sleep disorders seems to be present, with symptoms crossing over or occurring concomitantly. These parasomnias are thought to be associated with neurological immaturity. Symptoms most often begin in childhood and resolve spontaneously, although occasionally they persist into adolescence and adulthood. Manifestations are alarming, and injury often occurs.

Arousal disorders have bizarre, dramatic symptoms and share a number of features. All seem to occur during Stage 3 or 4 sleep; confusion, disorientation, and amnesia for the events are present; and episodes may be precipitated by forced arousal from slow-wave sleep. In contrast, forced arousal from REM sleep is most often followed by rapid awakening, clear thought processes, and dream recall.

Arousal disorders occur more frequently during periods of fever or stress, after sleep deprivation, and in patients with hypersomnolence syndromes. Stress increases the number and frequency of brief partial arousals in normal individuals, and this increase in frequency may account for stress-precipitating episodes. Slow-wave sleep rebound (increased volume of slow-wave sleep) occurs after sleep deprivation and may be an exacerbating factor.

Partial arousals normally occur at the end of slow-wave sleep periods during ascent to lighter sleep stages. Because of the depth of slow-wave sleep and the high arousal threshold in children, the manifestations of disorders of partial arousal may represent a conflict between the mechanisms generating slow-wave sleep and arousal. Chronobiological triggers that control sleep stage cycling may be more likely to result in a partial arousal if the sleep schedule is chaotic. There may be internal desynchronization, and the internal arousal stimulus may come at the "wrong time," resulting in incomplete arousal and manifesting internal characteristics of both states. As the child develops, these central nervous system mechanisms mature, synchronization occurs, and symptoms resolve spontaneously.

Confusional Arousals (Sleep Drunkenness)[25-28]

Confusional arousals or sleep drunkenness consists of partial arousals from slow-wave sleep during the first half of the sleep period. Episodes are sudden and startling and may be precipitated by forced awakenings. Children may appear awake during the episode but do not respond appropriately to commands and resist being consoled. They are confused and disoriented. Attempts to abort the "attack" may make the symptoms more severe and violent.

Factors that increase slow-wave sleep or those that impair arousal may precipitate or exacerbate confusional arousals. Hypersomnia resulting from rebound from sleep deprivation, narcolepsy, obstructive sleep apnea, or idiopathic hypersomnia, may exacerbate symptoms. Confusional arousals are often seen in patients with narcolepsy after prolonged daytime naps (those longer than 60 minutes and containing slow-wave sleep). Stress, anxiety, fever, and excessive exercise may precipitate attacks. Organic disease is rarely noted, although central nervous system lesions of the periventricular gray matter, reticular activating system, or posterior hypothalamus have been reported in some patients. Injuries during confusional arousals are common if the patient is displaced from the bed.

The exact prevalence of confusional arousals is not known. There appears to be an equal distribution between males and females. Although genetic mechanisms for transmission have not been defined, a strong familial pattern exists.

The onset of symptoms is usually before 5 years of age. Children arouse gradually from slow-wave sleep and may moan or mumble unintelligibly. Symptoms then crescendo: patients may thrash about in bed or fall from the bed to the floor. During the episode the child appears profoundly confused and disoriented. The child may be combative and aggressive, and consolation or restraint may only exacerbate the symptoms. Episodes may be as brief as a few minutes or may last for several hours. Patients usually have retrograde or anterograde amnesia for the event. There may be associated night terrors or somnambulism. Enuresis may occur during or following the episode.

Diagnosis is based on identification of confusion, disorientation, agitation, or combativeness on arousal, most often during the first half of the night, and on amnesia for the event. Rarely is a medical or psychiatric disorder found on clinical evaluation. Partial complex seizure disorders with confusional automatisms must be ruled out. Polysomnography findings may include sudden arousal from slow-wave sleep, brief periods of delta activity, Stage 1 theta patterns, recurrent microsleeps, and poorly reactive alpha activity. Focal, paroxysmal, or epileptiform activity are absent from the EEG. Evidence of obstructive sleep apnea or increased slow-wave sleep may be present. Although characteristics of other arousal disorders (e.g., sleep terrors and somnambulism) may occur, other manifestations of these disorders are usually absent. Symptoms may peak during middle childhood and then undergo spontaneous remission, deteriorate to more severe symptoms, or transform into other characteristic arousal disorders. The clinical course is usually benign (although frightening). Physical injury can occur, and the child must be protected from trauma during the episode.

Somnambulism (Sleep Walking)[28-35]

Somnambulism may vary in presentation from simple sitting up in bed to agitated running during sleep. A complex series of automatic behaviors are manifested and may appear purposeful on the surface. Like other partial arousal disorders, somnambulistic episodes occur out of slow-wave sleep, during the first third of the sleep period. Episodes may alarm family members. Patients are uncoordinated and clumsy during the walking episode. Injuries are common. Because of the high incidence of trauma during events, agitated somnambulism should be considered a potentially fatal disorder and the major goal of management should be to protect the child from harm.

Somnambulism has been reported to occur in 1% to 15% of the population. It occurs with greatest frequency during childhood, decreases significantly during adolescence, and is uncommon in adulthood. Episodes vary in frequency, intensity, and length, making parental reports inaccurate; the true incidence is therefore unknown. The sex distribution appears to be equal. A significant familial pattern has been recognized, although clear genetic transmission has not been identified. A 60% incidence when both parents were affected as children, 45% when one parent was affected, and 22% when no family history of sleep walking was reported.

Somnambulism usually begins between 4 and 8 years of age, although onset may occur at any time after the child learns to walk. Symptoms range from simple sitting up in bed to extremely agitated, semipurposeful automatisms and frantic running. The child usually wanders around the house and may perform complex tasks, such as unlocking doors, taking food from the refrigerator, and eating. At times children leave the house and roam the neighborhood. Often the behaviors are meaningless and unusual. Verbalizations may occur but are usually garbled, confused, and meaningless. Eyes are often open and the child may appear awake, but behaviors are only semipurposeful. Choreiform movements of the arms and head may occur. Enuretic episodes are common, and the child may urinate (or attempt to urinate) at unusual places around the house. During a somnambulistic episode the child is extremely difficult to wake, although complete arousal is possible. If awakened, the child is usually confused and disoriented.

The motor activity can cease spontaneously, and the child may lie down and return to sleep in an unusual place or may return to bed without ever becoming alert. Somniloquy may occur during episodes, but speech is usually incoherent.

A number of factors may precipitate somnambulistic events. Fever and sleep deprivation increase the frequency of sleep walking. Any disorder that significantly disrupts slow-wave sleep, such as obstructive sleep apnea, may precipitate events. In addition, sleep walking can be precipitated by urinary bladder distention in a susceptible patient. External noise may also trigger an event. A number of medications, including thioridazine, fluphenazine, perphenazine, desipramine, and chloral hydrate, can exacerbate the disorder.

Polysomnography typically reveals an arousal from Stage 3 or 4 sleep during the first half of the sleep period. Most of the background EEG activity is obscured by muscle artifact; however, seizure activity is absent.

Somnambulism should be differentiated from other disorders of arousal, such as confusional arousals and night terrors, although this may be difficult. Displacement from the bed and calm nocturnal wanderings are less common with confusional arousals. Night terrors more typically are associated with the appearance of intense fear and panic and are less likely to be associated with displacement from bed (although displacement from bed is more common with night terrors than with nightmares; see the next section). Intense autonomic discharges and an initial scream herald a sleep terror and are not present in somnambulism. Nocturnal seizure disorders typically reveal epileptiform discharges prior to and during the events; however, the interictal EEG may be normal. REM sleep behavior disorder has been rarely described in children; it characteristically occurs out of REM sleep in adults and is associated with clear verbalizations and more purposeful movements related to dream content.

Sleep Terrors (Pavor Nocturnus)[28,29,33-35]

Sleep terrors (or night terrors) are third in the continuum of partial arousals from slow-wave sleep. The term "sleep terror" is preferred to "night terror" to clearly differentiate this disorder from nightmares. Nightmares are "anxiety dreams" and differ significantly from sleep terrors in etiology and presentation. The onset of a sleep terror (in contrast to the gradual onset of confusional arousals) is abrupt, striking, and frightening. These arousals are associated with profound autonomic discharges and behavioral manifestations of intense fear. Table 10–3 shows how sleep terrors can be distinguished from nightmares.

As with other partial arousals, the exact prevalence of sleep terrors is unknown. They have been reported to occur in approximately 3% of prepubertal children and less than 1% of adults. Males are affected more frequently than females, and a familial pattern of occurrence has been noted.

Onset of symptoms is usually between 2 and 4 years of age, and they typically occur in children up to the age of 12 years. Although most common during childhood, sleep terrors can occur at any age. Symptoms tend to decrease during puberty and rarely persist into adolescence and adulthood. Precipitating factors include fever, bladder distention, sleep deprivation, and central nervous system depressant medication. Psychopathology is rare in children with sleep terrors but is more common in adults.

An event usually begins suddenly. The child sits upright in bed and emits a piercing scream. Severe autonomic discharge occurs. Eyes are wide open and pupils are dilated. Tachycardia, tachypnea, diaphoresis, and increased muscle tone are present. During the episode the child is unresponsive to consolation, and in fact such efforts often exacerbate autonomic and motor activity. The child may get out of bed and run hysterically around the house, colliding with walls, furniture, or windows. Frenzied fleeing episodes often result in injury to the child or to a parent who is trying to intercede. Unintelligible vocalizations and enuresis can occur. If awakened, the child is confused and disoriented and does not remember the event. In contrast to confusional arousals, episodes of sleep terrors usually last only a few minutes, subside spontaneously, and the child quickly returns to sleep. Figure 10–5 shows the characteristic pattern of sleep terrors.

Diagnosis is based on identification of the symptoms and exclusion of organic disorders. Polysomnography reveals sudden arousal from slow-wave sleep, usually during the first third of the major sleep period, although sleep terrors can occur at any time during the night. Partial arousals without motor manifestation occur more frequently in children with sleep terrors than in normal children. Autonomic discharges during these partial arousals are identified by the presence of tachycardia without full-blown symptoms.

Sleep terrors require differentiation from confusional arousals and sleep-related epilepsy with automatisms. In the latter condition the EEG may show abnormal discharges from the temporal lobe, although nasopharyngeal leads may be required to identify the focus of abnormal activity. Epileptic events may also be distinguished from disorders of partial arousal by the presence of a combination of clinical features, stereotypical behaviors, and their occurrence during any part of the sleep period and wakefulness. Identification of epileptiform activity does not rule out the presence of a partial arousal, since they may occur concomitantly.

Therapeutic Considerations

There is no clear consensus regarding when an arousal disorder requires treatment. Symp-

TABLE 10–3. Differentiation of Sleep Terrors from Nightmares

Characteristic	Sleep Terror	Nightmare
Name	Pavor nocturnus	Anxiety dream
Time of night	First third	Last third
Stage of sleep	Slow-wave sleep	REM sleep
Movements	Somnambulism common	Rare
Severity	Severe	Mild
Vocalizations	Common	Rare
Autonomic discharge	Severe/intense	Mild
Recall	Fragmented	Good
State on waking	Confused/disoriented	Function well
Injuries	75%	Rare
Violence	55%	Nonviolent
Displacement from bed	18% Run from house	None

toms are most often mild, occur less than once per month, and do not result in injury to either the child or the parents. In *mild* cases reassurance that the child is normal mentally and developmentally may be all that is necessary. A comprehensive explanation of the nature of these parasomnias should be provided. Parents should be encouraged to let the event run its course and to intervene minimally. Interventions should be focused on preventing injury and guiding the child back to bed. Too vigorous intervention may prolong the episode.

Parents can be warned of a somnambulistic episode by an alarm system (e.g., a bell placed on the doorknob of the child's room). Sleep deprivation should be avoided, and regular sleep-wake schedules should be maintained. Short daytime naps might be attempted. A period of quiet activity or relaxation techniques before bedtime should be instituted. Fluids after the nighttime meal should be limited, and the child should be encouraged to empty his or her bladder immediately before bedtime. Fever, if present, should be appropriately treated; the cause of the fever should be identified and attended to.

Severity of partial arousals is considered *moderate* when symptoms occur less than once per week and do not result in harm to the patient or to others. In these cases reassurance and a behavioral approach (including behavior training, sleep hygiene, psychotherapy, or hypnosis) have been successful.

In *severe* cases, when episodes occur almost nightly or are associated with injury, nondrug approaches are considered first. Drug treatment, when used, should be prescribed for a short time and should be used in conjunction with a behavioral approach. Medication should be discontinued when behavioral therapy begins to take effect. The most effective and most commonly used drug is diazepam, which is given in small doses at bedtime. Prolonged use of medication increases the potential for side effects and complications, as well as chronic disruption of sleep architecture. Young children generally respond well to both behavioral and medicinal approaches. Adolescent and adult patients with partial arousal disorders typically respond poorly to any form or combination of therapy.

PARASOMNIAS USUALLY ASSOCIATED WITH REM SLEEP

The parasomnias previously discussed are related to dysfunctions in sleep state transitions and partial arousal from NREM Stage 3 and Stage 4 sleep. Parasomnias have also been reported to occur during REM sleep. In most cases the manifestations of NREM and REM parasomnias are strikingly dissimilar and they can often be differentiated on clinical grounds alone. On occasion, certain REM sleep parasomnias may have symptoms similar to those of partial arousal disorders. Some REM sleep parasomnias occur frequently in children (e.g., nightmares), whereas others are extremely rare (e.g., REM sleep behavior disorder). Disorders rarely encountered during childhood are included because their importance to the practitioner may become clear when they are more completely understood and dysfunctions associated with the sleeping state are further delineated in children.

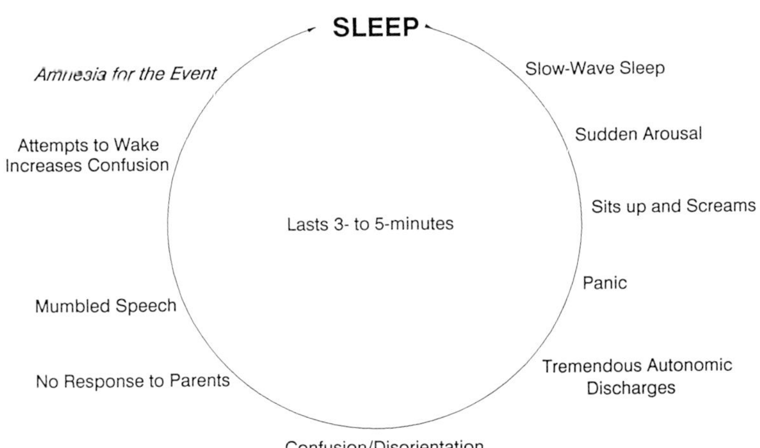

FIGURE 10–5. Characteristic pattern of sleep terrors.

Nightmares: Anxiety Dreams[1,36-41]

A nightmare is a long, frightening dream that awakens the individual from REM sleep (less commonly from Stage 1 sleep). The person clearly recalls the disturbing dream and may have anxiety and autonomic manifestations. After awakening the individual is oriented to the environment with clear sensorium. Dream content usually involves an immediate and credible threat to the individual's survival, security, or self-esteem. This threat differentiates the nightmare from "bad dreams," which tend to occur during states of depression. Bad dreams are disturbing to the individual but usually are not associated with an abrupt arousal or with autonomic manifestations.

"Dream anxiety attack" is a descriptor used to differentiate nightmares from sleep terrors. Sleep terrors are associated with considerably more intense autonomic discharge, arise out of slow-wave sleep, and usually are not recalled on awakening.

All children, adolescents, and adults experience occasional nightmares. Prevalence data are not clear, but an estimated 10% to 50% of children between 3 and 5 years of age experience dream anxiety attacks frequently enough to cause parental concern. The age of onset parallels the development of dreams, which are first noted between 3 and 6 years of age. There seems to be an equal sex distribution, and no clear familial pattern has been recognized.

Dream anxiety attacks are often associated with the longest, most intense REM period, during the last third of the night. Movements are rare because of REM hypotonia, but arousal from sleep with clear mentation is typical. Manifestations are generally mild, and vocalizations are rare. Although autonomic activity increases during nightmares, it is generally mild. There is good recall for the disturbing dream, and the child functions well on waking. Nightmares are generally not associated with violent outbursts, no displacement from the bed occurs, and injuries are uncommon. Return to sleep is generally delayed, but the child often responds well to parental intervention.

Diagnosis of dream anxiety attacks is based on identification of the mild manifestations of disturbing dreams occurring during the early morning hours, absence of intense autonomic activation, clear recall of the dream, appropriate functioning and alertness on awakening, and a good response to parental interventions. Polysomnography reveals an abrupt arousal from REM sleep. The REM period from which the child awakens is usually the longest and most intense period of the night. The attack typically occurs late in the sleep period, during early morning hours, and is associated with mild tachycardia, tachypnea, and heart and respiratory variability. Increased REM eye movement density is noted. Abnormal EEG activity is absent.

Nightmares must be differentiated from sleep terrors and REM sleep behavior disorder. Sleep terrors are usually more vivid, are frightening to the observer, occur during the first third of the sleep period, and are associated with severe autonomic discharges. The child has fragmented recall, is confused on waking, may sleep walk agitatedly, and may suffer injuries. REM sleep behavior disorder has been infrequently described in childhood and occurs most commonly in elderly patients. Adults have sudden, explosive, partial arousal from REM sleep and significant motor activity (apparently "acting out" their dream).

Sleep Paralysis[26,27,42-45]

Sleep paralysis is characterized by a period of inability to move voluntarily at the beginning of a sleep period (hypnogogic) or immediately after awakening from sleep (hypnopompic). The patient is conscious and vigilant to the environment but feels paralyzed. All muscle groups, except the diaphragm and extraocular muscles, are involved. Active inhibition of alpha motor neurons is present and similar to that seen in REM sleep and cataplexy. A sensation of difficulty breathing often occurs, and episodes can be frightening. Sleep paralysis lasts only several minutes and subsides spontaneously. The patient can sometimes abort attacks by being touched by another person or by rapid movements of the eyes. Hypnogogic or hypnopompic hallucinations are unusual but add to the person's anxiety when they occur.

Isolated episodes of sleep paralysis occur in healthy individuals. More frequent events occur in patients with narcolepsy and in "familial sleep paralysis." The sex distribution is equal in the isolated form of the disorder; the familial form shows a female preponderance. Sleep paralysis appears to be transmitted in an X-linked dominant pattern.

Onset usually takes place during adolescence, but symptoms may begin during childhood. Children often have difficulty describing the events and may appear asleep for the duration of the episode. Parents are frequently unaware of the occurrence, since the atonia can be aborted by touching or shaking.

The clinical course varies significantly between individuals. Most episodes are isolated and are provoked by sleep deprivation, excessive sleepiness, stress, irregular sleep-wake schedules, or acute changes in sleep phase. Sleep paralysis runs a more chronic course in patients with narcolepsy and in the familial form of the disorder.

Diagnosis is based on identification of the symptoms, which are usually obvious. Sleep paralysis associated with narcolepsy can be differentiated from the isolated form by the absence of chronic daytime sleepiness, sleep attacks, cataplexy precipitated by emotions, and hypnogogic hallucinations. Syncope also occurs during wakefulness and is commonly associated with altered levels of consciousness.

Polysomnography usually reveals a significant decrease in skeletal muscle tone in the presence of a normal waking EEG pattern and conjugate eye movements. Occasionally patients enter sleep during an episode of sleep paralysis and have an EEG pattern consistent with Stage 1 sleep. True sleep onset REM periods may occur. A Multiple Sleep Latency Test may be required to differentiate these episodes from sleep paralysis associated with narcolepsy.

Sleep-Related Painful Penile Erections[1]

Penile tumescence occurs during REM sleep at all ages. Rarely, penile pain occurs during these erections, resulting in arousal from sleep and REM sleep disruption. Symptoms of excessive daytime sleepiness and insomnia may occur. Although this disorder can occur at any age, it is exceedingly rare during childhood and is most common in middle-aged men. Interestingly, tumescence during the waking state is normal and painless. No specific abnormalities of the genitalia have been recognized, but the disorder has been noted in patients with Peyronie's disease, priapism, and sickle cell anemia. Polysomnography reveals arousal from REM sleep that is associated with penile tumescence, and the patient reports dream interruption and awakening because of pain. Differential diagnosis includes penile disorders, such as Peyronie's disease, balanitis, or phimosis. These disorders are usually evident clinically and are easy to differentiate from the sleep disorder. Other sleep disorders may be present but do not account for the symptoms.

REM Sleep Behavior Disorder[46-49]

REM sleep behavior disorder (RBD) has recently been described in adults, but only a few cases of a similar syndrome during childhood has been reported. RBD is an unusual disorder characterized by the appearance of elaborate, sometimes purposeful movement during REM sleep. Patients have a paradoxical increase in muscle tone and seem to be acting out their dreams. Violent behavior such as punching, kicking, leaping out of bed, and running is reported and often corresponds to dream mentation. Injuries to the patient and to bed partners are common. Episodes usually occur during the first REM period of the night, approximately 90 minutes after sleep onset.

RBD usually begins during late adulthood and progresses over a variable period. Although cases in pediatric patients have been rare, further understanding of this disorder may reveal the incidence and prevalence to be higher than current descriptions suggest. The majority of cases are idiopathic, but neurological disorders have been identified in approximately 40% of affected individuals.

Polysomnography reveals increased muscle tone that persists throughout sleep. Patients often have a paradoxical increase in muscle tone during REM sleep, increased phasic activity, and excessive limb or body jerking. Complex behaviors occur out of REM sleep, but no epileptiform activity is noted on EEG during the complex movements. Interestingly, REM sleep behavior disorder in adults responds well to benzodiazepines, especially clonazepam.

OTHER PARASOMNIAS[1]

The classification "other parasomnias" comprises a group of disorders that lack characteristics associated with REM sleep, slow-wave sleep, or sleep stage transitions. Future research in these disorders may reveal commonalities that are now obscure. The International Classification of Sleep Disorders identifies 11 such parasomnias, including nocturnal bruxism, sleep enuresis, sleep-related abnormal swallowing syndrome, nocturnal paroxysmal dystonia, sudden unexplained nocturnal death syndrome, primary snoring, infant sleep apnea, congenital central hypoventilation syndrome, sudden infant death syndrome, and benign neonatal myoclonus. A number of these disorders (e.g., enuresis, infant sleep apnea, sudden infant death syndrome) either occur exclusively in childhood or are frequently encountered by the pediatric practitioner. They are discussed in detail in other chapters and are mentioned here because of their nosological classification as parasomnias.

Sleep Bruxism: Tooth Grinding[50-54]

Sleep bruxism is forceful grinding or rhythmical clenching of the teeth during sleep. It is a result of involuntary, repetitive contractions of the masseter, temporalis, and pterygoid muscles. A loud, unmistakable grinding noise is produced without the patient's awareness. In contrast to sleep bruxism, diurnal bruxism consists of voluntary or habitual grinding of the teeth, is less profound (although dental damage may be similar), and produces minimal noise. Predisposing factors for the development of bruxism include minor abnormalities of the teeth, malocclusion, stress, and anxiety.

Although the true prevalence of sleep bruxism is unknown, an estimated 5% to 20% of children manifest symptoms. Bruxism has been reported in more than 50% of children with a mean age of onset of 10½ years. Dental evidence of bruxism can be identified in 10% to 20% of the general population. The disorder appears to have an equal sex distribution and is most commonly seen in children and young adults. As with many other parasomnias, a familial pattern without clear genetic transmission can be demonstrated. No longitudinal studies demonstrating the natural course of sleep bruxism have been published.

Sleep bruxism usually begins during late childhood and adolescence, although the disorder may begin at an earlier age. A loud, unpleasant sound is produced by violent grinding of the teeth. Episodes occur paroxysmally in bursts of 5 to 15 seconds or longer and are often repeated many times during the sleep period. The patient is typically unaware of the grinding noise, although it frequently arouses other members of the household. Daytime symptoms include jaw and face pain, painful teeth, morning headaches, chronic wear of the crowns of the teeth, periodontal tissue damage, and bleeding from the gums. Resorption of alveolar bone, hypertrophy of the masseter and temporalis muscles, and temporomandibular joint (TMJ) dysfunction can occur. Dental abnormalities are the most striking complication.

Diagnosis is made by identification of the loud, unmistakable sound of bruxism in the absence of other medical or psychiatric disorders that may produce abnormal movements during sleep. A comprehensive dental examination is essential. Abnormal wearing down of the crowns of the teeth is characteristic. Polysomnography reveals paroxysmal, rhythmical muscle activity of the chin, temporalis, and masseter muscle groups at approximately 1-second intervals for 5 to 15 seconds or longer. Episodes of bruxism occur most commonly during Stage 2 NREM sleep, although bruxism has been reported in all stages of sleep (including REM sleep). During the events the EEG may be obscured by muscle artifact, but no focal or epileptiform activity is noted.

A number of therapeutic approaches have been recommended, but the most important factor is appropriate dental management. A mouth guard (a rubber appliance fitted to the teeth) is worn at night to prevent damage to the teeth. It does not prevent episodes of bruxism, however, and is used primarily as a preventive dental intervention. If stress or anxiety is a prominent feature, efforts to alleviate the cause may be helpful. Treatment of dental or anatomical abnormalities, if present, may or may not alter the course of sleep bruxism.

Sleep Enuresis

Controversy over the classification of enuresis during sleep has existed for many years. In the International Classification of Sleep Disorders this disorder has recently been categorized as a parasomnia. Sleep enuresis is characterized by involuntary urination during sleep after 5 years of age. Persistent bedwetting in the absence of a urological, medical, or psychiatric disorder is considered *primary sleep enuresis*. *Secondary sleep enuresis* is the term used for the recurrence of bedwetting after a period of 3 to 6 months of dry nights has been achieved. Bedwetting is a symptom of a heterogeneous group of disorders ranging from organic disease (e.g., diabetes mellitus) to neurodevelopmental disorders (e.g., small functional bladder capacity, deficient nocturnal vasopressin secretion) to psychogenic problems. Figure 10–1 presents one proposed classification. A complete discussion of sleep enuresis may be found in Chapter 12.

Abnormal Swallowing Syndrome[1]

Abnormal swallowing syndrome is a disorder described in adults, but its symptoms are similar to those in children with swallowing abnormalities of unidentifiable cause. Further research and understanding of these sleep-related symptoms are needed to describe the syndrome in childhood.

Adult patients cough, choke, and awake from sleep because of inadequate swallowing and aspiration of pooled oral and pharyngeal secretions. The onset typically occurs during middle age and may include insomnia, excessive daytime sleepiness, and repeated pulmonary infections. Symptoms are often similar to those of obstructive sleep apnea syndrome, and polysomnography may be required to differentiate sleep-related swallowing abnormalities from sleep-disordered respiration. The sleep study reveals 5- to 10-minute arousals after a period of coughing or choking. There is typically evidence of restless sleep and noisy respiration. Slow-wave sleep may be absent. The patient does not have a true obstructive sleep apnea. Radiographic studies during sleep reveal abnormal patterns of swallowing, pooling of secretions in the hypopharynx, and tracheal aspiration.

Gastroesophageal reflux during sleep may present similar symptoms, but the complaints in adults generally center on chest pain, heartburn, or other symptoms of acid reflux. Endoscopy may be necessary to rule out other abnormalities of the larynx and esophagus.

Hypnogenic Paroxysmal Dystonia[55-58]

Hypnogenic paroxysmal dystonia is a rare disorder characterized by stereotypical choreoathetotic movements and dystonic posturing during NREM sleep. Symptoms may begin in infancy and be mistaken for normal (or abnormal) behavior patterns or other stereotypical movement disorders. Episodes may be brief, lasting less than a minute, or prolonged, persisting for hours. Eyes are often open, and vocalizations may occur. If episodes occur frequently or recur during a single sleep period, significant sleep disruption and insomnia may result. Rhythmical, stereotypical movements (e.g., kicking, thrashing) of the limbs or trunk are associated with dystonic posturing of the hands, feet, arms, legs, or face. At the termination of an episode patients are often coherent but rapidly return to sleep.

Polysomnography reveals episodes arising out of Stage 2 NREM sleep (although the disorder has been reported to occur in slow-wave sleep as well). An EEG pattern of arousal may occur a few seconds before an episode. Significant movement artifact is seen in the EEG, but clear epileptiform activity is absent. Results of radiographic studies and magnetic resonance imaging are normal. Whether hypnogenic paroxysmal dystonia is associated with central nervous system (or other) disease is unknown.

Symptoms generally run a chronic course and may persist for many years. Carbamazepine in small doses has ameliorated symptoms in some patients.

Sleep-Related Breathing Disorders

Sleep-related breathing disorders include primary snoring, infant sleep apnea, congenital central hypoventilation syndrome, and sudden infant death syndrome. They are comprehensively discussed in Chapter 11.

Benign Neonatal Sleep Myoclonus[59,60]

Benign neonatal sleep myoclonus consists of asynchronous twitching or jerking of the hands, feet, arms, legs, face, or trunk during quiet sleep. These jerking movements usually begin during the first week of life, occur in brief clusters lasting 1 second or less, and can vary in presentation (e.g., flexion/extension, abduction/adduction). Movements resolve spontaneously, but occasionally persist beyond the neonatal period. The cause is not identified, and the symptoms run a benign course. It is important to differentiate benign neonatal sleep myoclonus from significant pathological states, including primary convulsive disorders, seizures associated with anoxic encephalopathy, systemic or central nervous system infections, infantile spasms, and metabolical abnormalities.

REFERENCES

1. Association of Sleep Disorders Centers: Diagnostic classification of sleep and arousal disorders. Prepared by the Sleep Disorders Classification Committee, H.P. Roffwarg, Chairman. Sleep 1979;2:1-137.

2. Diagnostic Classification Steering Committee, Thorpy MJ, Chairman: International classification of sleep disorders: diagnostic and coding manual. Rochester, Minn, American Sleep Disorders Association, 1990.
3. Golbin AZ: Pathological sleep in children. Leningrad, Medicine Publishers, 1979.
4. deLissovoy V: Head banging in early childhood: a study of incidence. J Pediatr 1961;58:803.
5. Golbin AZ: Movements as an active factor in organization of sleep. Hum Physiol 1976;3:354.
6. Kravitz H et al: A study of head-banging in infants and children. Dis Nerv Syst 1960;21:203.
7. Lewis MH, Baumeister AA, and Mailman RB: Aneirobiological alternative to the perceptual reinforcement hypothesis of stereotyped behavior: a commentary on "self-stimulatory behavior and perceptual reinforcement." J Appl Behav Anal 1987;20:253.
8. Lourie RS: The role of rhythmic patterns in childhood. Am J Psychiatry 1949;105:653.
9. Lovaas I, Newsom C, and Hickman C: Self-stimulatory behavior and perceptual reinforcement. J Appl Behav Anal 1987;20:45.
10. Sallustro MA and Atwell CW: Body rocking, head banging, and head rolling in normal children. J Pediatr 1978;93:704.
11. Schwartz SS, Gallagher RJ, and Berkson G: Normal repetitive and abnormal stereotyped behavior of nonretarded infants and young mentally retarded children. Am J Ment Dis 1986;90:625.
12. Klackenburg G: Rhythmic movements in infancy and early childhood. Acta Paediatr Scand Suppl 1971;224:74.
13. Thorpy AJ and Glovinsky P: Jactatio capitis nocturna. In Kryger M, Roth T, and Dement WC (eds): Principles and practice of sleep medicine. Philadelphia, WB Saunders, 1989, pp 648-654.
14. Foulkes D: The psychology of sleep. New York, Scribner's, 1966.
15. Oswald I: Sudden bodily jerks on falling asleep. Brain 1959;82:92.
16. Carskadon MA and Dement WC: Normal human sleep: an overview. In Kryger M, Roth T, and Dement WC (eds): Principles and practice of sleep medicine. Philadelphia, WB Saunders, 1989, p 10.
17. Broughton R: Pathological fragmentary myoclonus, intensified sleep starts and hypnagogic foot tremor: three unusual sleep-related disorders. In Koella WP (ed): Sleep 1986. New York, Fischer-Verlag, 1988, pp 240-243.
18. Parkes JD: Sleep and its disorders. London, WB Saunders, 1985, p 195.
19. Rechtschaffen A, Goodenough D, and Shapiro A: Patterns of sleep talking. Arch Gen Psychiatry 1962;7:418.
20. Arkin AM: Sleep talking: a review. J Nerv Ment Dis 1966;143:101.
21. Klackenberg G: Incidence of parasomnias in children in a general population. In Guilleminault C (ed): Sleep and its disorders in children. New York, Raven Press, 1987, p 104.
22. Jacobsen JH et al: Familial nocturnal cramping. Sleep 1986;9:54.
23. Saskin P et al: Sleep and nocturnal leg cramps. Sleep 1988;11:307.
24. Weiner IH and Weiner HL: Nocturnal leg muscle cramps. JAMA 1980;244:2332.
25. Gastaut H and Broughton R: A clinical and polygraphic study of episodic phenomena during sleep. In Wortis J (ed): Recent Advances in Biological Psychiatry, vol 7. New York, Plenum Press, 1965, pp 197-223.
26. Guilleminault C: Narcolepsy and its differential diagnosis. In Guilleminault C (ed): Sleep and its disorders in children. New York, Raven Press, 1987, p 182.
27. Aldrich MS: Cardinal manifestations of sleep disorders. In Kryger MH, Roth T, and Dement WC (eds): Principles and practice of sleep medicine. Philadelphia, WB Saunders, 1989, p 314.
28. Ferber R: Sleepwalking, confusional arousals, and sleep terrors in the child. In Kryger MH, Roth T, and Dement WC (eds): Principles and practice of sleep medicine. Philadelphia, WB Saunders. 1989, p 641.
29. Broughton R: Sleep disorders: disorders of arousal? Science 1968;159:1070.
30. Gastaut H and Broughton R: A clinical and polygraphic study of episodic phenomena during sleep. Rec Adv Biol Psychiatry 1965;7:197.
31. Kales A et al: Somnambulism: psychophysiological correlates. I. All-night EEG studies. Arch Gen Psychiatry 1966;14:586.
32. Bawkin H: Sleep-walking in twins. Lancet 1970;2:446.
33. Kales A et al: Sleep walking and night terrors related to febrile illness. Am J Psychiatry 1979;136:1214.
34. Kales A et al: Hereditary factors in sleepwalking and night terrors. Br J Psychiatry 1980;137:111.
35. Broughton R: Childhood sleep walking, sleep terrors and enuresis nocturna: their pathophysiology and differentiation from nocturnal epileptic seizures. In Sleep 1978, Basel, S Karger, 1980, pp 103-111.
36. Fisher CJ et al: A psychophysiological study of nightmares. JAMA 1970;18:747.
37. Gastaut H and Broughton R: Paroxysmal psychological events and certain phases of sleep. Percept Mot Skills 1963;17:362.
38. Hartman E: The nightmare: the psychology and biology of terrifying dreams. New York, Basic Books, 1984.
39. Hartman E: Normal and abnormal dreams. In Kryger MH, Roth T, and Dement WC (eds): Priniciples and practice of sleep medicine. Philadelphia, WB Saunders, 1989, p 192.
40. Mack JE: Nightmares and the human conflict. Boston, Little, Brown, 1970.
41. Foulkes D: Children's dreams: longitudinal studies. New York, Wiley, 1982.
42. Guilleminault C: Narcolepsy syndrome. In Kryger MH, Roth T, and Dement WC: Principles and practice of sleep medicine. Philadelphia, WB Saunders, 1989, p 339.
43. Hishikawa Y: Sleep paralysis. In Guilleminault C, Dement WC, and Passouant P (eds): Narcolepsy. New York, Spectrum, 1979, pp 97-124.
44. Parkes JD: Sleep and its disorders. London, WB Saunders, 1985, pp 202-205.
45. Penn NE, Kripke DF, and Scharff J: Sleep paralysis among medical students. J Psychol 1981;107:247.
46. Schenck C et al: Chronic behavioral disorders of human REM sleep: a new category of parasomnia. Sleep 1986;9:293.
47. Schenck CH, Hurwitz TD, and Mahowald MW: REM sleep behavior disorder. Am J Psychiatry 1988;145:652.
48. Schenck CH et al: REM behavior disorder in a 10-year old girl and aperiodic REM and NREM sleep movements in an 8-year old brother. Sleep Res 1986;15:162.

49. Mahowald MW and Schenck CH: REM sleep behavior disorder. In Kryger MH, Roth T, and Dement WC (eds): Priniciples and practice of sleep medicine. Philadelphia, WB Saunders, 1989, pp 389-401.
50. Parkes JD: Sleep and its disorders. London, WB Saunders, 1985, pp 201-202.
51. Ramfjord S: Bruxism: a clinical and electromyographic study. J Am Dent Assoc 1961;62:21.
52. Yemm R: Variations in the electrical activity of the human masseter muscle occurring in association with emotional stress. Arch Oral Biol 1969;14:873.
53. Hartman E: Bruxism. In Kryger MH, Roth T, and Dement WC (eds): Principles and practice of sleep medicine. Philadelphia, WB Saunders, 1989, pp 385-388.
54. Ware JC and Rugh J: Destructive bruxism: sleep stage relationship. Sleep 1988;11:172.
55. Lugaresi E and Cirignotta F: Hypnogenic paroxysmal dystonia: epileptic seizure or a new syndrome? Sleep 1981;4:129.
56. Lugaresi E and Cirignotta F: Two variants of nocturnal paroxysmal dystonia with attacks of short and long duration. In Degen R and Niedermeyer E (eds): Epilepsy, sleep and sleep deprivation. Elsevier Science, 1984, pp 169-173.
57. Lee BI et al: Familial paroxysmal hypnogenic dystonia. Neurology 1985;35:1357.
58. Rosenberg RS and Pasternak JF: Nocturnal paroxysmal dystonia resembling tonic-clinic seizures. Presented at a meeting of the Association of Professional Sleep Societies, June 27 – July 1, 1990, Minneapolis.
59. Resnick RJ et al: Benign neonatal sleep myoclonus: relationship to sleep states. Arch Neurol 1986;43:266.
60. Coulter DL and Allen RJ: Benign neonatal sleep myoclonus. Arch Neurol 1982;39:191.

11

Sleep-Disordered Respiration in Childhood

Dysfunction of breathing during sleep has long been recognized as a major problem affecting the lives and well-being of children and their families. Extraordinary efforts have been focused on investigation of these problems. Although significant progress in description of various clinical abnormalities has been made, the exact causes of sleep-disordered respiration during infancy and childhood have not been determined. Disorders of breathing during sleep are known to be common. Loud snoring was once thought to be normal phenomenon, but it is actually a symptom of some degree of upper airway obstruction. Abnormalities of breathing during sleep also have profound influences on health and can result in significant morbidity. Sequelae range from sudden, unexpected death to school failure. This chapter is intended to provide the practitioner with an overview of what is known about breathing and sleep in infancy and childhood, an understanding of various methods of diagnosis, and an approach to treatment and long-term management of these common disorders. A careful, systematic evaluation of the child with suspected sleep-disordered breathing is essential for accurate diagnosis and appropriate management.

CONTROL OF BREATHING DURING SLEEP IN INFANTS AND CHILDREN

Changes in Respiratory Activity During Sleep

It has long been recognized that respiratory patterns differ during wakefulness and sleep. There is considerable variation of respiratory patterns between non–rapid eye movement (NREM) and REM sleep (Table 11–1), as well as between tonic REM and phasic REM sleep.

During NREM sleep, respiratory rate is decreased and follows a monotonously regular pattern when compared with those of wakefulness and REM sleep.[1-3] This breathing pattern appears to be due to a reduction in the number of active respiratory neurons and a decreased level of activity in those remaining active.[4] Resistance to airflow increases because of a decrease in upper airway muscle tone.[5,6] Minute ventilation decreases and tidal volume increases because of an increased duration of inspiration.[1] Other significant changes also occur: response to changes in carbon dioxide tension decreases, response

TABLE 11–1. Respiratory Activity in NREM and REM Sleep

NREM Sleep	REM Sleep
1. Respiratory rate is slower than in wakefulness or REM sleep.	1. Tidal volume decreases from wakefulness and NREM sleep.
2. Peak airflow and pressure developed against airway occlusion decreases from wakefulness.	2. Accessory muscles of respiration become hypotonic or atonic.
3. Upper airway resistance increases.	3. Upper airway muscles become hypotonic or atonic.
4. Tidal volume increases.	4. Irregular breathing occurs and apneas and hypopneas occur.
5. Minute ventilation decreases.	5. Ventilatory response to hypercapnia and hypoxia significantly decreases.
6. Response to hypercapnia decreases.	6. Laryngeal and diaphragmatic responses to occlusions are inconsistent and variable.
7. Response to hypoxia decreases.	7. Breathing is independent of variations in chemoreceptor, vagal, or thoracic afferent activity.
8. Ventilatory and muscle response to airway occlusion decreases.	

to changes in oxygen concentration is diminished, and ventilatory response to airway obstruction is lessened.[7-10]

During REM sleep a combination of reduced airflow rates[1,2] and shorter inspiratory times[1,11] results in tidal volumes that are less than those in NREM sleep and wakefulness. Because of skeletal muscle atonia the intercostal muscles do not participate in breathing.[12,13] Muscles of the upper airway further lose tone and become hypotonic or atonic,[14-16] and laryngeal and diaphragmatic responses to occlusion become inconsistent and variable.[17]

Breathing during REM sleep is controlled in part by processes that are state specific. Complex and even antagonistic effects at different levels of the nervous system occur, resulting in extreme variability of respiration. Apneas and hyperpneas are frequently noted. In addition, during phasic activity, *ventilatory response to chemical stimuli and the responses to other respiratory reflexes are significantly weakened.*[18,19]

Upper Airway During Sleep

Upper airway patency depends on the activity and tone of palatal, laryngeal, and genioglossal musculature. Motor neurons of these muscle groups are actively inhibited during REM sleep.[16,20,21] Clearly, therefore, muscle hypotonia and atonia that occur in REM sleep are deleterious to airflow, ventilation, and gas exchange.

Upper airway sensory stimuli are also important for maintenance of a patent pharynx. In the absence of pharyngeal stimulation by airflow, resulting from anesthesia of the pharyngeal mucosa or from bypass of the pharynx through a tracheostomy tube, a significant loss of genioglossal muscle activity can be demonstrated.[22] Maintenance of adequate respiratory function therefore depends on intact anatomy of the upper airway, is influenced by central neurophysiological mechanisms, and is state dependent.

Neonatal Ventilatory Patterns

Fetuses make episodic breathing movements.[23,24] Although the reason for the episodic nature of these breathing movements is obscure, they have been hypothesized to represent predecessors of postnatal breaths and may constitute an in utero "training program."[25] However, since fetal respiratory activity is extremely variable and since respiratory silence can occur for hours in the absence of pathology, absence of breathing movement cannot be used to predict the presence of distress.

Sleep states significantly modulate respiratory patterns and ventilation during postnatal life.[26-31] Control of respiratory timing is complex and apparently central in origin.[25] At 1 week of age, respiratory rates are higher in active sleep (REM) than in quiet sleep (NREM).[29,30,32] This increase in respiratory rate results in a higher minute ventilation during active sleep than during quiet sleep. In the first few months of life, inspiratory and expiratory times are longer during quiet sleep.[27] Shorter inspiratory and expiratory times during active sleep in newborns suggests that the termination of neural inspiratory and expiratory activities occurs earlier in this sleep state. In normal sleeping infants, tidal volume and the respiratory cycle time decrease with increasing frequency of rapid eye movements.[33] Variability in the respiratory cycle and tidal volume is two to four times greater in active sleep than in quiet sleep.[26,30] Variability of the respiratory cycle seems to be due primarily to variations in expiratory time, suggesting that central activation of inspiratory effort is highly irregular during active sleep and accounts for a majority of the breathing irregularities identified in that sleep state.

Respiratory Pauses During Sleep

Apnea is the cessation of respiratory airflow.[34] Respiratory pauses may be central or diaphragmatic (secondary to absence of respiratory effort), obstructive, or a combination of central and obstructive (mixed apnea). Short central apneas can be normal. During infancy, an apnea is considered pathological if it lasts more than 20 seconds or is shorter but accompanied by cardiovascular or neurological symptoms (cyanosis, abrupt marked pallor, hypotonia, bradycardia).

Periodic breathing is a breathing pattern characterized by three or more respiratory pauses of greater than 3 seconds' duration with less than 20 seconds of normal respiration between pauses (Fig. 11–1).[34] Periodic breathing can be normal, but if it constitutes more than 5% of the total sleep time, it is considered pathological. In premature infants periodic breathing with pathological apneas is termed apnea of prematurity. This usually resolves by 37 weeks' gestation but may persist several weeks past term.

Respiratory pauses in premature and term newborn infants are common. Three types of pauses are seen: central (Fig. 11–2), obstructive (Fig. 11–3), and mixed (Fig. 11–4). A study of the frequency distribution and ventilatory correlates of the various types of apneas[35] suggests that (1) apneas in the newborn and early infancy are primarily central in origin, and central apneas are more frequent in preterm than in term infants; (2) the higher rate of central apneas in healthy preterm infants accounts almost entirely for their higher rate of apnea; (3) a significant decrease in the rate of apnea occurs during the first 4 months after birth; and (4) preterm infants show longer respiratory pauses in both quiet sleep and active sleep when compared with term infants. A maturation pattern in respiratory pauses can be discerned by 3 months of age.

During sleep, premature infants breathe in a manner similar to Cheyne-Stokes breathing.[36] Periodic breathing occasionally resolves when the ambient oxygen concentration is increased. Central sensitivity to arterial oxygen tension (PaO_2) changes is apparently increased, possibly because the response to changes in arterial carbon dioxide tension ($PaCO_2$) is decreased.[37-39]

Additional factors can exacerbate respiratory center dysfunction and increase the risk for apnea in a preterm infant. Irregular breathing patterns occur (or worsen) when preterm infants

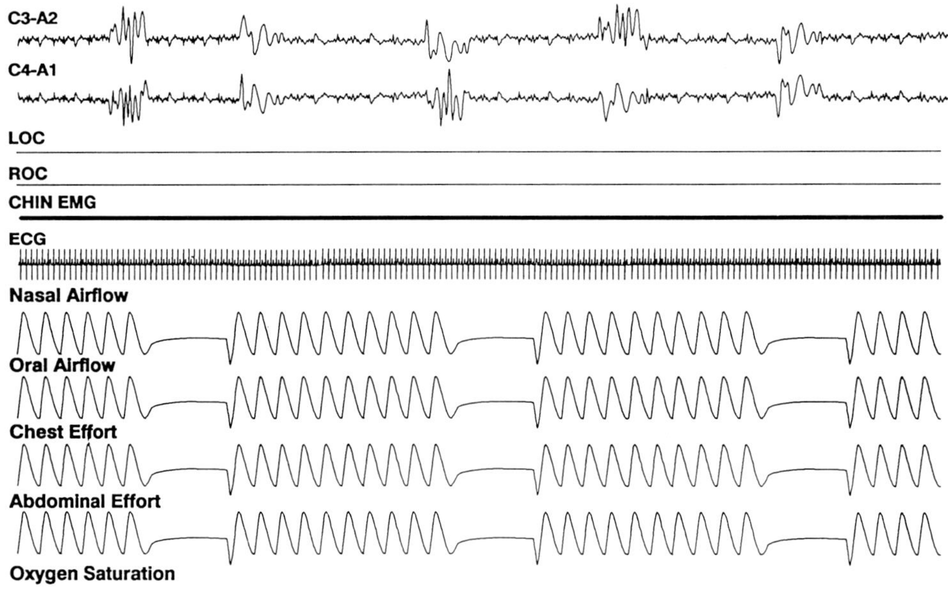

FIGURE 11–1. Periodic breathing in infants. Brief respiratory pauses (3 seconds or longer) are separated by periods of normal respiration (less than 20 seconds in length). A tracé alternant EEG pattern, tonic EMG, electromyography, and absence of eye movements characterize quiet sleep in this infant. Note that there are no significant oxygen desaturation or ECG changes during this episode of periodic breathing.

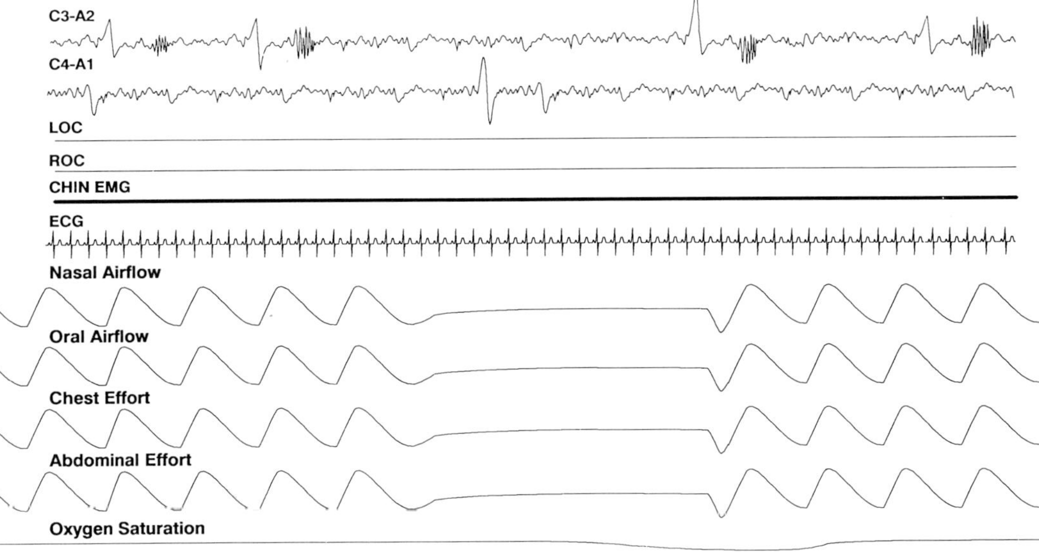

FIGURE 11–2. Central apnea. There is cessation of nasal and oral airflow with coincident absence of respiratory effort. Mild oxygen desaturation occurs. No arousal from the respiratory event is noted.

become anemic, and the pattern of respiration improves after correction of anemia. After transfusion the duration of periodic breathing decreases, the number of respiratory pauses lasting 5 to 20 seconds decreases, and the total duration of respiratory pauses (excluding pauses during periodic breathing) is significantly lower.[40]

In term infants periodic breathing occurs almost exclusively during active sleep.[41] Periodic breathing is rare after the age of 3 to 4 months in normal term infants, and those infants who exhibit periodic breathing rarely have cardiovascular or neurological abnormalities.[25] Respiratory pauses and irregularities are considered

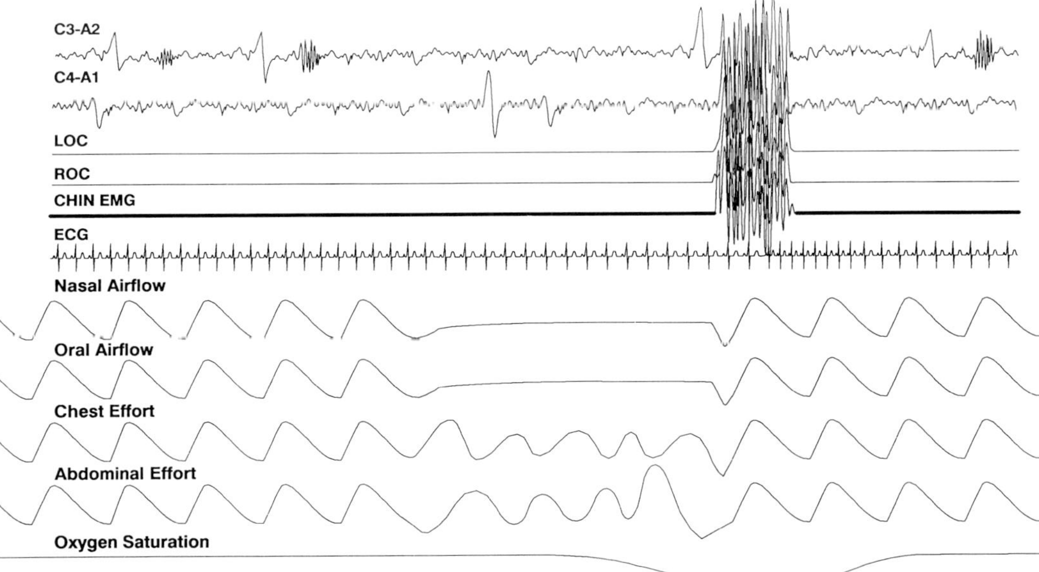

FIGURE 11–3. Obstructive apnea. There is cessation of nasal and oral airflow. Chest and abdominal respiratory efforts continue against the airway obstruction. Paradoxical breathing during the repiratory event is present (chest and abdominal effort are out of phase). Oxygen desaturation is significant. Note the arousal at the end of the apnea. EEG, EOG, and EMG patterns are obscured by movement artifact.

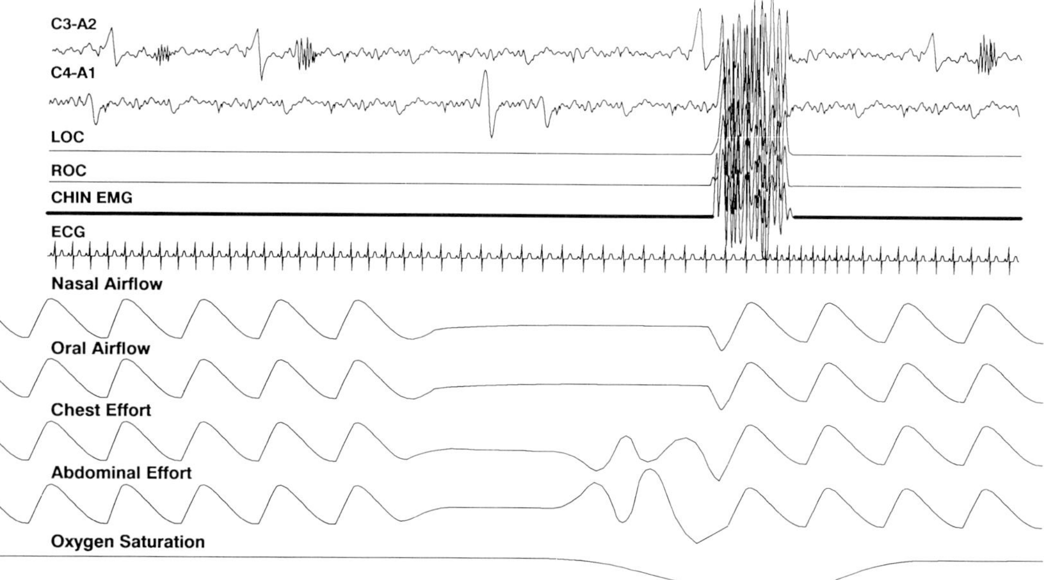

FIGURE 11–4. Mixed apnea. There is cessation of airflow from the nose and mouth. Effort tracings reveal an initial central component (effort absent), followed by at least two cycles of respiratory effort with continued absence of airflow. Significant oxygen desaturation is present. EEG, EOG, and EMG patterns are obscured by movement artifact.

normal, and the complete absence of such pauses during sleep may be indicative of abnormalities in the respiratory control system.

Although central apneas are common in premature and term infants, pathological apneas are of all types and a significant percentage are associated with airway obstruction.[42] During sleep the resting muscle tone of the buccopharyngeal muscles, including the genioglossus, decreases. Pharyngeal dilators, such as the stylopharyngeus and middle constrictor muscles, are active during inspiration in an awake person and normally contract before diaphragmatic movements.[43] If this antidiaphragmatic contraction fails to occur, the negative pressure related to the inspiratory diaphragmatic movement induces pharyngeal closure. In association with central apnea the normally preceding activation of pharyngeal muscles innervated by the superior laryngeal nerve may not occur at the proper time, leading to pharyngeal collapse. The combination of floppy genioglossal muscles during sleep and abnormal timing of contraction of pharyngeal dilators is cumulative. During REM sleep hypotonia the pharynx may collapse even further.[43,44]

Many neonates are considered to be obligate nasal breathers,[45] although oral breathing can occur. Premature infants, however, have rare episodes of spontaneous oronasal breathing during sleep.[46] The frequency of oral breathing in response to nasal occlusion increases with postconceptual age, but it is dissimilar to oronasal breathing seen in term infants. It is characterized by intermittent airway obstruction leading to a significant decrease in respiratory rate, tidal volume, minute ventilation, and transcutaneous oxygen pressure ($tcPo_2$).[46] Therefore the ability of preterm infants to use the oral route of breathing increases with postnatal maturation, but its effectiveness may remain limited by high oral airway resistance.

State Changes and Respiratory Control

Hemoglobin oxygen saturation varies considerably and may decrease to low levels during sleep.[21,47,48] Levels are lowest during tonic REM sleep. This decrease appears to be normal and can be demonstrated in healthy individuals and in premature infants.[48,49] Whereas ventilation during quiet sleep is only mildly altered from that during the waking state, active sleep is associated with consequential changes in ventilation and ventilatory patterns in infants.[26-30,50] Differences in heart rate, cardiac output, mean arterial blood pressure, and regional blood flow exist between active and quiet sleep, as well as between active sleep and wakefulness. Pulmonary blood flow and ventilation/perfusion ratio change with state of consciousness.[25] Along with a change in oxygen saturation, changes in Pa_{CO_2} occur. Simultaneous changes in Pa_{O_2} and Pa_{CO_2} indicate ventilation/perfusion inequalities in infants during active sleep.[51]

Ventilatory response to chemical stimuli undergoes significant maturational changes from fetal to adult life.[52-54] *In contrast to the brisk stimulation of ventilatory drive when hypoxia occurs in adults, fetuses exhibit suppression of this drive when Pa_{O_2} is lowered.*[54] Term newborns respond to hypoxia in a biphasic manner characterized by an increase in ventilation followed by a return to the baseline or a decrease in ventilation.[52] Although chemoreceptors are active in the fetus and newborn, carotid sinus nerve synapses within the central nervous system may not be fully mature and the hypoxic depression of the central nervous system may overwhelm excitatory carotid afferent stimulation.[25,55] No arousal response to moderate hypoxic challenges has been found in adults; experimental evidence of similar lack of arousal to hypoxia in the newborn is insufficient. Levels of oxygen saturation as low as 70% to 75% have been shown to be an ineffective arousal stimulus.[56]

TABLE 11–2. Causes of Apnea in Premature Newborns

Septicemia	Hypoxia
Metabolic abnormalities	Seizures
Right-to-left shunts	Anemia
Gastroesophageal reflux	Congenital abnormalities
Pharyngeal incoordination	Positioning and neck flexion
Increased beta-endorphin secretion*	Idiopathic

*Several authors have suggested a possible connection between sudden infant death syndrome (SIDS) and the respiratory depressant effects of opioids.[74-76] Postmortem examinations have suggested that beta-endorphin levels may be abnormal in some brain areas of SIDS victims when compared with adult values.[77] Others have reported supranormal levels of beta-endorphin in the cerebrospinal fluid of infants with apnea.[78-80] High levels of endogenous opioids have also been associated with respiratory difficulties in an infant with necrotizing encephalomyelopathy[81] and in infants with pickwickian syndrome.[82] Substantial improvement in the respiratory status of many of these infants after the administration of narcotic antagonists (such as naloxone) indicates the possible involvement of beta-endorphin or other endogenous opioids in the pathogenesis of apnea of infancy.

DIAGNOSING SLEEP-DISORDERED RESPIRATION IN INFANTS AND CHILDREN

Clinical Spectrum

Premature Newborns

As previously noted, apnea of prematurity (AOP) is defined as periodic breathing with pathological apnea in a premature infant. Periodic breathing is common in premature infants and can be identified in almost half of them during the neonatal period.[57-59] Periodic breathing occurs with greater frequency as gestational age decreases and is present in almost all newborns less than 28 weeks' gestation.[34] AOP develops in half of infants manifesting periodic breathing.[60] Although AOP is thought to be related to immaturity of brainstem respiratory centers, central and peripheral chemoreceptors, and pulmonary reflexes, the exact cause has not been fully elucidated.[61-66]

Many respiratory pauses are central in origin, but significant evidence suggests that more than half of the respiratory events may be obstructive or mixed in origin.[67-69] The complex neuromuscular events required to maintain pharyngeal patency during respiration are easily overwhelmed in these immature, and often ill, newborns.[70] In addition to central and peripheral immaturity, specific causes of apnea in the premature newborn include septicemia, hypoxia, metabolical abnormalities, seizures, significant right-to-left cardiovascular shunts, anemia, gastroesophageal reflux, pharyngeal incoordination, airway obstruction from positioning and congenital abnormalities of the upper respiratory tract, face, and mandible (Table 11–2).[59,67-69,71-73]

Infants

AOP resolves by 36 weeks' postconceptional age in most cases, but periodic breathing may persist for up to 3 months past 40 weeks' postconceptional age. Term infants (greater than 37 weeks' gestational age) may also have pathological apnea. Apnea of infancy (AOI) is present when breathing ceases for 20 seconds or longer or when breathing cessation is less than 20 seconds but is associated with one or more of the following systemic signs or symptoms:

- Bradycardia
- Cyanosis
- Abrupt marked pallor
- Profound hypotonia

Often no explanation for the apneic events can be found. Infants with apnea secondary to septicemia, seizures, metabolical abnormalities (e.g., hypoglycemia, hypocalcemia, electrolyte imbalance), maternal drug abuse or misuse, or identifiable anatomical defects are not classified in this diagnostic category.

Frequently parents or caretakers observe significant apneic episodes. These events are frightening to the observer and often result in resuscitative efforts. According to the 1986 National Institutes of Health Consensus Development (NIHCD) Conference Statement on Infantile Apnea and Home Monitoring,[34] these apparent life-threatening events (ALTEs) should not be termed aborted sudden infant death syndrome (SIDS) or near-miss SIDS because such labels imply a misleading association between ALTEs and SIDS. Most infants with ALTEs do not die of SIDS, some have not experienced apnea before an ALTE, and infants who die of SIDS most frequently do not have a history of ALTEs.[34] The term "ALTE" describes a clinical syndrome. A variety of identifiable diseases (e.g., gastroesophageal reflux, systemic infection, central nervous system tumors, and seizures) or conditions (e.g., upper airway obstruction, anemia, and central hypoventilation syndrome) can cause such episodes.

CHILDREN

Apnea during childhood differs significantly from AOP and AOI. Central apnea syndromes (e.g., congenital central hypoventilation syndrome) are most often diagnosed early in infancy. Ventilatory drive and effort are abolished during sleep, and the infant quickly becomes apneic and cyanotic. However, central hypoventilation syndrome is not always recognized at birth, and its principal features may be cyanosis and pulmonary hypertension.

Respiratory events during sleep in older children are primarily obstructive in origin. Whereas sleep-associated apnea in premature and term infants is noted primarily by health care workers or parents, apnea in older children is often overlooked.

The hallmark of obstructive sleep apnea (OSA) in older children is *snoring*. Sonorous breathing may be associated with perceptible pauses and snorts. Other nocturnal symptoms include difficulty breathing, restless sleep, heavy sweating, morning headaches, nightmares, sleep terrors, and enuresis.[83,84] Daytime symptoms include excessive daytime sleepiness, poor school performance, abnormal behavior, aggressiveness, hyperactivity, pathological shyness, and social withdrawal. Learning problems, morning headaches, frequent upper airway infections, failure to thrive, and obesity may occur. In the most severe cases, pulmonary hypertension and congestive heart failure (cor pulmonale) can occur. Table 11–3 lists the symptoms of OSA.

OSA in childhood is often associated with an anatomical abnormality of the airway. There are many causes, ranging from hypertrophied tonsillar and adenoidal tissue (the most common cause) to significant malformations of the mandible and maxilla. Neurological abnormalities may also result in OSA. Although obstructive apneas predominate, central and mixed apneas also occur and are thought to be due to central nervous system dysfunction.

Children may also have significant snoring and daytime symptoms suggestive of OSA without demonstrable apnea. This has recently been termed *upper airway resistance syndrome*. Excessive daytime sleepiness can be objectively demonstrated in these children by the Multiple Sleep Latency Test.[85-91] Nocturnal evaluations either fail to document significant apnea or find only a few central, mixed, or obstructive events. Esophageal balloon manometry has documented that these children have significantly increased effort of breathing during sleep, although oxygen tension and saturations remain normal. Therefore partial occlusion of the airway may lead to symptoms of OSA syndrome; complete airway obstruction is not necessary. The most important factor influencing the severity of symptoms appears to be the effort required to breathe during sleep and the amount of sleep disturbance caused by this additional effort, rather than the degree of apnea demonstrated by objective testing.[92]

TABLE 11–3. Symptoms of Obstructive Sleep Apnea During Childhood

NOCTURNAL	DIURNAL
Loud snoring	Performance deficits
Respiratory pauses and snorts	Excessive daytime sleepiness
Difficulty breathing	Hyperactivity
Restless sleep	School failure
Diaphoresis	Abnormal behavior
Nightmares	Unusual aggressiveness
Sleep terrors	Pathological shyness
Enuresis	Social withdrawal
	Learning disorders
	Attention span problems
	Morning headaches
	Failure to thrive
	Systemic hypertension
	Pulmonary hypertension
	Cor pulmonale
	Obesity

Diagnostic Methods

Definition of pathological apnea requires identification of cessation of airflow at the nose and mouth or of cardiovascular, physiological, or neurological consequences of the respiratory pause. Definitive diagnosis is based on continuous monitoring of cardiovascular, electroencephalographic (EEG), and respiratory parameters across the sleep period. Guilleminault and co-workers have shown that in infants with significant apnea, most episodes occur during the early morning hours.[93] Therefore diagnostic procedures should be performed at times when these events are most numerous. Continuous monitoring is most reliable when performed during the major sleep period at night. Premature newborns, because of clear ultradian sleep-wake rhythm and lack of entrainment to a 24-hour light-dark cycle, may be evaluated through several sleep-wake cycles during daytime hours.

Parameters to be continuously monitored include nasal and oral airflow, cardiac activity (electrocardiography [ECG]), respiratory effort (chest wall and abdominal movement), and oxygen saturation (Sa_{O_2}). Continuous pulse oximetry is a safe and reliable method of assessing Sa_{O_2} and approximating Pa_{O_2}.[94-96] In addition, continuous monitoring of the EEG is recommended for accurate identification of sleep stages during which respiratory events occur, as well as identification of apneas associated with significant central nervous system events such as seizure activity during sleep.

Pneumography should not be used to diagnose apnea.[34] The pneumogram has been widely used as a screening tool in asymptomatic premature and term infants, but there is no objective evidence that continuous recording of thoracic impedance and heart rate can be used to predict life-threatening apnea. Respiratory events recorded are those of central origin and those associated with significant cardiac events (tachycardia or bradycardia). Unfortunately, these events are only some of the respiratory events that might occur during the sleep period, and this type of recording can significantly underestimate the integrity of respiration during sleep. In addition, thoracic impedance may fail to detect obstructive apneas and can confuse cardiac artifact with respiratory impedance. Also, partial airway obstruction may cause false breath detection and breaths immediately following a sigh or biphasic large breath may be missed.[97] Pneumograms should be reserved for evaluation of infants who trigger frequent alarms during home apnea monitoring. Pneumography may help in these situations by differentiating true from false activation of the monitor. Polysomnography is the most reliable and effective method available for describing respiration during sleep.

Premature Newborns and Infants

Diagnosis of apnea in infants should begin with a comprehensive history and physical examination. A history of respiratory pauses with or without physiological consequences suggests the presence of AOP or AOI. Information sought in the history should include presence of prenatal and perinatal complications, Apgar scores, gestational age, drugs taken by the mother or infant, infant and environmental temperature before the episode, feeding tolerance, prior trauma, and a history of siblings with apnea or SIDS. Polysomnographic monitoring not only provides information about the presence of significant apnea, but also accurately classifies respiratory events.

Infants brought for medical attention after an ALTE should be hospitalized and evaluated for specific treatable conditions. Acute infection, chronic conditions, gastroesophageal reflux, pharyngeal incoordination, seizures, and anemia should be considered. In the absence of a clear cause after initial evaluation, two diagnostic approaches have been recommended.[34] A thoughtful, limited initial evaluation includes determination of serum bicarbonate or blood gas levels. Metabolic acidosis suggests an acute hypoxic episode and substantiates the history. A complete blood cell count permits evaluation for anemia or acute infection. Continuous cardiopulmonary monitoring during hospitalization may detect a cardiac arrhythmia. If the practitioner concludes that the apneic event was potentially dangerous, discharge with the use of a home monitor may be considered. If apneas continue at home and are thought to be real, further diagnostic evaluation may be indicated. This approach should be limited to infants whose initial history and results of physical examination do not suggest the presence of a treatable condition.

A second approach involves a more extensive initial evaluation and less liberal use of home monitoring.[34] In addition to obtaining serum bicarbonate concentration, arterial blood gas determinations, and a complete blood cell count (CBC), the practitioner obtains serum electrolyte measurements, serum chemistry profile (including blood glucose), ECG, chest x-ray, EEG, chalasia evaluation, neurological evaluation, and polysomnography. Polysomnography provides objective evidence distinguishing actual from artifactual alarms and discriminates central from obstructive or mixed apneic events.

Children

In older children evaluation also begins with a comprehensive history. The hallmark of OSA is loud snoring. Parents often do not consider snoring abnormal and therefore do not offer this information. Snoring is present in virtually all children with OSA.[83] Snoring may be associated with respiratory pauses, difficulty breathing, postpause snorts, restless sleep, frequent arousals, and diaphoresis. Morning headaches and dry mouth are common complaints. Recognized causes of childhood apnea are shown in Table 11–4.

The history must include a complete evaluation of daytime functioning. Excessive daytime sleepiness, behavioral abnormalities, unusual aggressiveness, school performance deficits, hyperactivity, and attention span problems often occur in the presence of significant sleep-disordered respiration. Brouilette and co-workers have suggested that calculation of a *clinical obstructive sleep apnea score* can correctly identify children without OSA as well as more than 95% of children with documentable apnea.[98] Calculation of the score requires observation by caretakers of difficulty breathing, apnea, and snoring. Difficulty breathing is scored on a 4-point scale (0 = never, 1 = occasionally, 2 = frequently, and 3 = always); apnea is scored either yes (0) or no (1); and snoring is scored on a 4-point scale (0 = never, 1 = occasionally, 2 = frequently, and 3 = always). The following formula was derived by discriminate analysis: OSA score = 1.42 (difficulty breathing) + 1.41 (apnea) + 0.71 (snoring) − 3.83. Scores greater than 3.5 were highly predictive of OSA requiring adenotonsillectomy, and no scores less than −1 were associated with OSA. Scores between −1 and 3.5 required polygraphic monitoring to determine the severity of sleep-related airway obstruction.

TABLE 11–4. Recognized Causes of Apnea During Childhood*

Hypertrophied tonsils and adenoids	Meningomyelocele
Micrognathia	Nemaline myopathy
Retrognathia	Congenital central hypoventilation
Long soft palate	Asthma
Post cleft palate repair	Burns to the head and neck
Macroglossia	Osteopetrosis
Malpositioned hyoid bone	Anemia
Anesthesia of the pharynx	Oropharyngeal papillomatosis
Central nervous system tumors	Obesity
Gastroesophageal reflux	Thyromegaly
Munchausen's syndrome by proxy	Acromegaly
Achondroplasia	Temporomandibular joint disease
Metabolic abnormalities	Myxedema
Drugs	Bulbar poliomyelitis
Fetal alcohol syndrome	Brainstem infarction
Respiratory syncytial virus infections	Spinal surgery
Myelodysplasia	Idiopathic

*All of the listed abnormalities have been associated with obstructive, central, or mixed apnea during childhood. The list is not intended to be all-inclusive.

Physical examination should focus on the integrity of the respiratory system, cardiovascular system, upper airway (including the nasopharynx, oropharynx, and tongue), maxilla, mandible, and neck (including the presence of masses, location of the trachea, characteristic of the submandibular soft tissue, and musculature). A comprehensive neurological examination should also be performed.

Failure to thrive, obesity, and cardiovascular compromise secondary to OSA may occur. Laboratory evaluations are seldom required, but CBC, waking blood gas determination, pulmonary function testing, radiographic evaluation of the chest, head, and neck, and ECG should be considered when clinical evidence warrants.

Polysomnography remains the definitive diagnostic technique. Significant sleep stage abnormalities can be identified. In severe cases of sleep apnea, Stage 2 NREM sleep is severely disrupted and slow-wave sleep and REM sleep volumes may be markedly decreased. During apneas sleep spindles may be rare and poorly defined. Low-amplitude theta activity may appear. Slow waves resembling repetitive K-complexes followed by slow alpha activity are often noted after 15 to 20 seconds of apnea.[83]

The apnea index is defined as the number of apneas per hour of sleep. An apnea index greater than 5 defines sleep-disordered respiration in adults. A similar definition of apnea has been suggested for children, although this level of apnea and the level requiring intervention are much less clear. Distinct sleep-disordered respiration can be present without documentable apneas. Sleepiness during the day and loud snoring at night, heavy sweating, restless sleep, and abnormal findings on the Multiple Sleep Latency Test have been documented in children[90] without apneas[89] or with few central, mixed, or obstructive events and normal oxygen saturation in combination during REM sleep. Esophageal balloon manometry revealed that intraesophageal pressure (reflecting intrathoracic pressure) was significantly higher than expected when compared with normal control values, particularly during REM sleep. Therefore sleep-disordered respiration resulting in nocturnal and diurnal symptoms may be caused by partial obstruction of the upper airway. The resulting increased respiratory resistive load increases the effort required to breathe during sleep, disrupts sleep continuity and architecture, and causes symptoms identical to those seen in children with documentable sleep apnea. Adenotonsillectomy, which decreases the respiratory resistive load, results in complete resolution of daytime and nighttime symptoms in most of these children. This response to treatment provides evidence that upper airway obstruction may be more significant in children with lower levels of documentable apnea.

TREATMENT

Apnea of Prematurity

Apnea of prematurity should be treated initially by appropriate management of any identifiable causes. For example, apnea secondary to seizure disorders may be appropriately treated by controlling seizure activity with anticonvulsants. Treatment of recurrent, clinically significant apnea in a premature infant should ensure adequate oxygenation and ventilation. Physical stimulation may be all that is necessary, provided that the infant is continuously monitored and under constant vigilance by the health care providers. Continuous positive airway pressure (CPAP),[99] supplemental oxygen therapy, and mechanical ventilation may be required. Stimulation by oscillatory water beds or air mattresses has been successful in some infants.[100] Intermittent oscillations seem to be more successful than continuous, rhythmical oscillation in alleviating apneic episodes.[101] Some conflicting evidence does exist that oscillating air mattresses have no value in preventing apnea and do not enhance growth and development. Oscillating water beds do, however, affect sleep and its staging.[102] While on a water bed, infants appear to have significantly more quiet and active sleep, shorter sleep latencies, fewer state changes, less restlessness during sleep, less waking activity, and fewer jittery movements.

Methylxanthines are currently the most widely used and successful medications in the treatment of apnea in premature infants.[103-107] Theophylline has been shown to reduce the number of apneic episodes and the development of respiratory failure[108] but does not appear to shorten the course of apnea of prematurity. Administration of theophylline is associated with a decrease in cerebral blood flow.[109]

Caffeine has been shown to induce a significant increase in ventilation, tidal volume, and mean inspiratory flow without changing inspiratory time, expiratory time, or total cycle duration.[105,107,110] Caffeine appears to increase ventilation mainly by increasing central inspiratory drive. This increase in ventilation associated with methylxanthine administration results in a substantial reduction in the Pa_{CO_2} and a concurrent reduction in cerebral blood flow.

Caffeine and theophylline have similar effects on episodes of apnea and bradycardia; however, caffeine seems to have an earlier effect on respiratory rate. Side effects of tachycardia, arousal, and gastrointestinal intolerance are more frequently observed with theophylline.[111] Both drugs have a natriuretic effect that appears to take place at the level of the distal tubule. According to Bairam and colleagues, caffeine provides stable plasma levels and has a significantly longer plasma half-life (65 to 100 hours versus 20 to 30 hours for theophylline), allowing the prescription of only one daily maintenance dose (2.5 mg/kg) and measurement of plasma levels only once a week.

When obstructive and mixed apneas are identified in a premature infant, CPAP may markedly reduce the incidence of these respiratory events. Central apneas, on the other hand, appear to be unaffected by CPAP, although tc_{PO_2} has been shown to increase during CPAP whether or not apnea is present.[112] In an infant who has predominantly central apneas, theophylline appears significantly superior to CPAP.[113] Patients treated with theophylline have fewer prolonged apneic attacks, fewer episodes of bradycardia, and less need for assisted ventilation than those treated with CPAP.

Doxapram, a potent respiratory stimulant in adults, has been used experimentally to treat AOP. It appears to affect both peripheral chemoreceptors and central respiratory centers.[114] Doxapram infusions have been used in preterm infants when therapeutic concentrations of theophylline had failed to control episodes of apnea.[115,116] Doxapram successfully controlled the apnea, and arterial blood P_{CO_2} values decreased significantly. When given in a dosage of 2 or 2.5 mg/kg per hour, doxapram increases minute ventilation, tidal volume, mean inspiratory flow, and airway pressure. Doxapram also has a wide margin of safety. Side effects are uncommon, mild, and reversible. However, at a rate of 2.5 mg/kg per hour, blood concentrations have been shown to be greater than 5 μg/ml, a level that may represent a narrower safety margin in very low birth weight infants. Hayakawa and co-workers have recommended that doxapram be administered initially at a rate of 1 to 1.5 mg/kg per hour and then decreased when control of apnea is achieved.[117] They consider an appropriate serum concentration to be less than 5 μg/ml. Doses of doxapram greater than 2 to 2.5 mg/kg per hour increase efficacy but also increase the risk of side effects. Additional investigations are needed before doxapram can be accepted as a routine treatment for AOP.

Apnea of Infancy and Apparent Life-threatening Events

AOP resolves spontaneously by 36 weeks postconceptual age in most cases. Periodic breathing may persist, however, up to 3 months after term.[118-120] Some periodic breathing and brief apneic events appear to be normal at almost any age, especially during active (REM) sleep. ALTEs, persistent and frequent periodic breathing, and respiratory instability may be associated with increased risk of sudden unexpected death.[34] It has been difficult to determine the exact epidemiology and outcome of patients with AOI and survivors of apparent life-threatening events. According to the NIHCD Conference on Apnea and Home Monitoring, there is evidence that apnea of prematurity is not a risk factor for SIDS. In the NIHCD Cooperative Epidemiological Study of SIDS Risk Factors, there was no difference in the incidence of reported apnea between the infants who died of SIDS and a control group.[34]

Mortality in ALTE subgroups is unknown, and certain infants who have had an ALTE may be at higher risk of sudden unexpected death than others.[121] Less than 4% of infants evaluated for an ALTE subsequently die of SIDS. Infants with ALTEs are a heterogeneous group, and some have a higher risk of sudden unexpected death than others. Even when the presence of an identifiable cause for the ALTE has been established, the infant must not be considered to have less risk of sudden unexpected death.

Not all children who suffer sudden unexpected death have SIDS. Only when criteria defining SIDS are established and stringently applied should the diagnosis be made. Because of the lack of continuity of data in the past, the relationship between ALTE and SIDS remains obscure.

Home monitoring has been recommended for certain infants at increased risk of sudden unexpected death.[34] Some data, however, suggest that infants with apnea during sleep who were perceived to require resuscitation may have a mortality rate as high as 10% *despite the use of home monitors*. Effectiveness of home monitoring depends on the proper choice of instrumentation, appropriate training of caretakers in acceptable intervention and in cardiopulmonary resuscitation, adequate compliance by caretakers, and continual professional support. Children who have had one or more episodes of ALTE requiring significant intervention (vigorous stimulation or mouth-to-mouth resuscitation), infants with AOP, siblings of two or more SIDS victims, and infants with certain conditions such as central hypoventilation syndrome should be monitored. Although monitoring does not guarantee prevention of unexpected death, evidence shows that lives of infants at extraordinarily high risk may be saved.

Decisions to discontinue home monitoring should be based on clinical criteria. When infants with ALTE have had 2 to 3 months free of significant apnea and have shown the ability to tolerate stress from intercurrent illness and immunizations, discontinuation of home monitoring should be considered. Many programs recommend discontinuing the home monitor at 6 months of age if the infant has been free of significant apnea events for at least 2 months. Requiring infants to have one or more normal pneumograms before discontinuing home monitoring may needlessly prolong the monitoring period. Use of home monitors is not without complications, and prolonged use may expose the infant to unnecessary risk,[122] testing, and hospitalization, and the parents to unnecessary stress. We emphasize, however, that recommendations for the duration of monitoring have not been based on conclusive data. The decisions to begin and discontinue monitoring should rest on clinical grounds and be made in close collaboration with the infant's parents.

Childhood Apnea

Upper airway obstruction is present in the majority of children with symptomatic apnea. Many therapeutic interventions are available. After a comprehensive evaluation of the patient for conditions that may lead to upper airway obstruction, an appropriate therapeutic approach can be developed. Since anatomical abnormalities of the upper airway play an important role, these factors must be identified. The practitioner must investigate such factors as the child's age, dental development, facial structure, and intellectual development before embarking on a treatment regimen.

Tonsillectomy or adenotonsillectomy is the treatment of first choice for children with uncomplicated OSA.[83,123-125] Treatment regimens that have not been overly successful in adults (e.g., uvelopalatopharyngeoplasty, tracheostomy, medication, and tongue-retaining devices) are generally avoided. Children with craniofacial or nuchal abnormalities (e.g., long soft palate, soft palate repair,[126] micrognathia,[127] and low-positioned hyoid bone) should be examined at frequent intervals and monitored polysomnographically to determine the need for other surgical procedures. Existence of significant increase in airway resistance during sleep without significant apnea may lead to as many clinical complaints as typical OSA and should be treated similarly.

Tracheostomy is an effective treatment for severe, complicated OSA when tonsillectomy and adenoidectomy were insufficient and always resolves the apnea.[92] Because of the complications and psychological impact of tracheostomy, this form of therapy should be avoided unless other forms of therapy have failed to resolve the apnea and its sequelae.

Nasal CPAP is well tolerated and effective in adults and children.[128-130] CPAP reduces airway resistance by splinting the pharynx[128] and by directly stimulating pharyngeal tissue.[22] Nasal CPAP is an effective alternative for the treatment of children with OSA syndrome who are too young for surgery, when surgical intervention is inappropriate, or when surgery would be too difficult to perform.[92] It may also be used for obstructive apnea that develops after soft palate repair[128] and for pubertal and postpubertal patients who require orthodontic preparation before undergoing maxillofacial surgery.[129] Successful long-term treatment has been reported,[129,131] but treatment failures do occur. Technical aspects of treatment are important and are usually responsible for treatment failures. Mask size and shape are critical factors in maintaining an effective mask seal. Air leaks at the edge of the mask may result in ocular trauma, dryness and irritation of the conjunctivae, and reappearance of apnea. An inappropriately fitting mask may also result in erosion of the skin over the bridge of the nose. The child's age and mental capacity, as well as compliance by the child and parents, are also critical factors when assessing appropriateness of nasal CPAP therapy.

An association between obesity and sleep apnea has long been recognized. The pathophysiological mechanism is not clear. Failure to thrive is more commonly associated with OSA than is obesity during childhood, but whenever obesity is present in association with OSA, it should be considered a contributing factor. Significant weight loss alleviates OSA in obese adults,[132] but a similar effect on obstructive apnea in childhood is speculative.

COMPLICATIONS OF APNEA IN CHILDHOOD

As previously noted, children with OSA may have failure to thrive.[133] Growth velocities may be subnormal for many months before apnea is suspected. Resolution of the apnea results in catch-up growth and subsequent normal growth velocity in these children.

Children with sleep apnea may develop persistent marked elevation of systemic blood pressure[83,134] and associated marked left ventricular hypertrophy. These significant cardiovascular sequelae are potentially reversible in adolescents[135] and adults[136,137] when the underlying apnea is effectively treated.

Other sequelae of sleep apnea are performance deficits during daytime hours. School failure, behavioral abnormalities, unusual aggressiveness, attention span problems, and learning disabilities may occur. These complications are significant because of the obscure etiology and considerable delay in diagnosis. This "new morbidity" may result in lifelong problems if not appropriately addressed and treated during childhood. Significant apnea should not be considered normal under any circumstances, and evaluation for sleep-disordered respiration should be part of any health maintenance regimen.

REFERENCES

1. Orem J, Netick A, and Dement WC: Breathing during sleep and wakefulness in the cat. Respir Physiol 1977;30:265.

2. Remmers JE, Bartlett D, and Putnam MD: Changes in the respiratory cycle associated with sleep. Respir Physiol 1976;28:277.
3. Bulow K: Respiration and wakefulness in man. Acta Physiol Scand 1963;59(suppl 209):1.
4. Orem J et al: Activity of respiratory neurons during NREM sleep. J Neurophysiol 1985;54:1144.
5. Megirian D and Sherrey JH: Respiratory functions of the laryngeal muscles during sleep. Sleep 1980;3:289.
6. Berger RJ: Tonus of extrinsic laryngeal muscles during sleep and dreaming. Science 1961;134:840.
7. Coccagna G and Lugaresi E: Arterial blood gases and pulmonary and systemic arterial pressure during sleep in chronic obstructive pulmonary disease. Sleep 1978;1:117.
8. Birchfield RI, Sieker HO, and Heyman A: Alterations in respiratory function during natural sleep. J Lab Clin Med 1959;54:216.
9. Birchfield RI, Sieker HO, and Heyman A: Alterations in blood gases during natural sleep and narcolepsy. Neurology 1958;8:107.
10. Phillipson EA et al: Ventilatory and waking responses to CO_2 in sleeping dogs. Am Rev Respir Dis 1977;115:251.
11. Phillipson EA, Murphy E, and Kozar LF: Regulation of respiration in sleeping dogs. J Appl Physiol 1976;40:688.
12. Parmeggiani PL and Sabattini L: Electromyographic aspects of postural, respiratory and thermoregulatory mechanisms in sleeping cats. Electroencephalogr Clin Neurophysiol 1972;33:1.
13. Tabachnick E et al: The behavior of the respiratory muscles during sleep. Physiologist 1980;23:1.
14. Orem J and Lydic R: Upper airway function during sleep and wakefulness: experimental studies on normal and anesthetized cats. Sleep 1978;1:49.
15. Sauerland EK and Harper RM: The human tongue during sleep: electromyographic activity of the genioglossus muscle. Exp Neurol 1976;51:160.
16. Remmers JE et al: Pathogenesis of upper airway occlusion during sleep. J Appl Physiol 1978;44:931.
17. Orem J, Dick TE, and Norris P: Laryngeal and diaphragmatic responses to airway occlusion in sleep and wakefulness. Electroencephalogr Clin Neurophysiol 1980;50:151.
18. Sullivan CE et al: Ventilatory responses to CO_2 and lung inflation in tonic versus phasic REM sleep. J Appl Physiol 1979;47:1304.
19. Sullivan CE: Breathing in sleep. In Orem J and Barnes CD (eds): Physiology in sleep. Academic Press, New York, 1980, pp 213-272.
20. Orem J, Netick A, and Dement WC: Increased upper-airway resistance to breathing during sleep in the cat. Electroencephalogr Clin Neurophysiol 1977;43:14.
21. Remmers JE, Anch AM, and deGroot WJ: Respiratory disturbances during sleep. Clin Chest Med 1980;1:57.
22. Abu-Osba YK, Mathew OP, and Thach BT: An animal model for airway sensory deprivation producing obstructive apnea with postmortem findings of sudden infant death syndrome. Pediatrics 1981;68:796-801.
23. Bowes G et al: Development of patterns of respiratory activity in unanesthetized fetal sheep in utero. J Appl Physiol 1981;50:693.
24. Dawes GS et al: Respiratory movements and rapid eye movement sleep in the foetal sheep. J Physiol (Lond) 1972;220:119.
25. Haddad GG: Control of breathing in children. In Edelman NH and Santiago TV (eds): Breathing disorders of sleep. New York, Churchill Livingstone, 1986, pp 57-80.
26. Haddad GG et al: Breath-to-breath variations in rate and depth of ventilation in sleeping infants. Am J Physiol 1982;243:R164.
27. Haddad GG et al: Maturation of ventilation and ventilatory pattern in normal sleeping infants. J Appl Physiol 1979;46:998.
28. Haddad GG et al: CO_2-induced changes in ventilation and ventilatory pattern in normal sleeping infants. J Appl Physiol 1980;48:684.
29. Bolton DPG and Herman S: Ventilation and sleep state in the newborn. J Physiol 1974;240:67.
30. Hathorn MKS: The rate and depth of breathing in newborn infants in different sleep states. J Physiol (Lond) 1974;243:101.
31. Hathorn MKS: Analysis of the rhythm of infantile breathing. Br Med Bull 1975;31:8.
32. Finer NN, Abroms IF, and Taeusch HW: Ventilation and sleep states in newborn infants. J Pediatr 1976;89:100.
33. Haddad GG, Lai TL, and Mellins RB: Determination of ventilatory pattern in REM sleep in normal infants. J Appl Physiol 1982;53:52.
34. National Institutes of Health Consensus Development Conference: Infantile apnea and home monitoring. Bethesda, Md, US Department of Health and Human Services, Oct 1, 1987, NIH Pub No 87-2905.
35. Lee D et al: A developmental study on types and frequency distribution of short apneas (3 to 15 seconds) in term and preterm infants. Pediatr Res 1987;22:344-349.
36. Cherniack NS: Respiratory dysrhythmias during sleep. N Engl J Med 1981;305:325.
37. Cherniack NS and Longobardo GS: Cheyne-Stokes breathing. N Engl J Med 1973;288:952.
38. Cherniack NS et al: Experimentally induced Cheyne-Stokes breathing. Respir Physiol 1979;37:185.
39. Cherniack NS et al: Animal models of Cheyne-Stokes breathing. In von Euler C and Lagercrantz H (eds): Central nervous control mechanisms in breathing. Oxford, Eng, Pergamon Press, 1979, p 417.
40. Joshi A et al: Blood transfusion effect on the respiratory pattern of preterm infants. Pediatrics 1987;80:79-84.
41. Haddad GG and Mellins RB: Cardiorespiratory aspects of SIDS: an overview. In Tildon T, Roeder L, and Steinschneider A (eds): Sudden infant death syndrome. New York, Academic Press, 1983, p 357.
42. Dransfield DA, Spitzer AR, and Fox WW: Episodic airway obstruction in premature infants. Am J Dis Child 1983;137:441-443.
43. Quera-Salva MA and Guilleminault C: Post-traumatic central sleep apnea in a child. J Pediatr 1987;110:906-909.
44. Kryger MH et al: Sleep and respiration: a postscript. Clin Chest Med 1985;6:713-718.
45. Nelson WE, Vaughn VC, and McKay RJ (eds): Textbook of pediatrics. Philadelphia, WB Saunders, 1987, p 868.
46. Miller MJ et al: Effect of maturation on oral breathing in sleeping premature infants. J Pediatr 1986; 109:515-519.
47. Block AJ et al: Sleep apnea, hypopnea and oxygen desaturation in normal subjects. N Engl J Med 1979;300:513.
48. Hanson N and Okken A: Transcutaneous oxygen tension of newborn infants in different behavioral states. Pediatr Res 1980;14:911.

49. Martin RJ, Okkew A, and Rubin D: Arterial oxygen tension during active and quiet sleep in the normal neonate. J Pediatr 1979;94:271.
50. Milic-Emili J and Grunstein MM: Drive and timing components of ventilation. Chest 1976;70:1341.
51. Martin RJ, Herrell N, and Pultusker M: Transcutaneous measurement of carbon dioxide tension: effect of sleep state in term infants. Pediatrics 1981;67:622-625.
52. Rigatto H: A critical analysis of the development of peripheral and central respiratory chemosensitivity during the neonatal period. In von Euler C and Langercrantz H (eds): Central nervous control mechanisms in breathing. Oxford, Eng, Pergamon Press, 1979, p 137.
53. Sankaran K et al: Immediate and late ventilatory response to high and low O_2 in preterm infants and adult subjects. Pediatr Res 1979;13:875.
54. Towell ME and Salvador HS: Intrauterine asphyxia and respiratory movements in the fetal goat. Am J Obstet Gynecol 1974;118:1124.
55. Lahiri S et al: Regulation of breathing in newborns at high altitude. J Appl Physiol 1978;44:673.
56. Berthon-Jones M and Sullivan CE: Ventilatory and arousal responses to hypoxia in sleeping humans. Am Rev Respir Dis 1982;126:632.
57. Rigatto H: Apnea. Pediatr Clin North Am 1982;29:1105.
58. Bouterline-Young HJ and Smith CA: Respiration of full-term and of premature infants. Am J Dis Child 1953;80:753.
59. Daily WJR, Klaus M, and Meyer HBP: Apnea in premature infants: monitoring incidence heart rate changes, and effect of environmental temperature. Pediatrics 1969;43:510.
60. Henderson-Smart DJ: The effect of gestational age on the incidence and duration of recurrent apnoea in newborn babies. Aust Pediatr J 1981;17:273.
61. Henderson-Smart DJ, Pettigrew AG, and Campbell DJ: Clinical apnea and brain stem neural function in preterm infants. N Engl J Med 1983;308:353.
62. Chernick V, Heldrich F, and Avery ME: Periodic breathing of premature infants. J Pediatr 1964;64:330.
63. Rigatto H, Brady JP, and de La Torre-Verduzco R: Chemoreceptor reflexes in preterm infants. II. The effect of gestational and postnatal age on the ventilatory response to inhaled carbon dioxide. Pediatrics 1975;55:614.
64. Cross KW and Oppe TE: The effect of inhalation of high and low concentrations of oxygen on the respiration of the premature infant. J Physiol 1952;117:38.
65. Rigatto H, Brady JP, and de La Torre-Verduzco R: Chemoreceptor reflexes in preterm infants. I. The effect of gestational and postnatal age on the ventilatory response to inhalation of 100% and 15% oxygen. Pediatrics 1975;55:604.
66. Johnson P, Robinson JS, and Salisbury D: The onset and control of breathing after birth: foetal and neonatal physiology. Proceedings of the Sir Joseph Barcroft Symposium, Cambridge, Eng, Cambridge University Press, 1973.
67. Dransfield DA, Spiter AR, and Fox WW: Episodic airway obstruction in premature infants. Am J Dis Child 1983;137:441.
68. Thach BT and Stark AR: Spontaneous neck flexion and airway obstruction during apneic spells in preterm infants. J Pediatr 1979;94:275.
69. Milner AD et al: Upper airway obstruction and apnea in preterm babies. Arch Dis Child 1980;55:22.
70. Wilson SL et al: Upper airway patency in the human infant: influence of airway pressure and posture. J Appl Physiol 1980;48:500.
71. Church NR et al: Respiratory syncytial virus-related apnea in infants, demographics and outcome. Am J Dis Child 1984;138:247.
72. Fenichel GM, Olson BJ, and Fitzpatrick JE: Heart rate changes in convulsive and nonconvulsive neonatal apnea. Ann Neurol 1980;7:577.
73. Perlstein DH, Edward NH, and Sutherland J: Apnea in premature infants and incubator air temperature changes. N Engl J Med 1970;282:461.
74. Kuich TE and Zimmerman D: Could endorphins be implicated in sudden-infant-death syndrome [letter]? N Engl J Med 1981;304:973.
75. McQueen DS: Opioid peptide interactions with respiratory and circulatory systems. Br Med Bull 1983;39:77-82.
76. Malcolm DS and Holaday JW: Opioid peptides and their antagonists: a role in respiratory function. Semin Respir Med 1985;7:81.
77. Pasi A et al: Regional levels of beta-lipotropin and beta-endorphin in the brain and the hypophysis of victims of sudden infant death syndrome [letter]. Arch Pathol Lab Med 1983;107:336.
78. Myer EC, Dewey W, and Colbert B: Endogenous opioids—a possible marker for infants at risk for sudden infant death (SIDS) [abstract]. Pediatr Res 1985;19:393.
79. Orlowski JP, Lonsdale D, and Denko CW: Beta-endorphin levels in infant apnea syndrome: a preliminary communication. Cleve Clin Q 1982;49:87.
80. Orlowski JP: Cerebrospinal fluid endorphins and the infant apnea syndrome. Pediatrics 1986;78:233.
81. Brandt NJ et al: Hyper-endorphin syndrome in a child with necrotizing encephalomyelopathy. N Engl J Med 1980;303:914.
82. Orlowski JP, Herrell DW, and Moodie DS: Narcotic antagonist therapy of the obesity-hypoventilation syndrome. Crit Care Med 1982;10:604.
83. Guilleminault C et al: Sleep apnea in eight children. Pediatrics 1976;58:28.
84. Guilleminault C and Winkle R: A review of 50 children with OSAS. Lung 1981;159:275.
85. Guilleminault C et al: Five cases of near miss sudden infant death syndrome and development of obstructive sleep apnea syndrome. Pediatrics 1984; 73:71.
86. Guilleminault C, Riley R, and Powell N: Sleep apnea in normal subjects following mandibular osteotomy with retrusion. Chest 1985;88:776.
87. Longobardo GS et al: Sleep apnea considered as a control system instability. Respir Physiol 1982; 50:311.
88. Guilleminault C: Diagnosis, pathogenesis and treatment of the sleep apnea syndromes. Ergeb Inn Med Kinderheilkd 1984;52:1.
89. Guilleminault C et al: Children and nocturnal snoring: evaluation of the effects of sleep related respiratory resistive load and daytime functioning. Eur J Pediatr 1982;139:165.
90. Carskadon MA and Dement WC: The Multiple Sleep Latency Test: what does it measure? Sleep 1982;5:565.
91. Cherniack NS: Respiratory dysrhythmias during sleep. N Engl J Med 1981;305:325.
92. Guilleminault C: Obstructive sleep apnea syndrome in children. In Guilleminault C (ed): Sleep and its disorders in children. Raven Press, New York, 1987, pp 213-224.

93. Guilleminault C: Sleep apnea in infancy. In Guilleminault C (ed): Sleep and its disorders in children. Raven Press, New York, 1987, p 213.
94. Yelderman N and New W: Evaluation of pulse oximetry. Anesthesiology 1983;59:349.
95. Deckardt R and Steward DS: Noninvasive arterial hemoglobin oxygen saturation versus transcutaneous oxygen tension monitoring in the preterm infant. Crit Care Med 1984;12:935.
96. Fait CD et al: Pulse oximetry in critically ill children. J Clin Monit 1985;1:232.
97. Brouillette RT et al: Comparison of respiratory inductive plethysmography and thoracic impedance for apnea monitoring. J Pediatr 1987;111:377.
98. Brouillette R et al: A diagnostic approach to suspected obstructive sleep apnea in children. J Pediatr 1984;105:10.
99. Miller MJ, Carlo WA, and Martin RJ: Continuous positive airway pressure selectively reduces obstructive apnea in preterm infants. J Pediatr 1985;106:91.
100. Korner AF et al: Effects of waterbed flotation on premature infants: a pilot study. Pediatrics 1975;56:361.
101. Saigal S, Watts J, and Campbell D: Randomized clinical trial of an oscillating air mattress in preterm infants: effect on apnea, growth, and development. J Pediatr 1986;109:857.
102. Korner AF, Ruppel EM, and Rho JM: Effects of water beds on the sleep and motility of theophylline-treated preterm infants. Pediatrics 1982;70:864.
103. Kelly DH and Shannon DC: Treatment of apnea and excessive periodic breathing in the full-term infant. Pediatrics 1981;68:183.
104. Shannon DC et al: Prevention of apnea and bradycardia in the low birth weight infant. Pediatrics 1975;55:589.
105. Aranda JV et al: Pharmacokinetic profile of caffeine in the premature newborn with apnea. J Pediatr 1979;94:663.
106. Rosen JP et al: Theophylline pharmacokinetics in the young infant. Pediatrics 1979;64:248.
107. Aranda JV et al: Efficacy of caffeine in treatment of apnea in the low birth weight infant. J Pediatr 1977;90:467.
108. Sims ME et al: Limitations of theophylline in the treatment of apnea of prematurity. Am J Dis Child 1985;139:567.
109. Rosenkrantz TS and Oh W: Aminophylline reduces cerebral blood flow velocity in low-birth-weight infants. Am J Dis Child 1984;138:489.
110. Aranda JV et al: Effect of caffeine on control of breathing in infantile apnea. J Pediatr 1983;103:975.
111. Bairam A et al: Theophylline versus caffeine: comparative effects in treatment of idiopathic apnea in the preterm infant. J Pediatr 1987;110:636.
112. Miller MJ, Carlo WA, and Martin RJ: Continuous positive airway pressure selectively reduces obstructive apnea in preterm infants. J Pediatr 1985;106:91.
113. Jones RAK: Apnoea of immaturity. I. A controlled trial of theophylline and face mask continuous positive airway pressure. Arch Dis Child 1982;57:761-765.
114. Hirsh K and Wang SC: Selective respiratory stimulating action of doxapram compared to pentylenetetrazol. J Pharmacol Exp Ther 1974;189:1-11.
115. Barrington KJ et al: Physiologic effects of doxapram in idiopathic apnea of prematurity. J Pediatr 1986;108:125.
116. Sagi E et al: Idiopathic apnoea of prematurity treated with doxapram and aminophylline. Arch Dis Child 1984;59:281.
117. Hayakawa F et al: Doxapram in the treatment of idiopathic apnea of prematurity: desirable dosage and serum concentrations. J Pediatr 1986;109:138.
118. Hoppenbrouwers T et al: Polygraphic studies of normal infants during the first six months of life. III. Incidence of apnea and periodic breathing. Pediatrics 1977;60:418.
119. Ariagno RL et al: Apnea and periodic breathing in control term infants. Clin Res 1984;32:120A.
120. Hoppenbrouwers T et al: Respiration during the first six months of life in normal infants. III. Computer identification of breathing pauses. Pediatr Res 1980;14:1230.
121. Oren J, Kelly D, and Shannon DC: Identification of a high-risk group for sudden infant death syndrome among infants who were resuscitated for sleep apnea. Pediatrics 1986;77:495.
122. Katcher ML, Shapiro MM, and Guist C: Severe injury and death associated with home infant cardiorespiratory monitors. Pediatrics 1986;78:775-779.
123. Guilleminault C: Obstructive sleep apnea syndrome and its treatment in children: areas of agreement and controversy. Pediatr Pulmonol 1987;3:429.
124. Brouillette RT, Ferbach SK, and Hunt CE: Obstructive sleep apnea in infants and children. Pediatrics 1982;100:31.
125. Eliaschar I et al: Sleep apneic episodes as indications for adenotonsillectomy. Arch Otolaryngol 1980; 106:492.
126. Dravath RE et al: Obstructive sleep apnea and death associated with surgical correction of velopharyngeal incompetence. Pediatrics 1980;96:645.
127. Coccagna R et al: Hypersomnia with periodic apneas in acquired micrognathia. Arch Neurol 1976;33:769.
128. Schmidt-Nowara WW: Continuous positive airway pressure for long-term treatment of sleep apnea. Am J Dis Child 1984;138:82.
129. Sullivan CE et al: Reversal of obstructive sleep apnea by continuous positive airway pressure applied through the nares. Lancet 1981;1:862.
130. Brouillette RT and Thach BT: A neuromuscular mechanism monitoring extrathoracic airway patency. J Appl Physiol 1979;46:772.
131. Rapoport DM et al: Reversal of the "pickwickian syndrome" by long-term use of nocturnal nasal-airway pressure. N Engl J Med 1982;307:931.
132. Charuzi I et al: Sleep apnea syndrome in the morbidly obese undergoing bariatric surgery. Gastroenterol Clin North Am 1987;16:517.
133. Everett AD, Koch WC, and Saulsbury FT: Failure to thrive due to obstructive sleep apnea. Clin Pediatr 1987;26:90.
134. Serratto M, Harris VJ, and Carr I: Upper airways obstruction: presentation with systemic hypertension. Arch Dis Child 1981;56:153.
135. Guilleminault C et al: Obstructive sleep apnea syndrome and tracheostomy: long-term follow-up experience. Arch Intern Med 1981;141:985.
136. Motta J et al: Tracheostomy and hemodynamic changes in sleep-induced apnea. Ann Intern Med 1978;89:454.
137. Burack B et al: The hypersomnia-sleep apnea syndrome: a reversible major cardiovascular hazard [abstract]. Circulation 1977;56:111.

12

Sleep-Related Enuresis

Sleep-related enuresis is an involuntary discharge of urine during sleep. It is a problem commonly seen by practitioners. Although biological sequelae are exceedingly rare, a comprehensive understanding of the causes, pathogenesis, diagnostic procedures, and treatment efforts is important in preventing significant long-term psychological sequelae.

Development of urinary continence is related to integration of neurological, physiological, anatomical, and behavioral maturation. It is difficult to determine when during the developmental process sleep-related enuresis becomes abnormal and requires intervention. In the progression of neurological development of the child, daytime continence becomes possible between 1 and 2 years of age. Nocturnal enuresis is still present in 30% of 4-year-olds, 15% of 5-year-olds, 10% of 6-year-olds, 3% of 12-year-olds, and 1% of 15-year-olds.[1,2] Indeed, the highest incidence of nocturnal enuresis occurs between the ages of 4 and 5 years, after which a considerable decrease occurs.[1,3] Some authors recommend therapeutic intervention after the age of 3 years.[4,5] However, most authorities agree that 5 years of age is the developmental level at which concern over bedwetting should be raised. This age has been chosen because most children spontaneously and finally become dry at night between the ages of 3 and 5 years and entry into the school system occurs at approximately 5 years of age. The lack of a precise age for all children is a manifestation of normal variations in human development.

The frequency of wetting at night has also been a point of controversy in the definition of sleep-related enuresis. Some have used a frequency of one episode per month to establish a diagnosis,[6] whereas others have used a frequency of one to two episodes per week.[7] Requiring a specific frequency of episodes for diagnosis may be inappropriate, since poor self-esteem, guilt, and anxiety, which often occur in enuretic children, can be identified even at a very low frequency of bedwetting. The uncertainty, unpredictability, and powerlessness that children feel may be damaging to their psychological and social development. Therefore diagnosis and treatment should be provided for the child regardless of the frequency of episodes of wetting.[8]

Sleep-related nocturnal enuresis is differentiated from daytime incontinence (diurnal enuresis). Approximately 80% of enuretic children wet only at night, 5% wet only during daytime waking hours, and about 15% experience both nocturnal and diurnal enuresis.[9] Differentiation is important because these types have different etiological implications. For example, organic and psychological causes (e.g., chronic urinary tract infection and stress) are significantly more common for diurnal or mixed enuresis than for nocturnal enuresis alone.

Sleep-related enuresis is subdivided into primary and secondary forms. *Primary sleep-related nocturnal enuresis* describes a pattern of incontinence that occurs at night, has been present since birth, and has no significant dry intervals. *Secondary nocturnal enuresis* refers to a pattern of incontinence occurring at night in children who have achieved nocturnal continence for a period of at least 3 months, followed by recurrence of nocturnal wetting.[4,8,10] Again, organic and psychological factors are more common in patients with secondary nocturnal enuresis than in those with primary enuresis.

Although direct physical complications of nocturnal enuresis are virtually nonexistent, this condition has caused consequential injuries because of parents' reactions, folk remedies, and medical treatments. Remedies used by parents have included tying the penis, placing a clothespin to obstruct the urethral meatus, placing the buttocks on a hot stove, cold streams of water directed onto the child's lower spine, beatings, shaming or ridiculing the child, severe physical punishment, making the child wear the wet pajamas around the neck, and hanging the wet sheets out of the window as a means of shaming the child.[4] Children have been burned with hot pokers and threatened with further mutilation if the wetting continued.[11] Other children have been made to sleep in a bathtub with a rope knotted around the waist.[12] During the 17th century some parents required the enuretic child to drink a pint of his or her own urine.[4] These forms of therapy are clearly abusive and risk causing significant physical and psychological trauma. Unfortunately, some are still inappropriately practiced today.

Throughout history, physicians have also treated nocturnal enuresis with harsh, abusive methods. Since 1500 BC physicians had prescribed inappropriate treatments including ground hedgehog and white hyacinthamum flowers, viscera of pigs, urine of spayed swine,[4] thermal blistering of the presacral skin to "heat" the sacral nerves,[13] mattresses with steel spikes, frames for pelvic elevation, cauterization of the urethral meatus with silver nitrate, and rubber balloons inserted into a girl's vagina to compress the bladder neck and urethra.

Fortunately, the vast majority of remedies have been discarded because of their ineffectiveness and inappropriateness. Newer methods of treatment are effective and appropriate and provide most enuretic children with a long-lasting cure and improved self-esteem.[14]

EPIDEMIOLOGY

The absence of universally accepted criteria for the diagnosis of primary nocturnal enuresis has resulted in restricted research designs, heterogeneous data, and varied conclusions. Data should therefore be viewed in this context, and generalizations to large populations should be accepted as approximations rather than a reflection of the true incidence and prevalence of this disorder.

Sleep-related nocturnal enuresis is common during childhood. It is estimated that between 3 million and 7 million school-age children in the United States suffer from this problem.[4] Prevalence data are similar in all societies whether they are industrialized or primitive,[15] attesting to the neurodevelopmental hypothesis of the disorder's origin.

The incidence of nocturnal enuresis rapidly and steadily declines with age as shown in Figure 12–1.[16] Approximately 80% of 2-year-old children wet the bed at night, about 50% at age 3,[17] 30% at age 4, 10% at age 6, 3% at age 12, and 1% after age 15.[1]

Based on these data and data from a study of more than 1,100 enuretic children,[2] spontaneous resolution of symptoms occurs at a rate of about 14% to 19% per year. However, a 5-year-old who continues to wet the bed at night has only about a 50% chance of spontaneous remission by the age of 10 years, and it may take several years for the remission to occur.

Primary nocturnal enuresis also appears to be familial in origin. The highest incidence of bedwetting occurs when both the child's mother and father were enuretic as children.[18] More than 77% of offspring of parents who both were enuretic will develop the disorder. If neither parent was enuretic, the incidence falls to approximately 15%.

Boys are affected nearly twice as often as girls before the age of 11 years. After this age the sex distribution seems to be equal.[19] Enuresis has been shown to be more common among families from lower socioeconomic groups and lower educational backgrounds.[3,20] Living in foster care,[21] residing in an institution,[22] inadequate toilet training, and birth order (firstborn) also have been shown to affect the incidence of nocturnal enuresis.

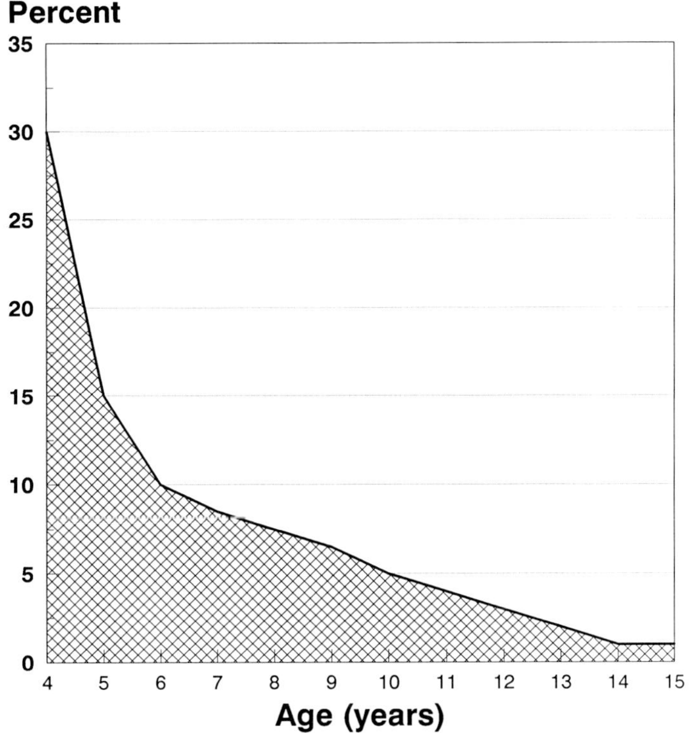

FIGURE 12–1. Frequency of nocturnal enuresis by age group. (Modified from Crawford JD: Introductory comments. J Pediatr 1989;114[Part 2]:687-690; and Novello AC and Novello JR: Enuresis. Pediatr Clin North Am 1987;34:719-730, with permission.)

PATHOPHYSIOLOGY

Sleep enuresis has many, varied causes. Appropriate management is based on accurate diagnosis. When an identifiable cause (e.g., urinary tract infection, diabetes mellitus) cannot be found, the symptom is termed *functional*. Although the exact cause of functional sleep enuresis remains obscure, it is thought to be due to delayed or inadequate maturation of the bladder (and perhaps delayed development of portions of the central nervous system). An understanding of a proposed pathophysiological scheme is important for the development of a rational approach to diagnosis and management. Appreciation of the physiological mechanism of bladder continence and bladder emptying is seminal (Fig. 12–2).

The infant begins life with an "automatic" bladder and sleeps nearly 60% to 70% of the day. Approximately 40% of voidings occur during sleep in this stage of development.[23] The number of voidings per day remains fairly constant in the first year of life but decreases during the next 2 years.

By 1 to 2 years of age, neurophysiological development progresses to a point at which the sensation of bladder fullness can be perceived. When the child is able to communicate the desire to void, a protocol of toilet training begins (a stepwise, *learned* process in which the child becomes able to hold urine for a period beyond the desire to void and then becomes able to initiate the urinary stream when the bladder is full). By 4½ years of age most children have acquired complete diurnal and nocturnal urinary control. If the maturation process that takes place between 2 and 4½ years is incomplete, the child will be left with a bladder that retains some of its infantile characteristics.[24]

Contrary to previously accepted mechanisms, normal voiding does not begin with bladder detrusor muscle contraction.[25] The first step in voluntary initiation of the urinary stream involves causing descent of the bladder neck by increasing intraabdominal pressure. This increase in pressure is directed toward the bladder by coordinated contraction of voluntary muscles (diaphragm and lower abdominal musculature).[24] In addition, the pubococcygeus muscle (anterior

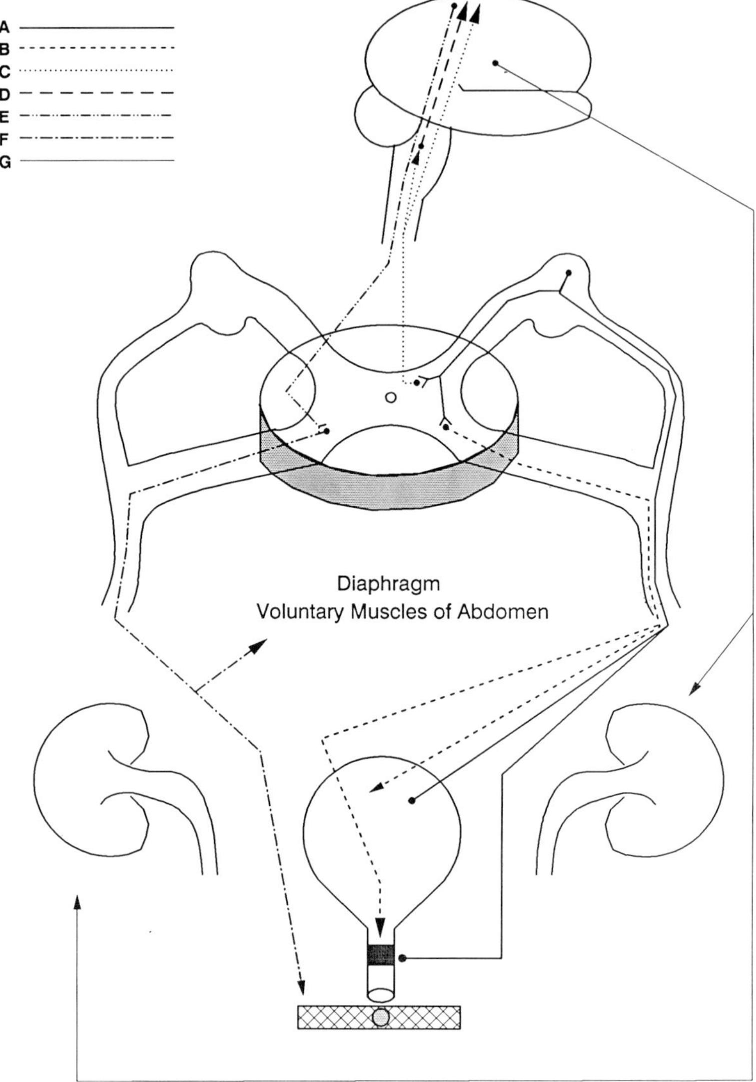

FIGURE 12–2. Bladder control pathways. Autonomic afferent pathways *(A)* from the bladder musculature and vesicle sphincter enter the spinal cord through sacral nerve roots (and some by pelvic splanchnic nerves). These neurons synapse on interneurons (not shown), autonomic efferent neurons *(B)*, and neurons that ascend to higher centers for conscious perception of the need to urinate. A proposed pathway through the reticular activating system *(D)* may cause arousal from sleep when bladder volume has reached its maximum functional capacity and arousal threshold is exceeded. Conscious control of bladder function is accomplished through descending impulses from the cortex *(E)* to lower motor neurons that control the voluntary musculature of the abdomen, levator ani, and diaphragm *(F)*. In addition, there appears to be a nocturnal peak of antidiuretic hormone secretion *(G)* that decreases urine volume, increases urine osmolality, and decreases serum osmolality during sleep. (Modified from Muellner SR: Development of urinary control in children: some aspects of the cause and treatment of primary enuresis. JAMA 1960;172:1259, with permission. Copyright 1960, American Medical Association.)

portion of the levator ani muscle) relaxes. Descent of the vesicle neck is the main stimulus for detrusor muscle contraction. Contraction of the detrusor muscle results in the opening of the internal vesicle sphincter and urination occurs. Although there is no voluntary control over the involuntary muscle of the bladder, continence and voluntary control of micturition involves mastery of large skeletal muscle groups that directly influence the smooth muscle of the bladder.

Development of urinary continence in a child begins with recognition of bladder fullness. Autonomic afferent impulses ("visceroception") from the bladder are most likely responsible for the sensation of vesicle distention. Once

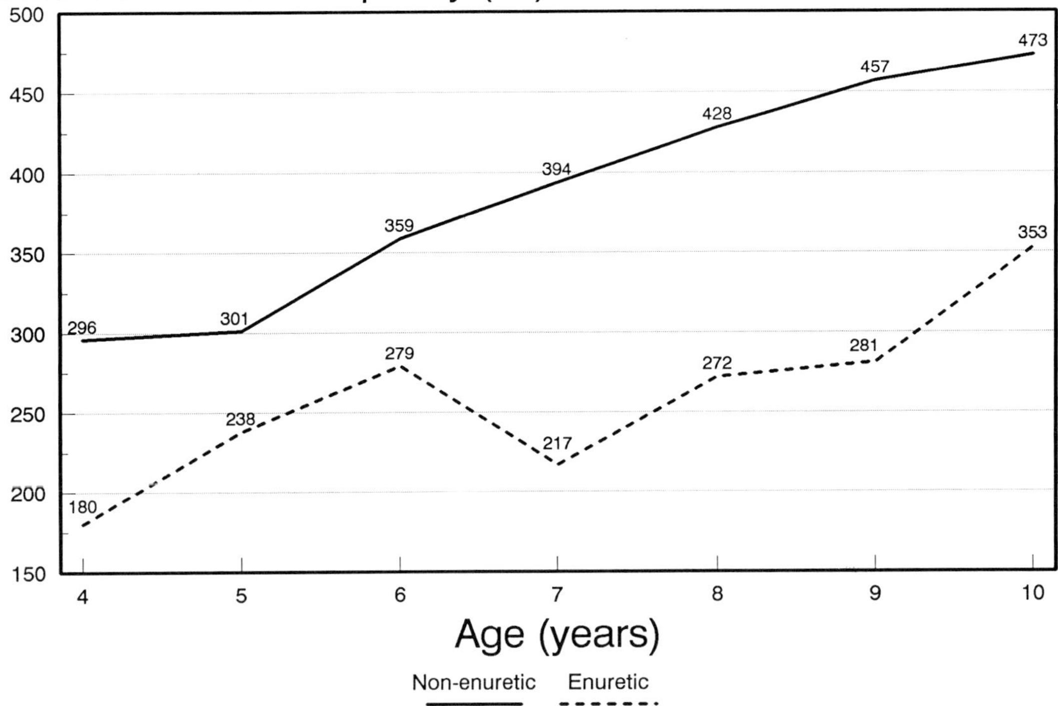

FIGURE 12–3. Functional bladder capacity across late and middle childhood. (Reprinted from, by permission of the publisher, Esperanca M and Gerrard JW: Nocturnal enuresis: studies in bladder function in normal children and enuretics. *CMAJ*, Vol. 101, September 20, 1969.)

this perception is possible, the child must be developmentally capable of communicating this new awareness. The next step is the development of an ability to withhold urination briefly beyond the point of perception. Inhibition of reflex contraction of the detrusor muscle is accomplished through prevention (or reversal) of descent of the vesicle neck by voluntary contraction of the levator ani muscle. Through trial and error the child next learns to initiate the urinary stream when the bladder is full by voluntary contraction of the diaphragm and abdominal musculature. At the outset of acquisition of this skill there are many false starts, since direction of the pressure into the pelvis toward the bladder is a highly coordinated, learned maneuver. According to Muellner, "Parental training constitutes at most an artificial urinary frequency which succeeds in catching the urine in the toilet bowl before the child wets its diaper. It is not possible for any parent to teach a child the complex use of the various muscle groups or to coordinate them in such a fashion as to develop mastery over the voluntary mechanism."[24]

Nocturnal continence depends on several interacting factors. First, *functional bladder capacity* must increase to a volume that can adequately maintain urine throughout the entire sleep period without contracting reflexively. Functional bladder capacity is defined as the volume of urine voided when the child has the normal sensation to urinate and is differentiated from anatomical bladder capacity as measured by cystometry. An infant's bladder has a small functional volume that increases as the child grows, develops, and matures. Once voluntary waking control of bladder function has been achieved and the child has established a functional urine volume of approximately 300 to 360 ml, nocturnal enuresis ceases. An adequate functional volume is reached between the ages of 2 and 7 years in most children. Studies of enuretic children have shown that their development of an adequate functional bladder capacity (a volume sufficient to maintain continence throughout the night) is significantly delayed when compared with nonenuretic children who have a normal bladder capacity for age, as shown in Figure 12–3. Enuretic children tend to maintain a capacity close to that of a 2-year-old.[10] This small volume is insufficient to maintain urine output throughout the night in a child 4½ years or older.[24]

Second, a clear nocturnal circadian peak of antidiuretic hormone secretion occurs in most nonenuretic children, resulting in decreased free water clearance and a diminution in the volume of urine production at night, a decrease in serum osmolality, and an increase in urine osmolality during the sleep period. This peak in secretion is significantly blunted in some children with nocturnal enuresis.[26] The increased volume of urine produced during the night often exceeds the functional bladder capacity and results in reflex emptying of the bladder.

Third, in nonenuretic children and adults, arousal from sleep occurs when the functional bladder capacity reaches its maximum. Arousal is most likely mediated by autonomic, afferent visceroceptive impulses originating in the bladder detrusor muscle. Although the exact mechanism of arousal is obscure, it may involve an increase in neuronal activity of the ascending reticular activating system, resulting in cortical activation, awakening, conscious perception of the need to void, and subsequent activation of voluntary muscle groups to maintain continence and to void at will.

Probably none of these mechanisms functions in isolation. Maintenance of continence during sleep and arousal when functional bladder capacity is exceeded most likely result from an interaction between these (and possibly other) factors related to ongoing development of the bladder, endocrine system, autonomic nervous system, and cortex.

ETIOLOGY

Psychological Causes

A psychological cause for primary nocturnal enuresis is unusual, occurring in less than 1% of prepubertal children with this disorder. However, signs of emotional disorders can be found with approximately 10% to 15% greater frequency in enuretic children than in nonenuretic children.[27,28] Thumb sucking, nail biting, poor school adjustment, temper tantrums, sibling rivalry, short attention span, poor self-esteem, eating disorders, negativism, fire starting, and stuttering have all been described.[29,30] Whether these signs of emotional distress are the cause or the result of bedwetting is not clear. Indeed, when the enuresis resolves, so do the emotional signs and symptoms in many enuretic children.[12]

Secondary nocturnal enuresis is more frequently associated with psychological factors, anxiety, and stress. In a study of 82 abused and

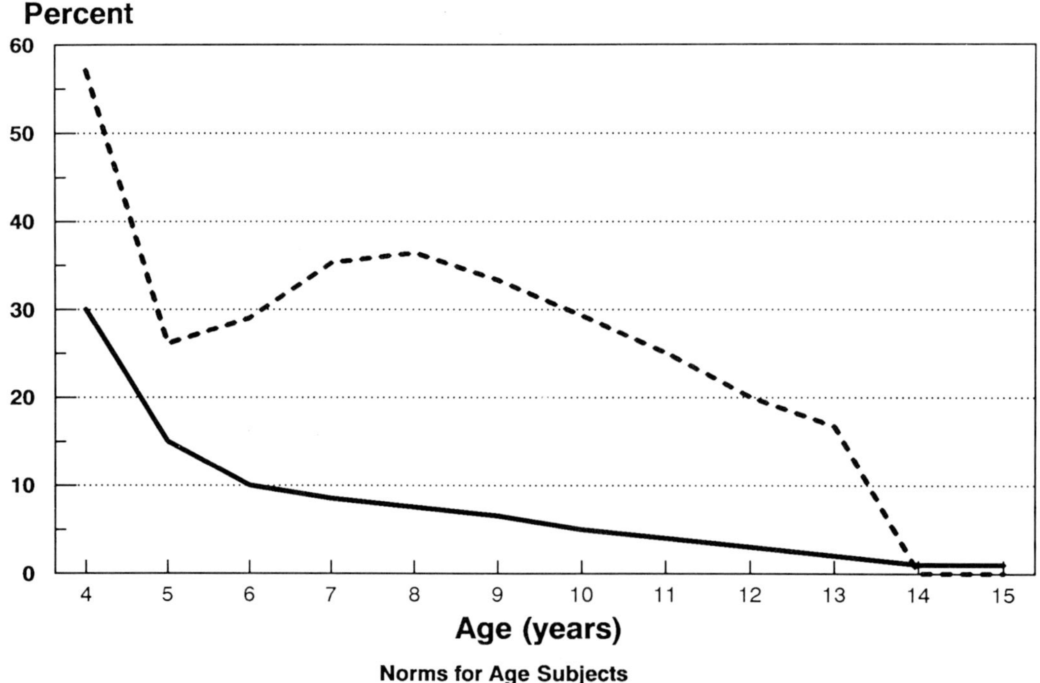

FIGURE 12–4. Frequency of sleep enuresis in abused and neglected children compared with norms for age.

neglected children between the ages of 3 and 6 years, the incidence of nocturnal enuresis was significantly greater than those reported for the general population in each age group (Fig. 12–4). Situational stress such as hospitalization or separation from parents, high levels of anxiety during periods of toilet training, and birth of a sibling has been associated with the recurrence of bedwetting after a significant dry period.[4,29,32,33]

Dysfunctional Toilet Training Practices

Physiological development of diurnal and nocturnal continence cannot be "taught" by parents. Maturation of many interacting systems and "learning" by trial and error are required before diurnal and nocturnal continence can be achieved. Yet many parents mistakenly believe that rigid, strict, or early introduction of toilet training regimens can be successful. Several investigations have shown that inappropriately rigid and early toilet training practices are associated with an increased incidence of sleep enuresis.[5,34,35] However, significant conflicting evidence does exist showing no correlation between parental toilet training efforts and the development of enuresis.[36,37] If maturation of bladder control can be affected by anxiety, fear, and stress, precipitation of these emotions by dysfunctional toilet training practices may contribute to the development of sleep enuresis. Further research is needed to determine the relationship, if any, between toilet training practices and the development of sleep enuresis.

Maturational Delay

Primary sleep enuresis most likely represents a delay in development of maturation of the systems and feedback loops responsible for the maintenance of continence. Although clear documentation is lacking, this hypothesis is attractive and supported by a number of clinical observations. First, functional bladder capacity increases as maturation progresses. As previously stated, functional bladder capacity reaches approximately 300 to 360 ml by the mean age of 4½ years, a volume that should allow the child to spend the night without wetting. Enuretic children, however, have been shown to have a much smaller functional bladder capacity and to maintain volumes more consistent with those observed at 2 years of age. The bladder is not anatomically small, since total bladder capacity when measured under anesthesia is not significantly different from the capacities of normal control subjects.[38] Second, uninhibited bladder contractions occur much more frequently in children with nocturnal enuresis, though almost one third of children with uninhibited bladder contractions have no symptoms of nocturnal or diurnal enuresis.[39,40] These urodynamic abnormalities, which are common in enuretic children, tend to improve as the child matures and resolve spontaneously. Third, coordinated diaphragm and skeletal muscle contractions are necessary to initiate the urinary stream, as well as to inhibit urination. Development of control over, and coordination of, these muscle groups follows patterns of maturation similar to the development of other motor skills such as walking. Fourth, development of arousal from sleep in response to autonomic afferent ("visceroceptive") impulses from the bladder is necessary for conscious control over mechanisms that inhibit detrusor muscle contraction. Therefore it appears that achieving nocturnal continence is a part of the child's general development.

Sleep Factors and Stages

Sleep enuresis was once thought to be a disorder of sleep or an abnormality of partial arousal from slow-wave sleep. This idea was supported by observations that enuretic children appeared to be deep sleepers, were difficult to arouse from sleep, and seemed to experience enuretic episodes during deep sleep.[41-44] Although depth of sleep may be an important factor in some children (enuresis is commonly associated with parasomnias), enuretic children sleep no more soundly than normal control children and their sleep architecture is not appreciably different. Enuretic episodes are not associated with deep sleep, a transition between sleep stages, or arousal. They are noted throughout the sleep period and occur in all sleep stages. Episodes appear to be random or related to time of night.[45,46]

Arousal thresholds for various stimuli differ considerably between sleep and wakefulness and between sleep stages, and there is substantial diversity between individuals. If autonomic afferent stimuli from a functionally full bladder are important in generating arousal to maintain continence, individual differences in threshold response may be significant in the development of enuresis.

Genetics

A familial occurrence of primary enuresis has long been recognized. Studies have shown that parents of almost half of enuretic youngsters were enuretic themselves as children.[47-49] In one study, when both parents had had enuresis, three fourths of their children were enuretic. When one parent had been enuretic, 44% of children were bedwetters. These data are compared with a 15% incidence of enuresis in children from nonenuretic parents. Evaluation of twins has indicated that when one sibling has enuresis, the other is predisposed to bedwetting.[50]

Organic Factors

Organic factors cause nocturnal enuresis in less than 10% of enuretic children.[2,51]

Urinary Tract Infection

Urinary tract infection is relatively common among enuretic children,[52] especially girls. Among girls who experience enuresis nightly, there is a 10-fold greater incidence of urinary tract infection.[28] Typical symptoms of urinary tract disorders (e.g., dysuria, frequency) may be absent. Controversy exists, however, regarding cause and effect. Whether enuresis in these patients is a symptom or a result of the enuresis is unknown. After adequate treatment and sterilization of the urine, many patients continue wetting the bed.[2] One explanation for enuresis as a contributing factor in urinary tract infection involves voluntary constriction of the levator ani muscle in an attempt to maintain continence during periods of uninhibited bladder contraction.[2,23] This produces a functional bladder outlet obstruction with high intravesical pressures comparable to those in patients with an anatomical urinary tract obstruction. In contrast to girls, enuretic boys do not seem to be prone to urinary tract infection, even in the presence of uninhibited bladder activity.[39,40,53]

Anatomical Abnormalities

Numerous anatomical abnormalities of the genitourinary tract have been associated with nocturnal enuresis. Urethral obstruction caused by posterior urethral valves can result in difficult or hesitant micturition, urinary frequency, and dribbling. In fact, any distal obstruction (e.g., meatal stenosis, juxtameatal stricture, and bladder neck contracture) may be linked to the development of bedwetting in some children.[7,54,55] Enuresis may occur with wide bladder neck anomaly.[54,56] Other associated abnormalities have included ectopic ureters, epispadias, hypospadias, postoperative state (iatrogenic), and ectopic bladder. Although the incidence of these abnormalities is low and invasive urological studies are usually unnecessary in evaluation of enuretic children, anatomical defects should be considered when symptoms such as difficulty starting and stopping the urinary stream, dysuria, or excessive frequency are present in addition to enuresis.

Severe Constipation

Extrinsic pressure on the bladder from a large fecal mass can decrease anatomical bladder capacity and result in long-term disorders of bladder control.[4] Resolution of the fecal mass and relief of constipation often alleviate the bladder control problem.

Conditions Causing Polyuria

Diabetes mellitus and diabetes insipidus are often associated with enuresis, and bedwetting may be the primary symptom. Clearly, any condition causing polyuria (whether produced by osmotic diuresis or intrinsic renal disease such as acquired renal insufficiency and renal tubular disease) can result in enuresis. A higher incidence of enuresis in patients with sickle cell anemia, sickle cell trait, or other hemoglobinopathies has also been noted. This symptom may be due to increased fluid intake in combination with a decreased concentrating ability of the kidney, causing hyposthenuria.[8]

Allergy

In some children enuresis may be a manifestation of atopic disorders.[57,58] The mucosal lining of the bladder may react in a manner similar to the mucosal lining of the respiratory tract when exposed to an allergen. Although no clear evidence exists, the mechanism has been postulated to be irritation from atopic inflammation.

Neurological Disorders

Abnormalities involving the spinal cord, such as meningomyelocele, spinal cord tumors, spina bifida occulta, diastematomyelia, sacral lipoma, sacral agenesis, and nerve root irritation, may result in enuresis. Enuresis has been reported with neurofibromatosis of the bladder. Nocturnal seizure disorders may also result in incontinence during sleep.

OBSTRUCTIVE SLEEP APNEA

Children with obstructive sleep apnea have a high incidence of nocturnal enuresis. The exact mechanism for this association is unknown. In adults with obstructive sleep apnea syndrome there appears to be an increase in the concentration of atrial natriuretic peptide,[59] abnormal plasma renin activity, and decreased plasma aldosterone levels[60] that are not normalized by treatment with nasal CPAP. It is unknown whether similar abnormalities occur in children with obstructive sleep apnea syndrome. Sleep enuresis may be secondary to increased intraabdominal pressure from paradoxical respiration associated with increased respiratory resistive load or may be due to a combination of factors. Auxiliary symptoms of restless sleep, significant snoring, daytime hypersomnolence, short attention span, hyperactivity, and school failure should suggest obstructive sleep apnea as a possible cause of enuresis.

Medications and Drugs

Prescribed medications, such as diuretics, may cause enuresis. Enuresis secondary to medications and drugs should be suspected in children on long-term regimens of medication that could increase urinary output and decrease urine osmolality. Accidental or unintentional ingestion should be suspected when secondary enuresis occurs with other signs or symptoms suggestive of side effects or toxic effects of a particular drug.

DIAGNOSIS

Diagnosis begins with a comprehensive history and physical examination. The presence of dysuria, hematuria, hesitancy, urgency, frequency, polyuria, polydipsia, polyphagia, seizure disorders, severe snoring, prior urinary tract infections, genitourinary surgery, allergies, or diurnal enuresis should raise the suspicion of an organic cause. Evaluation for possible psychopathology and assessment of family dynamics by the practitioner should be included in the initial workup. Family history should be evaluated for prior enuresis in family members. A complete assessment of past and current sleep patterns and habits should be obtained. Physical examination should include a comprehensive examination of the child's genitalia and a complete neurological examination.

A sleep log (kept for 2 weeks) documenting the child's sleep habits and pattern of wetting provides insight into the accuracy of the sleep-wake history and yields a graphic and longitudinal description of the child's sleep and waking behaviors. In addition, measurement of the child's functional bladder capacity over a period of 2 weeks provides information about the degree of bladder distention present when the child senses the need to urinate. Functional bladder capacity is measured simply by having the child urinate into a graduated container each time the child has the urge to void. Each void is recorded and averaged over a 1-week period. Urine volume should be measured only while the child is at home, and parents should be instructed that the urine need not be saved. Embarrassment from carrying the container to the washroom in school or during other activities should be avoided. If the functional bladder capacity is normal, a search for other causes for the symptom should be continued. A urinalysis for evaluation of urine specific gravity, presence of glycosuria or proteinuria, and presence of casts and cells in the sediment should be performed. A urine culture should also be obtained, especially in female patients, to rule out an occult urinary tract infection. Figure 12–5 illustrates an algorithm for evaluating an enuretic child.

TREATMENT

Treatment of nocturnal enuresis is based on a rational approach to diagnosis and initial management of any underlying organic or pathological condition. If a psychological or psychiatric disorder is suspected, this issue must be addressed before or in conjunction with institution of any developmental, maturational, or behavioral management program. If a primary sleep disorder (e.g., parasomnia, obstructive sleep apnea) is suspected, polysomnographic testing should be conducted and treatment protocols should be based on the results of this evaluation. Treatment and resolution of obstructive sleep apnea often result in resolution of the bedwetting.

Motivational Counseling and Behavior Modification

Once an organic cause has been ruled out, a *positive* approach to the problem should be created for the child. Plans should be appropriate for the child's age and developmental level.

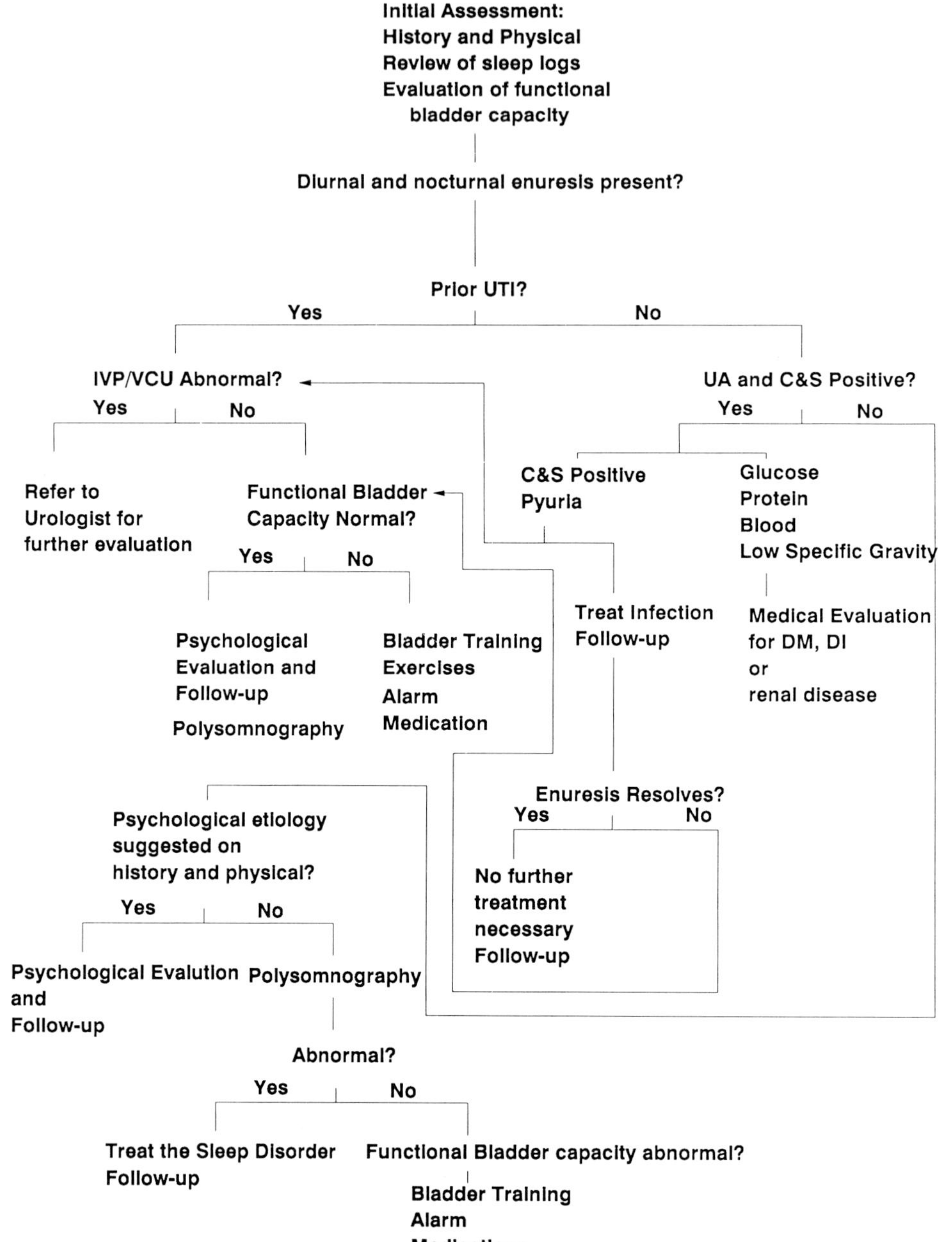

FIGURE 12–5. Algorithm for evaluation of the enuretic child. (Modified from Nino-Murcia G and Keenan SA: Enuresis and sleep. In Guilleminault C [ed]: Sleep and its disorders in children. New York, Raven Press, 1987, p 260, with permission.)

Children between 3 and 5 years of age may be managed by reassurance, motivational counseling, and simple bladder training exercises (described later in this section). Support from the health care professional during treatment and close follow-up are important for maintenance of compliance. *Persistency* and *consistency* in application of recommendations must be encouraged and supported. Complete resolution is usually a slow process, and the possibility of the child and family becoming discouraged is high. If parents and patients receive little support and follow-up, they are likely to discontinue the program and persistence of the problem will be inevitable.

For children over the age of 5 years a sequential management plan should be constructed. At the outset of treatment, sufficient time should be spent advising the parents and child about suspected developmental and mat-

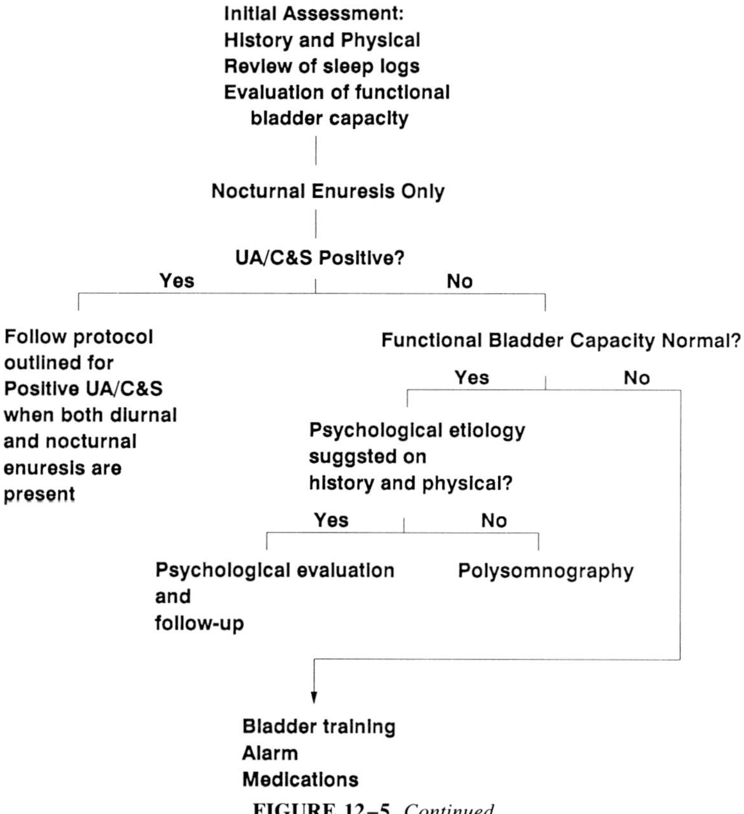

FIGURE 12–5. *Continued*

urational causes of enuresis, *expectations* of the program, and the time required for complete resolution of the problem. Here again, support from the health care professional is vital. If the family understands the therapeutic protocol and has appropriate expectations, the likelihood for success is greater. The tone of counseling should be positive. Although resolution of symptoms may take months, persistently working toward that goal should be the focus (and stimulus for reward) of intervention, rather than instantaneous cure of the problem. The parents must not inflict punishment or become angry or disappointed with the child's progress. Previously attempted interventions (such as waking the child several times each night to attempt to urinate) should be discontinued. Such approaches generally do not help and may in fact prolong the problem. *Management should focus on treatment of the child and not treatment of the bed.*

Initially parents and children should agree on a reward system (respondent conditioning). As with any behavior modification program, the reward should be readily achievable by the child (reward only for a dry bed in the morning is beyond the child's capacity and becomes more discouraging than supportive). Rewards should be simple, something that the child really wants to obtain, and within the family's means. Rewards should be given to the child for compliance with each behavior and immediately after completion of each task. Consistency in provision of rewards and the power of the reward significantly increase compliance with the regimen and the chance for a successful outcome.

The enuresis regimen begins with *bladder training exercises*. During daytime hours fluids should be encouraged to increase diurnal urine output. During the day the child should be encouraged to withhold urination as long as possible without the development of pain or incon tinence. This assists in increasing functional bladder capacity to an appropriate developmental volume (a process that may take up to 6 months). During this time, volumetric analysis of each void should continue in order to document increases in functional volume. It must be noted, however, that in the presence of diurnal enuresis and suspected bladder instability with uninhibited bladder contractions, withholding urination should be avoided. It is possible that this exercise might result in a functional outlet obstruction–like condition and increase the possibility of development of a urinary tract infection.

After the child learns to withhold micturition (usually after 1 week), attempts at *stream interruption* should begin. When urination cannot be delayed any longer, the child should begin to void into the toilet. Approximately halfway through the void the child should try to stop the urine stream. Initial attempts may be unsuccessful. With practice, however, the child is able to interrupt the void. When this is accomplished, the child should be instructed to interrupt the void for a count of 5 and then again begin voiding to empty the bladder. In this way the child learns mastery over the large skeletal muscles responsible for inhibition of detrusor muscle contraction (and voluntary initiation of micturition), promoting the maintenance of continence. Each of these tasks should be appropriately rewarded. If these behavioral-maturational interventions are successful, the regimen may be discontinued. Intermittent follow-up visits to the practitioner should continue. If a relapse occurs, the bladder training exercises may be reinstituted. In this case remission of symptoms usually occurs much more rapidly than at the initiation of the process. Support from the practitioner is vital during this time. Counseling the child and family beforehand that exacerbation of symptoms may occur prepares them for immediate intervention and decreases the likelihood of discouragement.

Bladder training and exercises should continue for 2 weeks to 3 months (depending on the child's response) before other regimens are introduced. Resolution of the symptom occurs at a rate of approximately 35% per year with use of this regimen alone.

Enuresis Alarm Systems

If no change in the nocturnal wetting pattern occurs after the initial therapeutic period, addition of an *enuresis alarm system* should be considered (operant conditioning). The alarm system is an open-circuit buzzer that is placed on the shoulder of the child's bedclothes, with connection wires that lead to open metallic contacts worn in a pouch on the outside of the undergarment in the area of the external urethral meatus (Figs. 12–6 and 12–7).* When the pouch becomes wet, the circuit closes and the alarm sounds. The sound should be loud enough to exceed the child's arousal threshold. Occasionally a child sleeps through the alarm but the buzzer awakens the parents. *It is important that the parents then attempt to wake the child and lead the child to the toilet to complete the void.* After a while the child will awaken with the buzzer. Gradually a perceptible decrease in the volume of urine voided into the bed and an increase in the volume of urine emptied into the toilet take place. The child progresses to a point at which only a small spot of urine (just enough

*The description of the system should not be interpreted as an endorsement for this product. Many different alarm systems are available. Some are worn on the patient's shoulder, others on the patient's wrist, and still others are placed on a night-table at the patient's bedside. Systems vary in price and complexity. The alarm system described here is used at the Center for Childhood Sleep Disorders Studies, Mount Sinai Hospital Medical Center, Chicago, exclusively because it has been very successful, is relatively inexpensive, and is safe (virtually without complications). All systems function in the same manner. Figures 12–6 and 12–7 are intended for demonstration purposes only. They do not represent an endorsement of any particular alarm system. To the best of our knowledge, no controlled trials of efficacy of various alarm systems have been published.

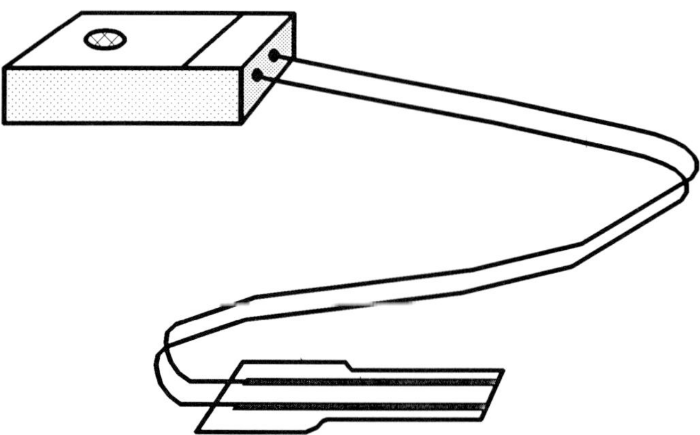

FIGURE 12–6. Diagram of an enuresis alarm. (From Palco Labs: Help for bedwetting. Santa Cruz, Calif. [See footnote above.])

to activate the alarm) is released. The bed remains dry. Appearance of dry nights occurs next. If the child initially had occasional dry nights, these increase in frequency and become strung together into a series of dry nights. The child should continue to wear the alarm system until 21 consecutive dry nights are achieved, after which time the alarm may be discontinued. Change in the wetting pattern is typically seen after 3 to 6 weeks. Using an alarm system, some children achieve nocturnal continence within several weeks. Other children require treatment for as long as a year. The resolution rate for alarm systems is about 70% per year. A sample of instructions for use of the bedwetting alarm system to be given to parents is shown in Figure 12–8.

As with all other forms of therapy, exacerbations occur when alarm systems are used. Parents and children should be forewarned of this possibility and should not be discouraged if it occurs. They should be instructed to reinstitute the alarm and to discontinue treatment when 21 consecutive dry nights are again achieved. Resolution in these cases occurs much more rapidly than at the outset of treatment. Bladder training exercises as previously described may be continued during treatment with the alarm system.

Several conditions may preclude use of an alarm system. The child must be able to hear the alarm, and it must exceed the child's arousal threshold. Children with congenital or acquired hearing loss often are not responsive to alarm systems. Children (as well as their parents) must

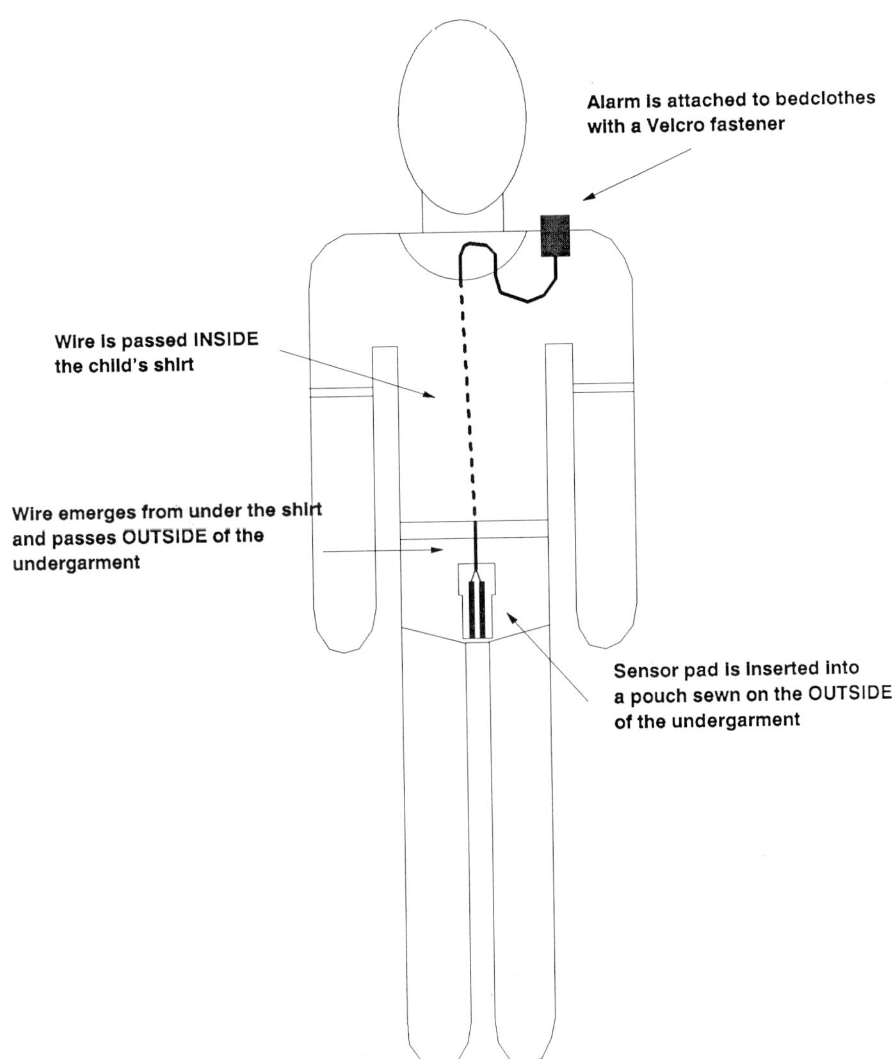

FIGURE 12–7. Diagram of proper placement of an enuresis alarm. (From Palco Labs: Help for bedwetting. Santa Cruz, Calif. [See footnote on p. 162.])

CENTER FOR CHILDHOOD SLEEP DISORDERS STUDIES
INSTRUCTIONS FOR PARENTS
Bedwetting Alarm Instructions

- ☐ DEMONSTRATION OF THE ALARM.
  - ☐ At first your child may not wake up when the alarm goes off.
  - ☐ It is important that you still attempt to wake your child and immediately take him/her to the bathroom to urinate.
  - ☐ After a time, you will notice your child waking with the alarm.
  - ☐ At about the same time, you will notice that the amount of urine in the bed has decreased and the amount of urine voided in the bathroom has increased.
  - ☐ The decrease in urine in the bed will continue until there is just a small spot of urine on your child's underwear (just enough to trigger the alarm).
  - ☐ At this time, the bed should be dry.
  - ☐ Dry nights will then appear and the alarm will not go off.
- ☐ YOUR CHILD SHOULD CONTINUE WEARING THE ALARM UNTIL THERE ARE 21 DRY NIGHTS IN A ROW.

If you have any questions, please call the Sleep Center

FIGURE 12–8. Written instructions for use of an enuresis alarm system.

be motivated to use the alarm and assume some responsibility in management of the problem. A child who is resistant to its use or fearful of the regimen has a greater likelihood of failure. The child must be developmentally capable of responding to the alarm system. Children younger than 4 years may not be able to coordinate control of the voluntary musculature required for nocturnal continence. Last, the alarm system should not be used in a toilet training regimen. Conditioning of the multiple reflexes involved in maintenance of nocturnal continence requires time and persistence. The alarm system should not be considered a quick fix for nocturnal enuresis. Parents' expectations should be appropriate to the system used.

Medication

DESMOPRESSIN

If the child continues to wet the bed without appreciable change in the pattern of wetting after sufficient time has elapsed (3 to 6 months in our clinic), *medication* may be considered. We have used desmopressin (DDAVP) as the first drug of choice in management of alarm failures. We have also used desmopressin as first-line treatment of primary enuresis in adolescents. Embarrassment associated with using the alarm (especially when the patient has younger "dry" siblings) and the many social obligations of adolescents make desmopressin a more acceptable initial treatment modality. Some authorities use desmopressin as the treatment of choice for all children with primary enuresis.[61] This is based on the assumption (and some observations) that nocturnal secretion of antidiuretic hormone is blunted in many enuretic children. Desmopressin decreases urine production throughout the night, and urine volume falls to levels commensurate with the functional bladder capacity. Desmopressin has been used for many years in the treatment of diabetes insipidus[62] and has been found safe and efficacious. Although side effects are few and are rarely seen in clinical practice, there exists the potential for significant irritation of the nasal mucosa, epistaxis, hypersensitivity reactions, hyponatremia, and water intoxication. In high doses desmopressin may cause slight elevation of blood pressure, transient headache, nausea, nasal congestion, rhinitis, mild abdominal cramps, and flushing. These uncommon side effects and adverse reactions generally resolve once the dosage has been decreased or the medication discontinued. Since enuresis alarm systems have no known side effects or adverse reactions, we have chosen alarms as the treatment of choice and use desmopressin only for selected patients and when the alarm system has failed to achieve a significant change in bedwetting pattern after 3 to 6 months or to resolve the enuresis after 1 year.

Desmopressin is administered as a nasal spray, available in 2.5 and 5 ml bottles with a spray pump delivering 10 μg doses. The usual starting dose is 40 μg administered at bedtime (20 μg/nares). Response to the medication is generally rapid, and symptoms of nocturnal enuresis generally respond in 1 to 2 weeks. A response has been defined as a decrease in the frequency of wet nights by 50% or a decrease in the degree of wetness (perceptibly smaller volume of urine).[61] If there is an initial response to desmopressin, the medication should be continued until the patient is completely dry. The medication can then be tapered by 10 μg every 2 weeks until it is discontinued. If there is relapse, the medication may be reinstituted and weaning attempted at a later date.

In Miller's study of 55 enuretic children treated with desmopressin,[61] medication was discontinued if there was no response in 2 weeks (nonresponders were 15% of the subjects). Fifteen percent of the subjects were partial responders (had an initial response but did not progess to total dryness); 24% had an initial response and progressed to total dryness with long-term therapy but relapsed when the medication was discontinued; and 27% had an initial positive response, progressed to total dryness with long-term therapy, and remained dry when the medication was discontinued.

Other Medications

In the past, imipramine has been recommended in the treatment of nocturnal enuresis. The response rate is variable and relapses are frequent. Because imipramine, a tricyclic antidepressant medication, significantly affects the sleep cycle and is a powerful REM suppressant, because of the narrow therapeutic window, and because of the possibility of cardiac arrhythmias, we avoid prescribing this medication for primary nocturnal enuresis.

REFERENCES

1. DeJonge GA: Epidemiology of enuresis: a survey of the literature. In Kolvin I, MacKeith RC, and Meadows SR (eds): Bladder control and enuresis. Clin Dev Med 48/49, London, Heinemann, 1973, pp 39-46.
2. Forsythe WI and Redmond A: Enuresis and spontaneous cure rate: study of 1129 enuretics. Arch Dis Child 1974;49:259.
3. Gross RT and Dornbusch SM: Enuresis. In Levine MD et al (eds): Developmental-behavioral pediatrics. Philadelphia, WB Saunders, 1983, p 573.
4. Schaefer CE: Childhood encopresis and enuresis. New York, Van Nostrand Reinhold, 1979, p 89.
5. Powell NB: Urinary incontinence in children. Arch Pediatr 1951;68:151.
6. Starfield B: Enuresis: its pathogenesis and management. Clin Pediatr 1972;11:343.
7. McLain IG: Childhood enuresis. Curr Probl Pediatr 1979;9:4.
8. Nino-Murcia G and Keenan SA: Enuresis and sleep. In Guilleminault C (ed): Sleep and its disorders in children. New York, Raven Press, p 253.
9. Campbell MF: Clinical pediatric urology. Philadelphia, WB Saunders, 1951, p 848.
10. Wyker AW: Standard diagnostic considerations. In Gillenwater JY et al (eds): Adult and pediatric urology. Chicago, Year Book, 1987, p 62.
11. Smith S: Bedwetting: its cause, effect, and remedy. Valley Stream, NY, HR Press, 1974.
12. Baller WR: Bed-wetting: origin and treatment. New York, Pergamon Press, 1975.
13. Glicklich LB: A historical account of enuresis. Pediatrics 1951;8:859.
14. Moffatt MEK, Kato C, and Pless IB: Improvement in self-concept after treatment of nocturnal enuresis: a randomized controlled trial. J Pediatr 1987;110:647.
15. Schmitt BD: Nocturnal enuresis: an update on treatment. Pediatr Clin North Am 1982;29:21.
16. Jones HG: The behavioral treatment of enuresis nocturna. In Eysenck HJ (ed): Behaviour therapy and the neuroses. Oxford, Eng, Pergamon Press, 1960.

17. Chamberlin RW: Management of preschool behavior problems. Pediatr Clin North Am 1974;21:33.
18. Cohen MW: Symposium on behavioral pediatrics. Pediatr Clin North Am 1975;22:3.
19. Meadow SR: Enuresis. In Edelman CH (ed): Pediatric kidney disease. Boston, Little, Brown, 1978, p 1176.
20. Bloomfield JM and Douglas J: Enuresis: prevalence among children aged 4-7 years. Lancet 1956;1:850.
21. Stein ZA and Susser MW: Nocturnal enuresis as a phenomenon of institutions. Dev Med Child Neurol 1966;8:677.
22. Dittman KS and Blinn KA: Sleep levels in enuresis. Am J Psychiatry 1955;12:913.
23. Koff SA: Enuresis. In Walsh PC et al: Campbell's urology. Philadelphia, WB Saunders, 1986, p 2179.
24. Muellner SR: Development of urinary control in children: some aspects of the cause and treatment of primary enuresis. JAMA 1960;172:1256.
25. Muellner SR: Physiology of micturition. J Urol 1951;65:805.
26. Norgaard JP, Rittig S, and Djurhuus JC: Nocturnal enuresis: an approach to treatment based on pathogenesis. J Pediatr 1989;114(Part 2):705.
27. Rutter M, Yule W, and Grahm P: Enuresis and behavioral deviance. In Kolvin I, MacKeith RC, and Meadow SR: Bladder control and enuresis. Clin Dev Med 48/49, London, Heinemann, 1973.
28. Taylor PD and Turner RK: A clinical trial of continuous, intermittent and overlearning "bell and pad" treatment for nocturnal enuresis. Behav Res Ther 1975;13:281.
29. Benjamin LS et al: The relative importance of psychopathology, training procedure and urological pathology in nocturnal enuresis. Child Psychiatry Hum Dev 1971;1:215.
30. Faschingbauer TR: Enuresis: its nature, etiology, and treatment; a review of the literature, 1924-1970. JSAS Catalog of Selected Documents for Psychology 1975;5:194.
31. Sheldon SH et al: Sleep disorders in abused and neglected children. Unpublished data.
32. Werry JS: Enuresis—a psychosomatic entity? Can Med Assoc J 1967;97:319.
33. Douglas JW: Early disturbing events and later enuresis. In Klovin I, MacKeith RC, and Meadows SR (eds): Bladder control and enuresis. Clin Dev Med 48/49, London, Heinemann, 1973.
34. Bindelglas PM, Dee GH, and Enos FA: Medical and psychosocial factors in enuretic children treated with imipramine hydrochloride. Am J Psychiatry 1968;124:125.
35. Despert J: Urinary control and enuresis. Psychosom Med 1944;6:294.
36. Benjamin LS, Serdahely W, and Geppert TV: Night training through parents' implicit use of operant conditioning. Child Dev 1971;42:963.
37. Klackenberg G: Primary enuresis: when is a child dry at night? Acta Paediatr Scand 1955;44:513.
38. Troup CW and Hodgson NB: Nocturnal functional bladder capacity in enuretic children. J Urol 1971;129:132.
39. Lapides J and Diokno AC: Persistence of the infant bladder as a cause of urinary infection in girls. J Urol 1970;103:243.
40. Koff SA, Lapides J, and Piazza DH: The uninhibited bladder in children: a cause for urinary tract infection, obstruction, and reflux. In Hodson J and Kincaid-Smith P (eds): Reflux nephropathy. New York, Masson, 1979.
41. Broughton RJ: Sleep disorders: disorders of arousal? Science 1968;159:1070.
42. Lowy FH: Recent sleep and dream research: clinical implications. Can Med Assoc J 1970;102:1069.
43. Anders TF and Weinstein P: Sleep and its disorders in infants: a review. Pediatrics 1972;50:312.
44. Kales A and Kales JD: Sleep disorders: recent findings in the diagnosis and treatment of disturbed sleep. N Engl J Med 1974;290:487.
45. Kales A et al: Effect of imipramine on enuretic frequency and sleep stages. Pediatrics 1977;60:431.
46. Mikkelsen EJ et al: Childhood enuresis. I. Sleep patterns and psychopathology. Arch Gen Psychiatry 1980;37:1139.
47. Hallgren B: Enuresis: a clinical and genetic study. Acta Psychiatr Neurol Scand [suppl] 1957;114:1.
48. White M: A thousand consecutive cases of enuresis: results of treatment. Child Fam 1971;10:198.
49. Young GC: The family history of enuresis. J R Inst Pub Health 1963, August, pp 197-201.
50. Bawkin H: Sleep walking in twins. Lancet 1970;2:446.
51. McKendry JBJ and Stewart DA: Enuresis. Pediatr Clin North Am 1974;21:1019.
52. Dodge WF et al: Nocturnal enuresis in 6 to 10 year-old children: correlation with bacteriuria, proteinuria and dysuria. Am J Dis Child 1970;120:32.
53. Koff SA and Murtagh DS: The uninhibited bladder in children: effect of treatment on recurrence of urinary infection and on vesicoureteral reflux resolution. J Urol 1983;130:1138.
54. Williams DI: Urinary incontinence. In Williams DI et al (eds): Urology in childhood. New York, Springer-Verlag, 1974, p 238.
55. Murphy S and Chapman W: Adolescent enuresis: a urologic study. Pediatrics 1970;45:426.
56. Stanton S and Williams DI: Wide bladder neck anomaly. Br J Urol 1973;45:60.
57. Esperanca M and Gerrard JW: Nocturnal enuresis: comparison of the effect of imipramine and dietary restrictions on bladder capacity. Can Med Assoc J 1969;101:721.
58. Gerrard JW: Allergy and urinary infections: is there an association? Pediatrics 1971;48:994.
59. Baruzzi A et al: Atrial natriuretic peptide and catecholamines in obstructive sleep apnea syndrome. Sleep 1991;14:83-86.
60. Follenius M et al: Obstructive sleep apnea treatment: peripheral and central effects on plasma renin activity and aldosterone. Sleep 1991;14:211-217.
61. Miller K, Goldberg S, and Atkin B: Nocturnal enuresis: experience with long-term use of intranasally administered desmopressin. J Pediatr 1989;114(Part 2):723.
62. Harris A: Clinical experience with desmopressin: efficacy and safety in central diabetes insipidus and other conditions. J Pediatr 1989;114(Part 2):711.

APPENDIX 1

Introduction to Polysomnography

Polysomnography is the term used to describe a procedure of objective, simultaneous recording of many different physiological parameters during sleep. Practitioners who treat children with sleep problems should be familiar with the general methods and techniques employed in the sleep laboratory. Practical issues such as patient preparation before the study, techniques used to monitor physiological parameters, and components of the polysomnogram report should be understood.

PHYSIOLOGICAL PARAMETERS MONITORED DURING SLEEP

Electroencephalographic Activity

Information obtained from the electroencephalogram (EEG) forms the basis for differentiating stages of non–rapid eye movement (NREM) sleep. Continuous monitoring of the EEG throughout the night also provides ongoing information about the development and integrity of the central nervous system. Therefore use of standard methods is necessary for accurate and reliable recording.

The EEG is generated by fluctuations of electrical potentials of cortical neurons. These fluctuations are induced by impulses arriving from other cells and centers of the brain and are transmitted through the coverings of the brain to the scalp. Scalp electrodes record mainly the summated potential changes of neurons in the underlying cortex, favoring slow potential changes generated in large areas near the recording electrodes.

Use of the standard *International 10-20 System* allows symmetrical, reproducible lead placement (Fig. A1–1); comparison of EEGs from the same patient and from different patients; and comparison of recordings from the same or different laboratories. Improper electrode placement on the scalp can lead to problems with overall validity, evaluation, and scoring of sleep stages.

Sleep stage scoring has been standardized with the use of a limited, referential EEG montage. In most sleep laboratories a central recording site (C3 or C4) is coupled with a referential site (usually the opposite earlobe or mastoid process). Although only one channel of EEG is deemed sufficient for identification of NREM stages, many laboratories employ other derivations to obtain a more complete assessment. Addition of an occipital recording channel is helpful in demonstrating alpha activity (Fig. A1–2). A coronal (Fig. A1–3) or parasagittal (Fig. A1–4) bipolar montage will be helpful in identifying nocturnal seizure disorders. A complete EEG montage and recording strategy may be useful in localizing abnormal EEG activity.

Application of EEG electrodes begins with accurate measurement and marking of proper electrode positions on the head. The skin surface is cleansed and prepared to minimize impedance. Cup-shaped electrodes may be filled with conductive paste or jelly. All electrodes are affixed to the scalp with cotton or gauze. Many cup-shaped electrodes have a hole in the center

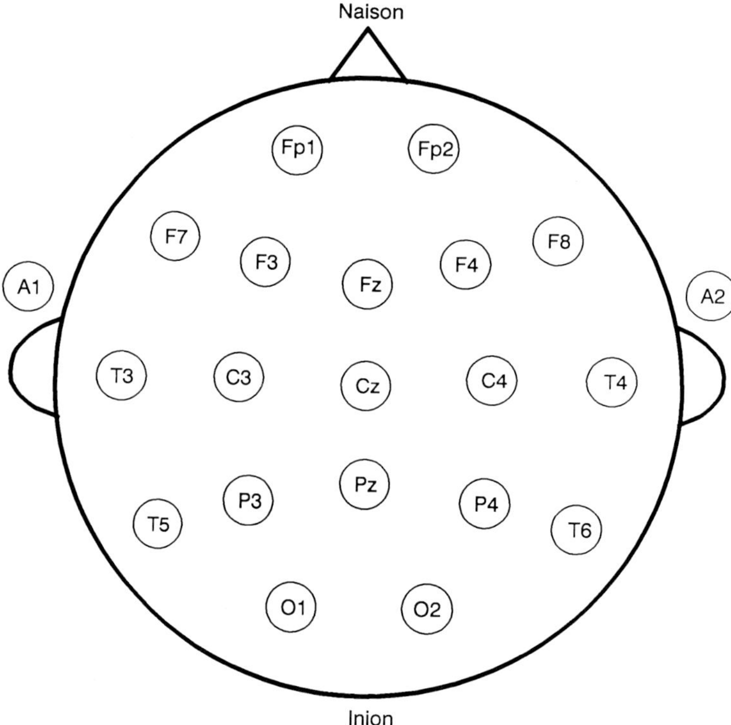

FIGURE A1–1. International 10-20 system of electrode placement. (Redrawn with permission from Jasper HH: The ten-twenty electrode system of the International Federation. Electroencephalogr Clin Neurophysiol 1958;10:371-375.)

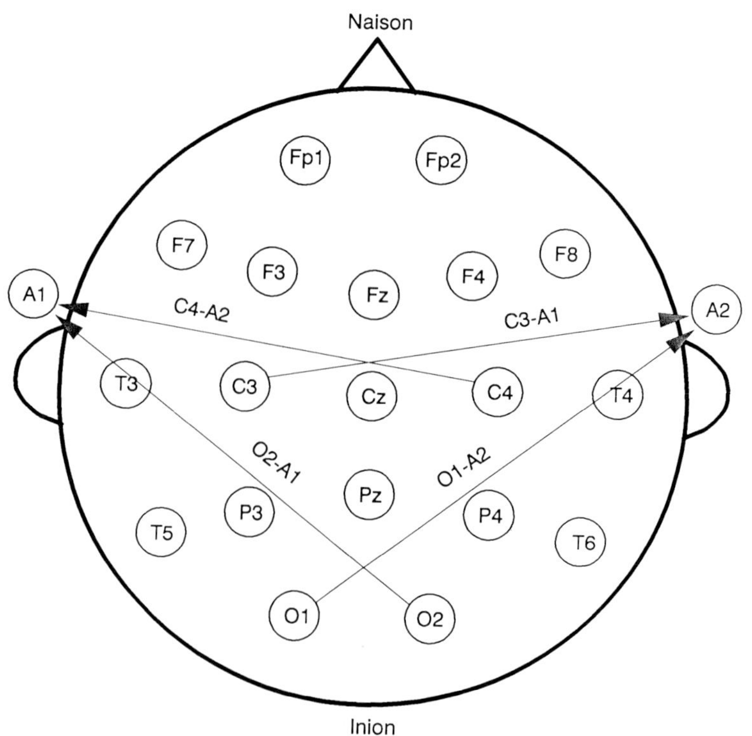

FIGURE A1–2. Standard polysomnographic EEG montage. Standards of sleep stage scoring have been developed using C3-A2 or C4-A1 referential montage (or both). Occipital electrode monitoring is recommended, since alpha EEG activity is preponderant in the occipital leads and sleep onset may be more easily determined. Only one EEG channel is required for sleep stage scoring, but many laboratories use other channels as backup. In the event that an electrode is displaced during the recording period, the patient need not be disturbed. Laboratories may also use a more complete referential or bipolar montage to assess EEG activity more completely during sleep (see Figs. A1–3 and A1–4).

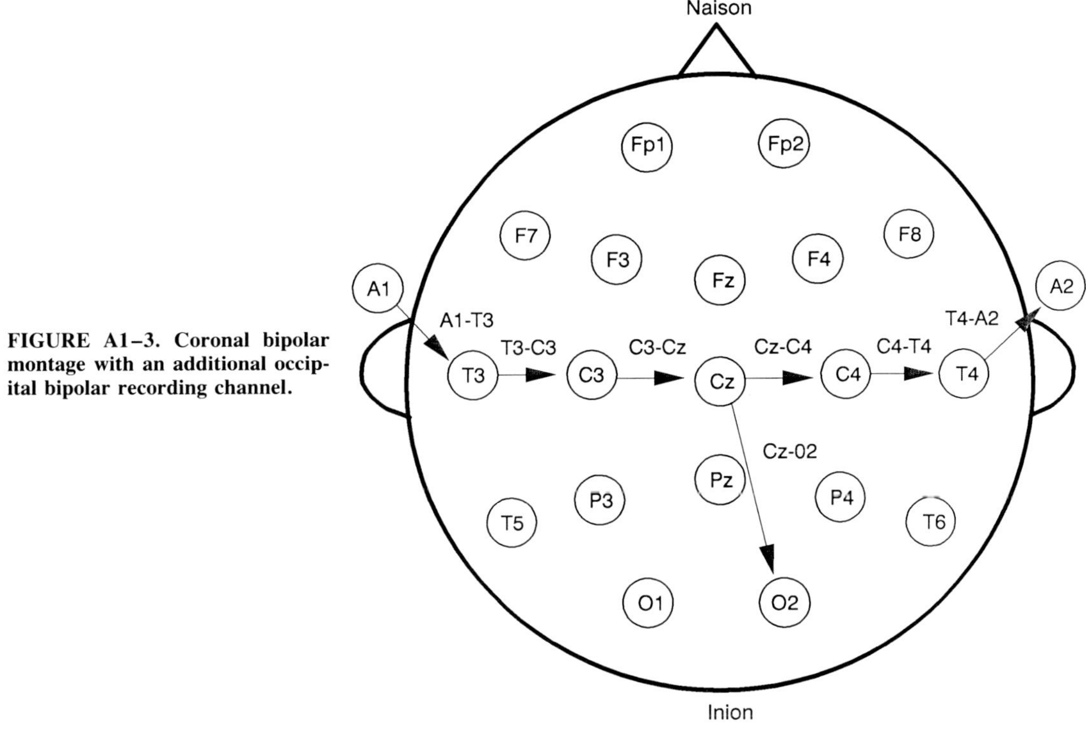

FIGURE A1–3. Coronal bipolar montage with an additional occipital bipolar recording channel.

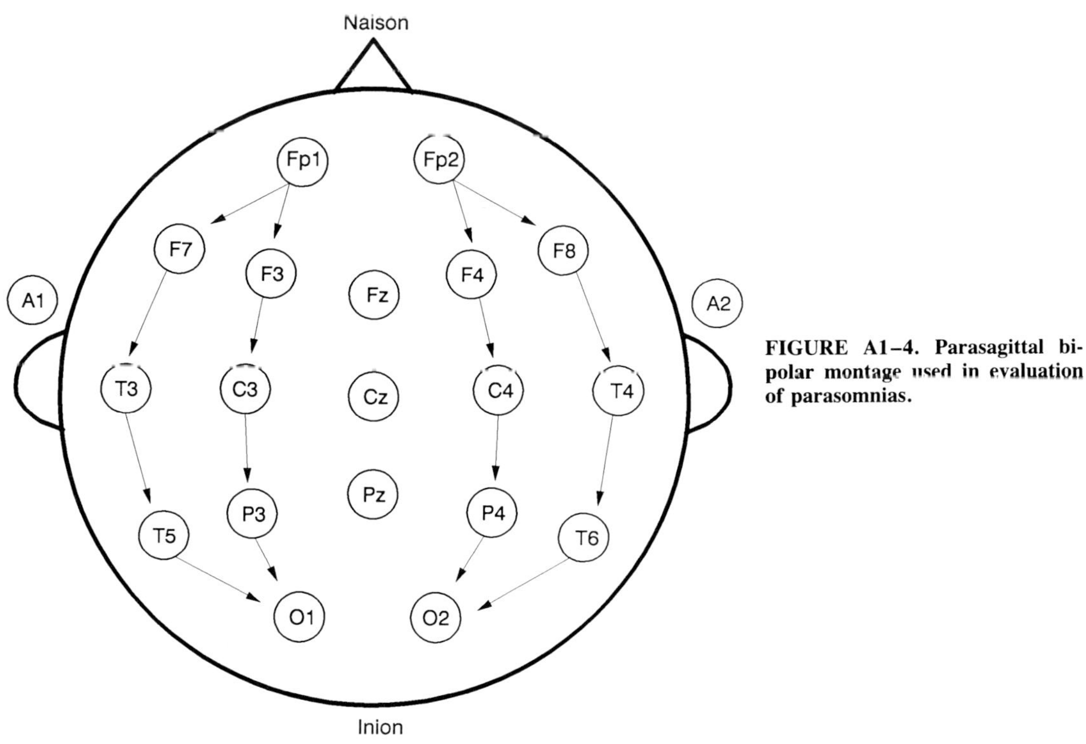

FIGURE A1–4. Parasagittal bipolar montage used in evaluation of parasomnias.

for instillation of a conductive medium after the electrode has been fixed to the scalp. Alternatively, a gauze pad may be soaked with collodion, placed over the electrode, and dried with compressed air. This technique has the advantage of providing excellent contact with the scalp for extended periods in active patients. Prolonged, stable placement is especially helpful if the all-night recording is followed by a Multiple Sleep Latency Test (MSLT). Few if any complications are associated with the use of collodion. Rarely irritation or allergic reactions occur. Some children find the aroma of the adhesive (and the acetone used to remove it) initially bothersome.

Electrooculographic Activity

The electrooculogram (EOG) is recorded during the course of a sleep study to identify the slow, rolling eye movements that are characteristic of Stage 1 sleep and herald sleep onset, as well as to record the rapid, conjugate eye movements associated with REM sleep. Because of the small electrical potential difference between the cornea (positive) and retina (negative), movement of the eyes can be recorded from electrodes placed on the skin surface in the periorbital region. Electrodes are generally taped 1 cm lateral to the outer canthi of the eyes, are offset from horizontal (one above and the other below) by about 1 cm, and are referred to one ear or mastoid process (Fig. A1–5). Offsetting the leads from the horizontal permits recording of horizontal, vertical, and oblique eye movements (Fig. A1–6). As the eyes move with respect to the fixed electrodes, potential changes register as pen deflections on the polygraph. If separate channels are used for each eye, the pens move in opposite directions when conjugate deviation occurs.

Electromyographic Activity

Although electromyographic (EMG) activity during sleep can be assessed from any number of skeletal muscle groups, recording muscle tone from the chin has become customary. Certain sleep disorders (e.g., bruxism, REM sleep behavior disorder) are associated with unusual muscle activity that can be recorded by surface EMG. EMG recording also provides information about the patient's sleep-wake behavior and permits quantification of arousal responses and sleep movements.

In general, three recording electrodes are applied to the chin, although recording is obtained from only two. The extra electrode provides a backup in the event of electrode failure during the recording. Because the electrodes are simply taped to the skin, without the use of collodion, electrode failures are common, especially if the patient is active, awake, eating, or talking.

EMG activity from other muscles (e.g., tibialis anterior) may be simultaneously recorded for evaluation of abnormal or paroxysmal movements during sleep.

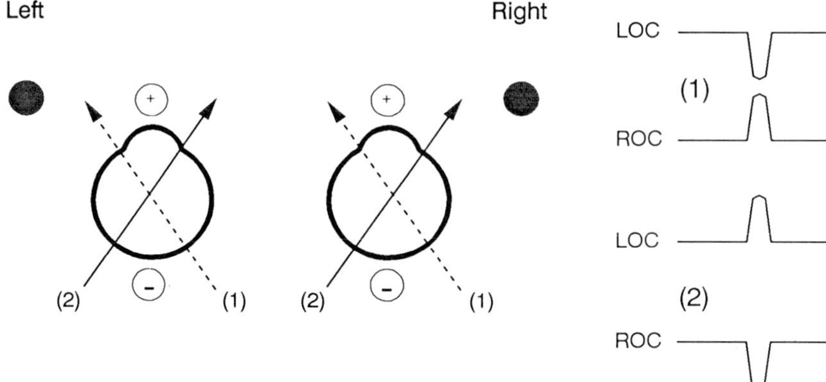

FIGURE A1–5. Generation of the EOG. The globe of the eye is a functional dipole with an anterior positive charge (cornea) and a posterior negative charge (retina). Potential differences between the left outer canthus and right outer canthus are detected when the eyes move toward or away from each electrode. With movement of the eyes to the left (*1*), there is a positive (downward) deflection of the pen recording from the left outer canthus and a negative (upward) deflection of the pen recording from the right outer canthus. When the eyes move to the right (*2*), there is a negative deflection of the pen recording from the left outer canthus and a positive deflection of the pen recording from the right outer canthus.

Electrocardiographic Activity

At least one channel of the polysomnogram must record the patient's electrocardiogram (ECG). Cardiac activity is generally monitored for rate and rhythm, since only a limited, single channel is used. Only relative information about cardiac electrical function is provided by polysomnography, and clinical conclusions regarding a patient's ECG are not possible. If comprehensive evaluation of cardiac activity is necessary, Holter monitoring may be requested.

Respiratory Activity

Three respiratory parameters are typically monitored during polysomnographic assessment: nasal-oral airflow, respiratory effort, and oxygen saturation. Nasal and oral airflow is most commonly recorded by the placement of thermistors or thermocouples in the stream of air. This method of measurement is simple, comfortable, and highly reliable in most patients. However, it can be imprecise because of positional factors and may require that the technician frequently adjust the sensors and alter the

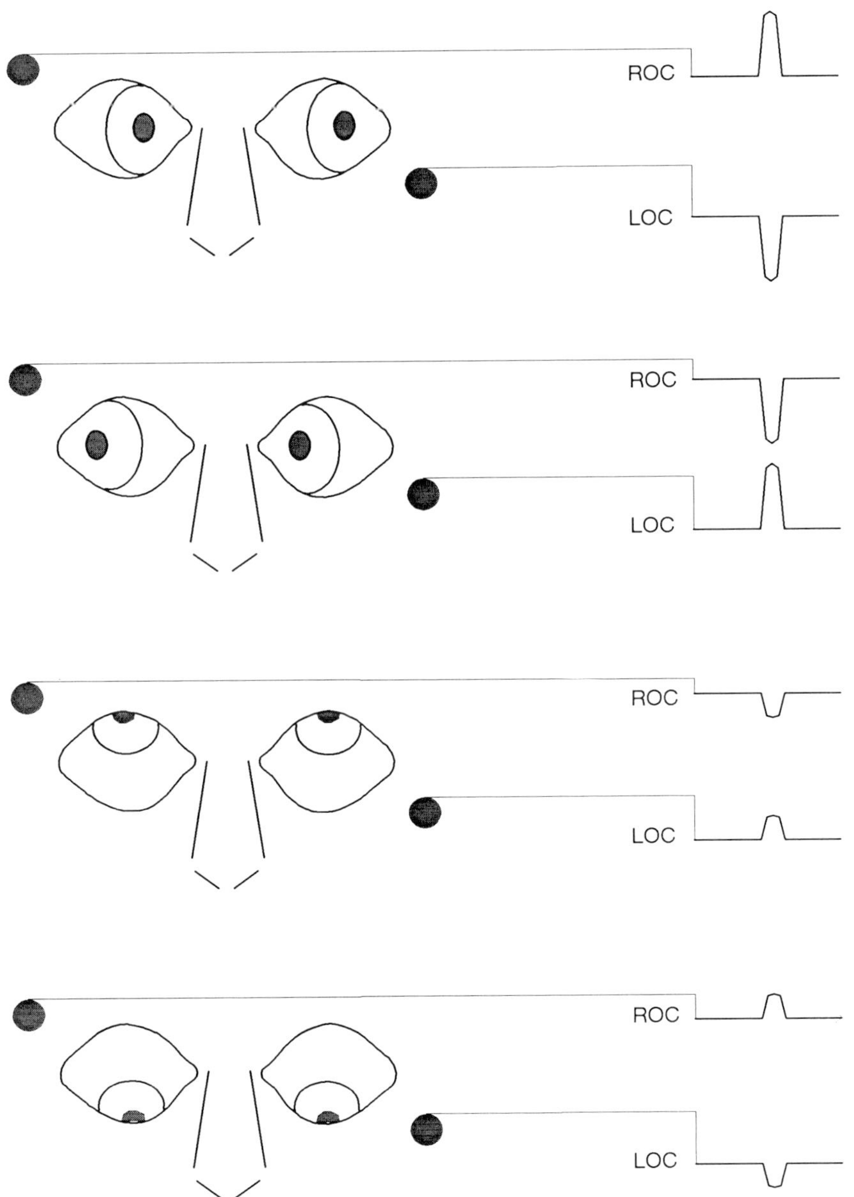

FIGURE A1–6. EOG electrode position. The electrodes are displaced from the horizontal to identify vertical eye movements.

amplifier sensitivity. Pneumotachograph recording is less commonly used, requires that the patient sleep with a large face mask, and may be impractical for many patients.

Respiratory effort may be measured with strain gauges, chest wall impedance, intercostal EMG, inductance plethysmography, and pneumatic transducers. All of these methods provide reliable qualitative information about the patient's breathing by monitoring movement of the chest and abdomen. In children and adults the least restrictive methods are preferable because they minimize discomfort and promote compliance with the all-night procedure.

Pulse oximetry is the standard method for noninvasive, continuous monitoring of arterial oxygen saturation. The probe may be placed on an earlobe, finger, toe, or foot (in a young infant). Because the pulse oximeter uses spectrophotoelectric principles for recording, it circumvents complications associated with transcutaneous measurement of the partial pressure of oxygen or the use of an indwelling arterial catheter. It provides reliable information about the respiratory function and has excellent correlation with simultaneous blood gas determinations.

Tibialis Anterior Electromyographic Activity

If periodic leg movements during sleep or nocturnal myoclonus is suspected, EMGs from the left and right tibialis anterior muscles are recorded. Two surface electrodes are taped approximately 3 cm apart on each leg to monitor leg muscle activity during the sleep period. Leg muscle EMG can also provide information about limb and body movements during the recording period.

Audio and Video Monitoring

Continuous audio and video monitoring and recording of the patient during the sleep period is mandatory and provides significant details about underlying sleep disorders. Somnambulistic episodes can be chronicled, seizure activity can be documented, and some symptoms of sleep apnea (e.g., loud snoring) can be recorded. Continuous monitoring provides a safety function as well as detailed observational data about the patient's sleeping positions at the time of normal or abnormal physiological events.

POLYSOMNOGRAPHIC TECHNIQUES

Calibration Signals

The polysomnograph is calibrated before the electrodes are affixed to the patient. Square pulses of known voltage (20, 50, and 100 μV) are sent to the amplifiers. These pulses are recorded to assess (and adjust) vertical and horizontal pen alignment, degree of pen deflection (sensitivity) for each voltage input, polarity, and time constant, as shown in Figure A1–7. In general, EEG and EOG channels are set with a high-frequency filter at 35 Hz and a low-frequency filter at 0.3 Hz. The *high-frequency filter* reduces the size of fast waves. Filtering of high frequencies affects mainly the rise time of the calibration pulses. The *low-frequency filter* specifies the frequency at which sine waves are reduced in amplitude by a fixed fraction. The *time constant* describes the effect of the low-frequency filter on square pulses and is defined as the time it takes for the pen to fall 37% of the peak deflection produced when a steady voltage is applied to the input of the amplifier. The two filters help to eliminate distortion of and interference with the recording.

Sensitivity for the chin muscle EMG channel varies among individuals. Initially, however, the high-frequency response and low-frequency settings are 75 Hz and 10 Hz, respectively. Recommendations for calibration signals for the channels devoted to ECG and respiratory monitoring are not distinct, since the sensitivity varies considerably among patients and with the technique used.

Patient Calibration

Before retiring, patients complete their usual bedtime ritual. Electrodes are applied, and an impedance check is conducted. For all active electrode sites the impedance must be less than 5000 Ohms to minimize artifacts.

Presleep patient calibration is conducted before the recording is begun. This provides a baseline reference for the awake EEG, eye movements, muscle tone, ECG, and respiratory variables. It also provides an opportunity to identify and correct electrode, amplifier, and paper transport malfunction before the study begins.

With the chart recorder operating, the patient is asked to open and close the eyes, look to the

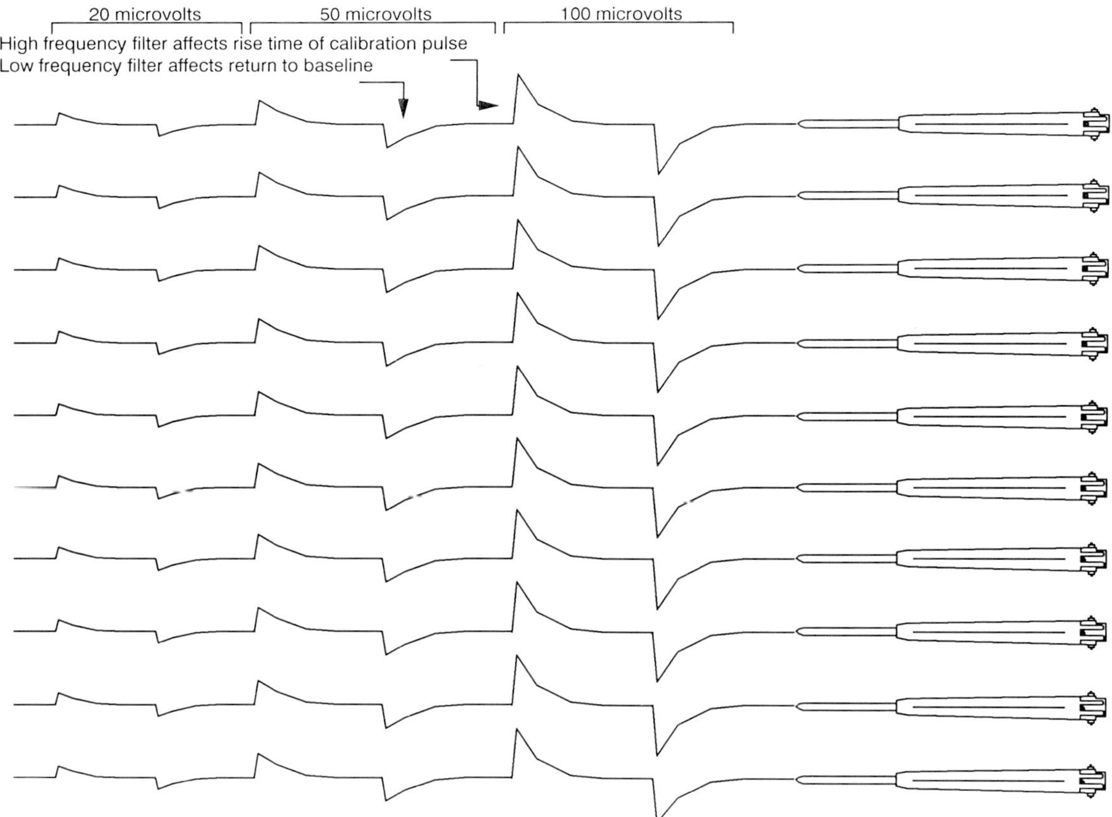

FIGURE A1–7. EEG calibration pulses. Recording pens are checked for degree of deflection, timing of upstroke and return to the baseline (settings of the high- and low-frequency filters), and alignment when square pulses of known voltage are sent to the amplifiers. (Modified from Spehlmann R: EEG primer. Amsterdam, The Netherlands, Elsevier, 1981, p 473, with permission.)

right and then left, take a deep breath, and grit the teeth several times. If this calibration is successful, the technician checks on the patient once again, bids him or her goodnight, and turns out the lights. The time of "lights out" is documented on the record; this signals the beginning of the study.

Considerations for All-Night Recordings

From a procedural viewpoint, alertness of the technician is the most important component in conducting an acceptable sleep study. Although some patients demonstrate few pathological events during the course of the sleep period, the technician must be vigilant in order to operate the recording instruments properly, correct technical problems (e.g., pen clogs, computer failure, electrode malfunction) during the study, mark any changes in the preselected recording protocol, and respond to brief pathological events if they occur. Time of night, patient's sleeping position, and any observed behaviors are also recorded. The technician can provide extremely valuable behavioral information about physiological events occurring while the patient is asleep.

A paper speed of 10 mm/sec is most often used for polysomnographic recording. This speed is one-third the speed of traditional EEG recordings. Although some sensitivity in EEG analysis is lost at this speed, abnormalities in multiple physiological parameters can still be clearly identified and economy of paper is obtained (800 to 1,000 pages for a typical sleep study, compared with 2,400 to 3,000 at the usual EEG speed).

Morning Procedure

After the patient awakens in the morning, the technician turns on the lights and records the time (representing the end of the recording time). Additional patient and polysomnograph calibrations are then conducted. Electrodes and sensors are removed from the patient. Depending on the type of evaluation, other measures (e.g., blood pressure, temperature) may be necessary. The technician conducts a poststudy interview, documents the patient's perception of the night's sleep, and records technical comments. The sleep study is then completed, and the record is analyzed.

POLYSOMNOGRAM REPORT

Following completion of the sleep study, the record is analyzed and a detailed report is generated, as shown in Figure A1–8. Patient demographic data, the reason for referral and testing, and the procedures used in the course of study are presented. Although polysomnogram reports vary considerable, the following objective parameters are typically included:

1. Time of *lights out* and *final wake*
2. Number of minutes spent in each sleep stage and amount of time spent awake after sleep onset
3. Percentage of the total recording time and percentage of the sleep period time for each sleep stage
4. *Total recording time*—number of minutes from the time of lights out to the time of final wake
5. *Sleep period time*—number of minutes from the time of sleep onset to the time of final wake
6. *Sleep efficiency*—calculated percentage of the total time spent sleeping during the total recording time
7. *Sleep onset latency*—number of minutes from lights out to the first three consecutive 30-second epochs of Stage 1 sleep, or the first 30-second epoch of any other sleep stage
8. *REM latency*—number of minutes from sleep onset to the first 30-second epoch of REM stage sleep
9. *Wake after sleep onset*—number of minutes spent awake after sleep onset
10. *Movement time*—number of minutes of recording obscured by body movement artifact
11. *Apneas*—total number of central, obstructive, and mixed apneas (lasting 10 seconds or longer) during the sleep period time. The total number of apneas during each stage of sleep and the total number of apneas when the patient is prone, supine, or on his or her side may also be presented.
12. *Apnea index*—total number of apneas per hour of sleep
13. *Hypopneas*—total number of hypopneic events recorded during the sleep period
14. *Apnea + hypopnea index*—number of apneas and hypopneas per hour of sleep
15. *Longest apnea*
16. *Average apnea length*
17. *Oxygen saturation*—highest, lowest, and average oxygen saturation recorded. A graphic representation of the continuous monitoring of oxygen saturation may also be provided.
18. *Mean heart rate*
19. *Mean respiratory rate*

Some laboratories also provide a *hypnogram,* a graphic depiction of the progression of sleep stages across the recording time (see Fig. A1–8).

Presentation of the objective parameters is followed by an interpretation of each physiological variable, including the following:

1. *Technical quality* of the study and patient compliance
2. *Latencies,* including evaluation of the sleep onset latency and REM latency
3. *Sleep architecture,* including the adequacy of progression of sleep stages across the recording time and adequacy of volumes of each sleep stage (when compared with age-appropriate norms)
4. *EEG,* including an assessment of any focal, paroxysmal, or epileptic activity
5. *EOG,* including an evaluation of the quality and quantity of eye movements during REM sleep
6. *EMG,* including an evaluation of chin muscle activity and evaluation of the presence (or absence) of periodic leg movements or nocturnal myoclonus
7. *ECG,* assessed for rate, rhythm, and changes associated with respiratory events
8. *Respiratory variables,* including the average respiratory rate, quality of respiratory effort, presence of paradoxical respiratory movements, apneas, and hypopneas, oxygen saturation, and respiratory indices

Provided with these measures of sleep, the clinician integrates them with the history and physical findings to arrive at an accurate diagnosis. Without the comprehensive use of polysomnographic data, sleep disorders cannot be diagnosed with accuracy.

PATIENT'S NAME: XXXXXXXX, Xxxxxxx **STUDY DATE:** 4/16/91
MEDICAL RECORD #: 123456 **SDC#:** 91-1234

Objective Findings

	MINUTES	% REC TIME	% SPT
AWAKE:	17.50	4.07	xxxx
STAGE 1:	11.50	2.68	2.79
STAGE 2:	223.50	52.04	54.25
STAGE 3:	16.00	3.73	3.73
STAGE 4:	111.00	25.84	25.84
STG. REM:	50.00	11.64	12.14

TOTAL RECORD:	429.50 min
TOTAL SLEEP:	412.00 min
SLEEP EFFICIENCY:	95.93 %
SLEEP LATENCY:	2.00 min
REM LATENCY:	170.00 min
STAGE CHANGES:	45

Mean Respiratory Rate: 12/min
Mean Heart Rate: 76/min

RESPIRATORY VARIABLES

Obstr. Apneas:	2
Cent. Apneas	4
Mixed Apneas:	0
Hypopneas:	0
APNEA INDEX:	0.87
AHI:	0.87
High SaO2:	100%
Low SaO2:	91%
Average SaO2:	97%

Study Date: 4/16/91
REM represented by Stage 1.5

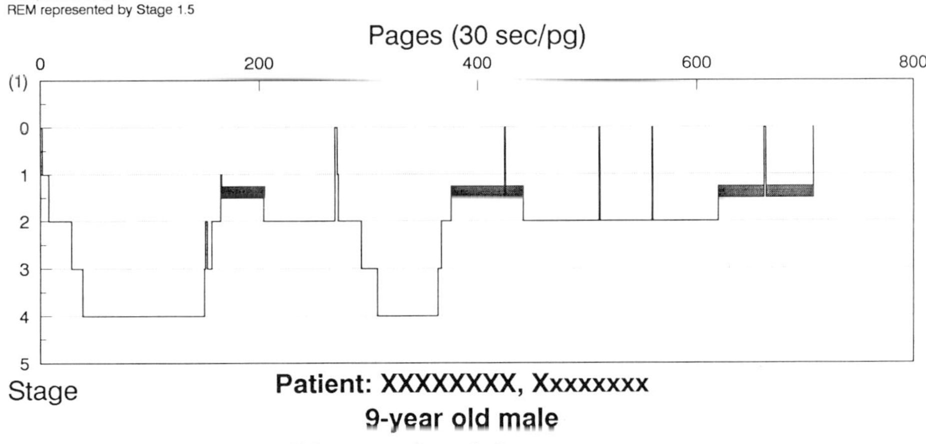

Sleep Architecture

FIGURE A1–8. Report of polysomnographic objective findings. Reports from different laboratories may vary significantly. Information on movement time, arousal index, periodic leg movement index, respiratory events during various stages of sleep, and body position during respiratory events is not shown in this example.

OTHER CONSIDERATIONS

Several other issues are important in understanding the processes of polysomnography. These include patient preparation by the practitioner for the sleep study, patient safety, and the physical layout of the laboratory.

Patient Preparation

Proper preparation of the patient for the study decreases anxiety about the procedure and increases compliance. Before the study, the practitioner should discuss with the patient the reason for the testing, the procedures that will be used, and what the patient can expect from the laboratory staff. Directly addressing these issues alleviates the anxiety associated with sleeping in the strange laboratory environment and results in a more representative night's sleep. The extra effort and additional time spent with younger patients and their families can significantly ease tensions. Most laboratories permit a tour of the facilities before the study, to familiarize the child with the equipment that will be used. Parents are encouraged to spend the night in the laboratory with their child, and a suitable cot, bed, or fouton should be available for their use.

Often patients and families think that the presence of multiple electrodes, sensors, and monitoring equipment will surely interfere with sleep. Although the potential for this exists, children (and adults) usually sleep surprisingly well in the laboratory, and the sleep recorded is generally satisfactorily representative of the patient's typical sleep physiology. The laboratory staff may note a discrepancy between sleep measurements on the first night and those on consecutive nights. Sometimes two or more nights of polysomnography may be required for an accurate assessment. This can frequently be anticipated from historical information before the study night, and many sleep laboratories require a clinical evaluation in the sleep center before the study. The sleep center's staff can determine the appropriate polysomnographic montage and the number of nights required for an accurate diagnosis.

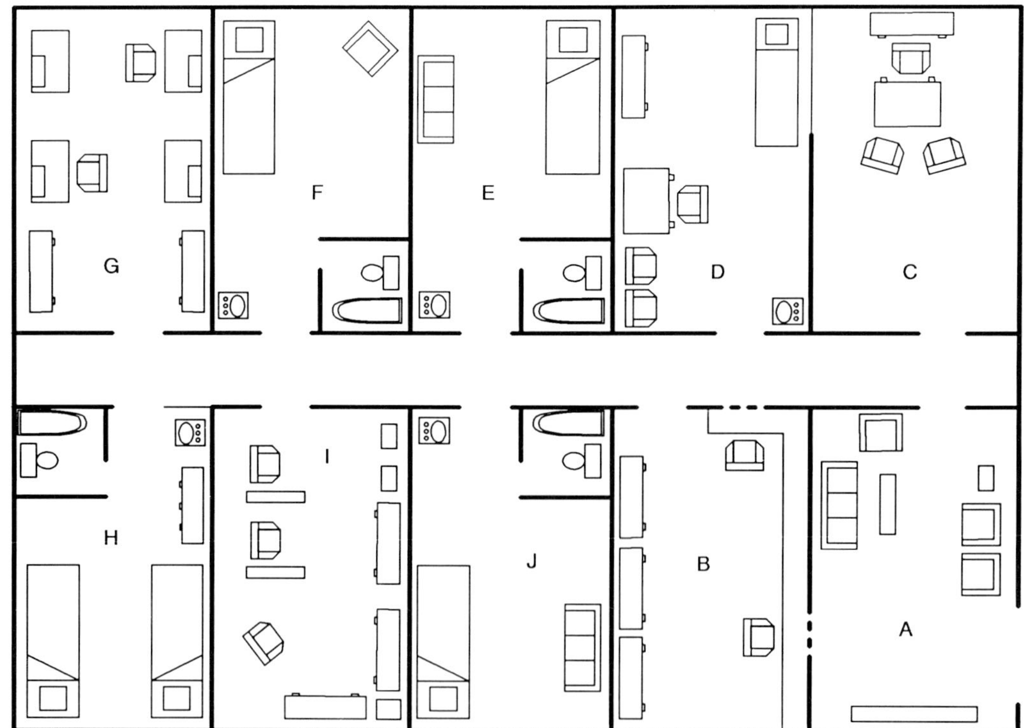

FIGURE A1–9. Schematic floor plan of a four-bed sleep disorders center. *A,* Reception and waiting room. *B,* Receptionist, secretary, and file area. *C,* Consultation-conference room. *D,* Patient examination room. *E, F, H,* and *J,* Monitored sleeping rooms. *G,* Control room. *I,* Patient preparation room. Areas for record storage and staff washroom are not shown.

Patient Safety

Patient safety in the sleep laboratory is of primary importance. Because the patient is connected to complex electrical equipment, the potential for exposure to incoming electrical currents and shock is minimized by compulsive inspection and maintenance of the recording apparatus. A *single* electrical ground is affixed to the patient. If more than one are used, the possibility of creating a "ground loop" is greatly enhanced.

The technician must observe the patient and the recording continuously throughout the recording period. Patients may require prompt medical attention during the sleep study, and the laboratory and staff must be prepared for these situations.

Sleep Laboratory Environment

Although sleep laboratories differ markedly in layout, design, and decor, they generally consist of one or more bedrooms for monitoring patients, an adjacent control room, a restroom, and a storage area. To reduce the probability of one patient disturbing the sleep of another, each patient is provided with a private room. The sleeping rooms should simulate a home environment, be painted a neutral color, and attenuate light and sound. The rooms must be easily accessible to the technician. Some laboratories have a separate patient preparation room. Keeping the supplies needed in patient setup in this area obviates the need to interrupt patients who are relaxing and attempting to sleep in the bedrooms. Furthermore, it maximizes efficiency because time-consuming clean-up procedures can be performed in areas other than the sleeping rooms.

The control room should be large enough to accommodate the equipment required for recordings and should be safe and comfortable for the technician. The room must be constructed in a manner that minimizes electrical interference and artifact intrusion. Since polysomnographic records consist of voluminous pages of data, an adjacent reading and storage room is helpful.

Design of sleep laboratories is geared both to patient comfort and safety and to the technician's needs. A typical floor plan of a four-bed sleep disorders center is shown in Figure A1–9. With appropriate management strategies the physical laboratory environment can ensure efficient patient care and accurate, reproducible recordings.

APPENDIX 2

Normal Values

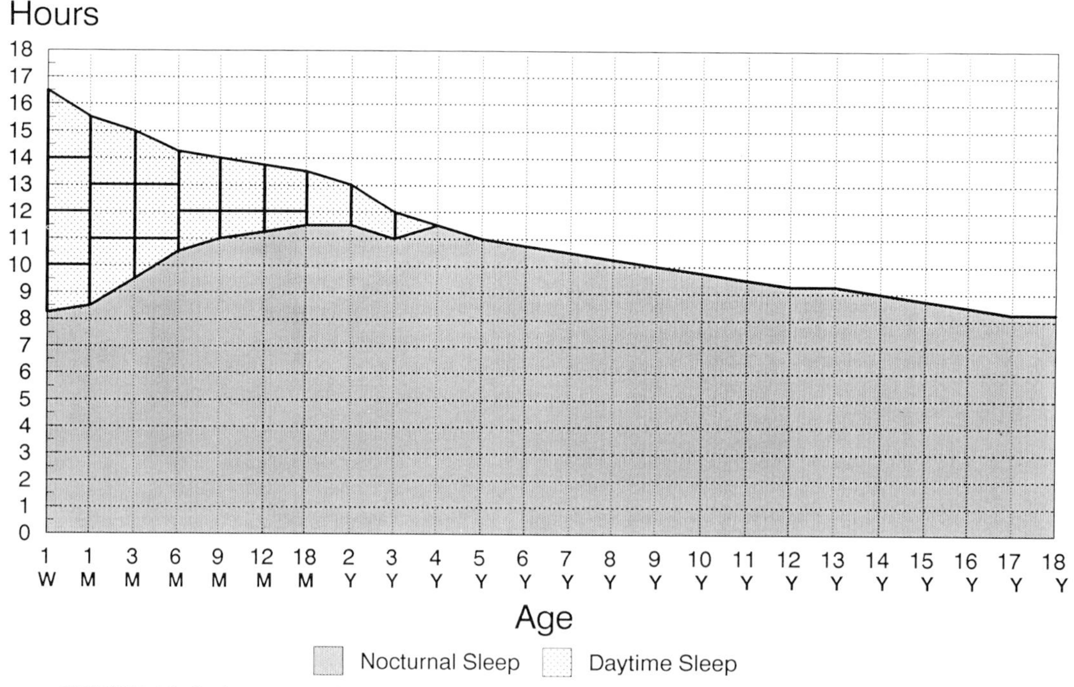

FIGURE A2–1. Average total sleep times during childhood. During infancy, normal daytime sleep is broken into several discrete naps that decrease in frequency and length as the child ages. (Modified from Ferber R: Solve your child's sleep problems. New York, Simon & Schuster, 1985, p 19, with permission.)

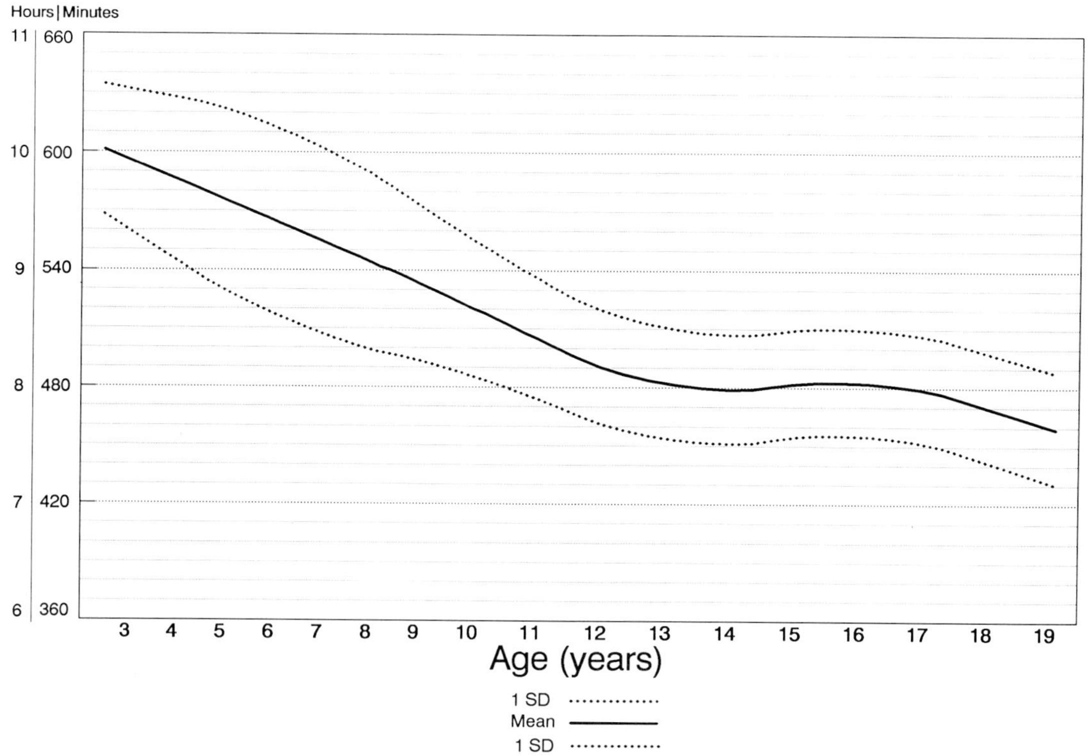

FIGURE A2–2. Polysomnographic variables: sleep period time. (Data derived and modified from Williams RL, Karacan I, and Hursch CJ: Electroencephalogram (EEG) of human sleep. New York, Wiley, 1975, pp 35-45; and Cobel PA et al: EEG sleep of healthy children 6 to 12 years of age. In Guilleminault C [ed]: Sleep and its disorders in children. New York, Raven Press, 1987, pp 32-33, with permission.)

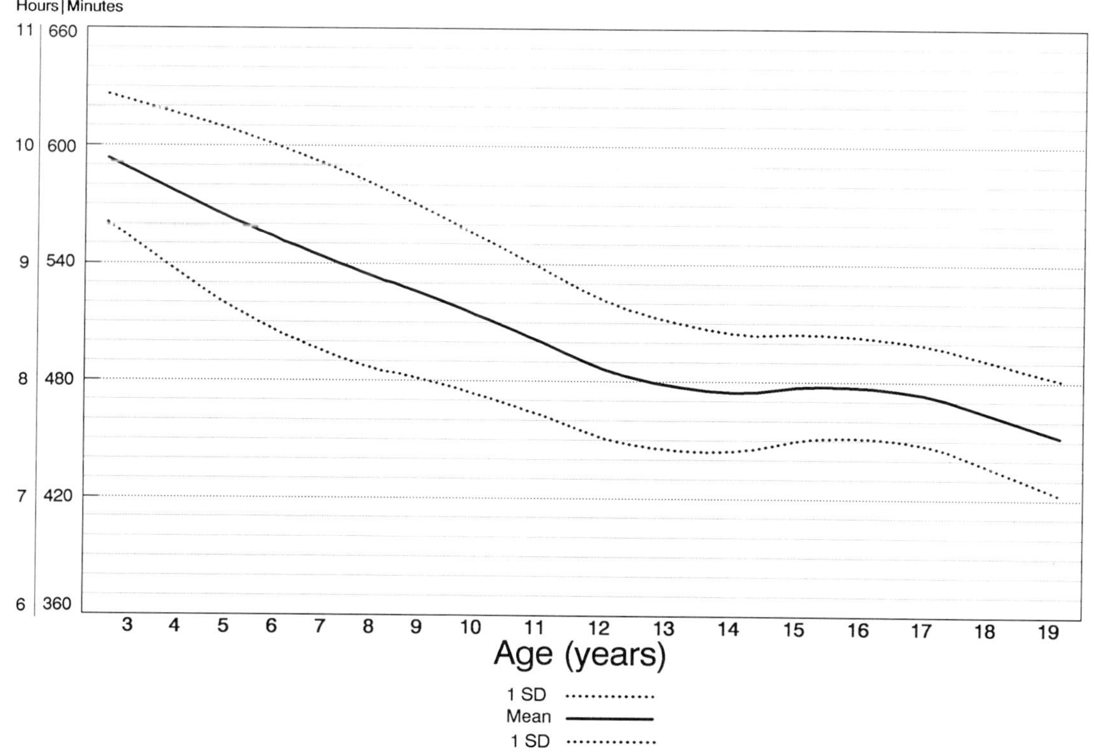

FIGURE A2–3. Polysomnographic variables: total sleep time. (Data derived and modified from Williams RL, Karacan I, and Hursch CJ: Electroencephalogram (EEG) of human sleep. New York, Wiley, 1975, pp 35-45; and Cobel PA et al: EEG sleep of healthy children 6 to 12 years of age. In Guilleminault C [ed]: Sleep and its disorders in children. New York, Raven Press, 1987, pp 32-33, with permission.)

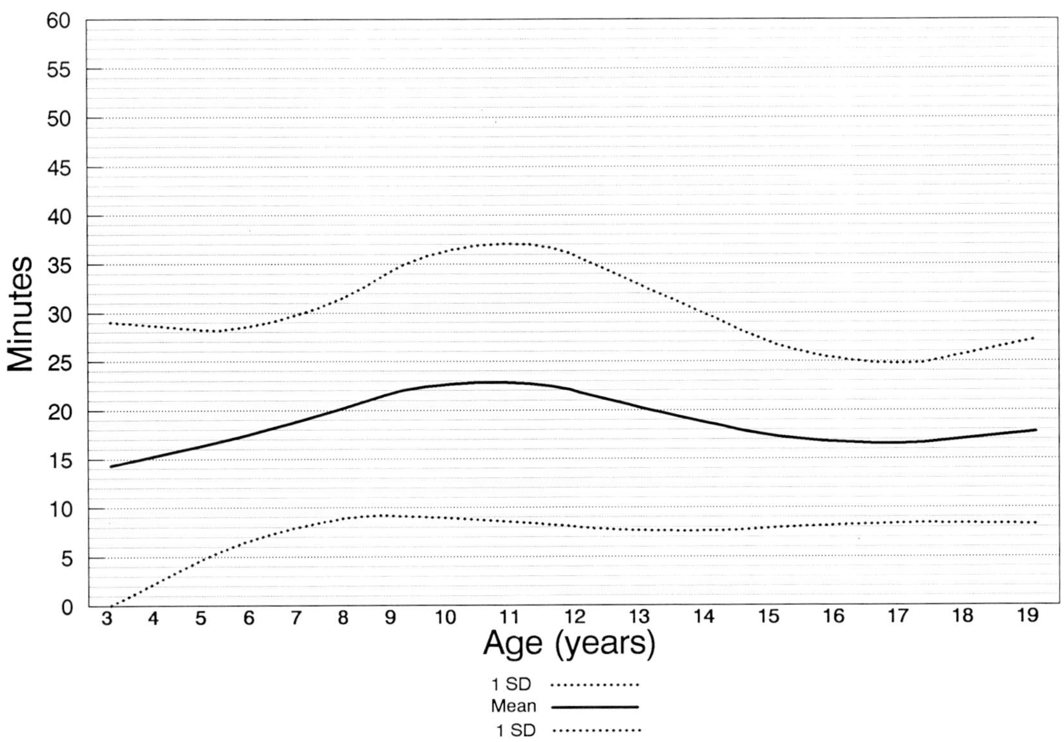

FIGURE A2–4. Polysomnographic variables: nocturnal sleep onset latency. (Data derived and modified from Williams RL, Karacan I, and Hursch CJ: Electroencephalogram (EEG) of human sleep. New York, Wiley, 1975, pp 35-45; and Cobel PA et al: EEG sleep of healthy children 6 to 12 years of age. In Guilleminault C [ed]: Sleep and its disorders in children. New York, Raven Press, 1987, pp 32-33, with permission.)

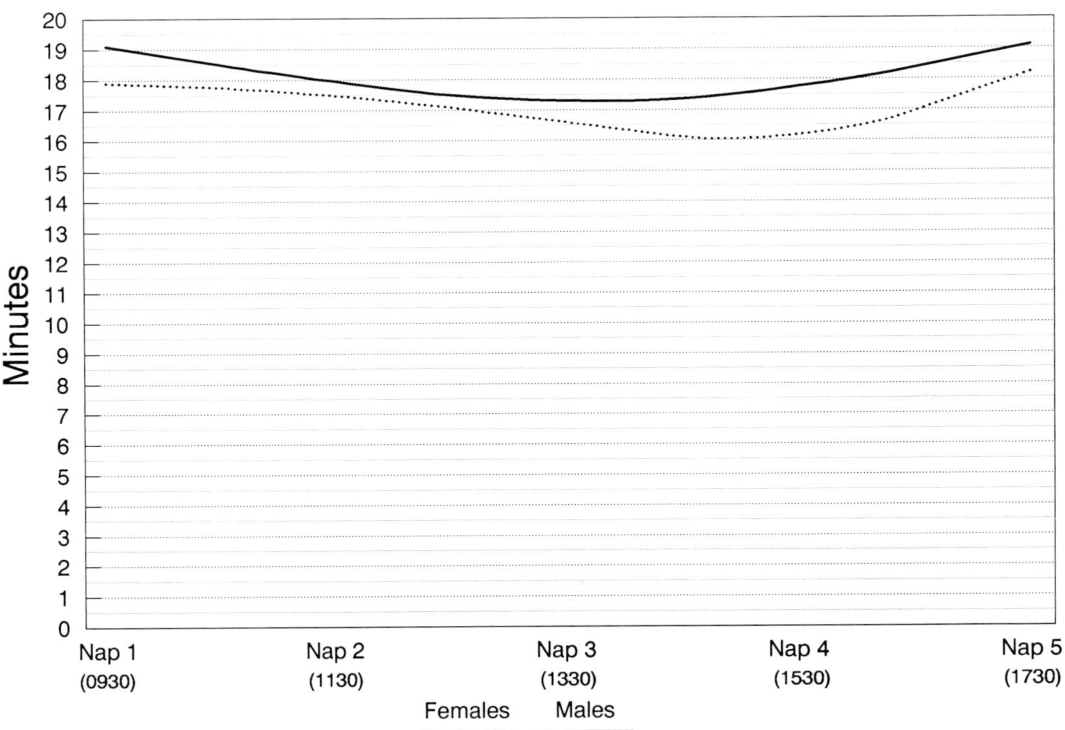

FIGURE A2–5. Polysomnographic variables: diurnal sleep onset latency (MSLT means). (Data derived and modified from Carskadon MA, Keenan S, and Dement WC: Night time sleep and daytime sleep tendency in pre-adolescents. In Guilleminault C [ed]: Sleep and its disorders in children. New York, Raven Press, 1987, p 50, with permission.)

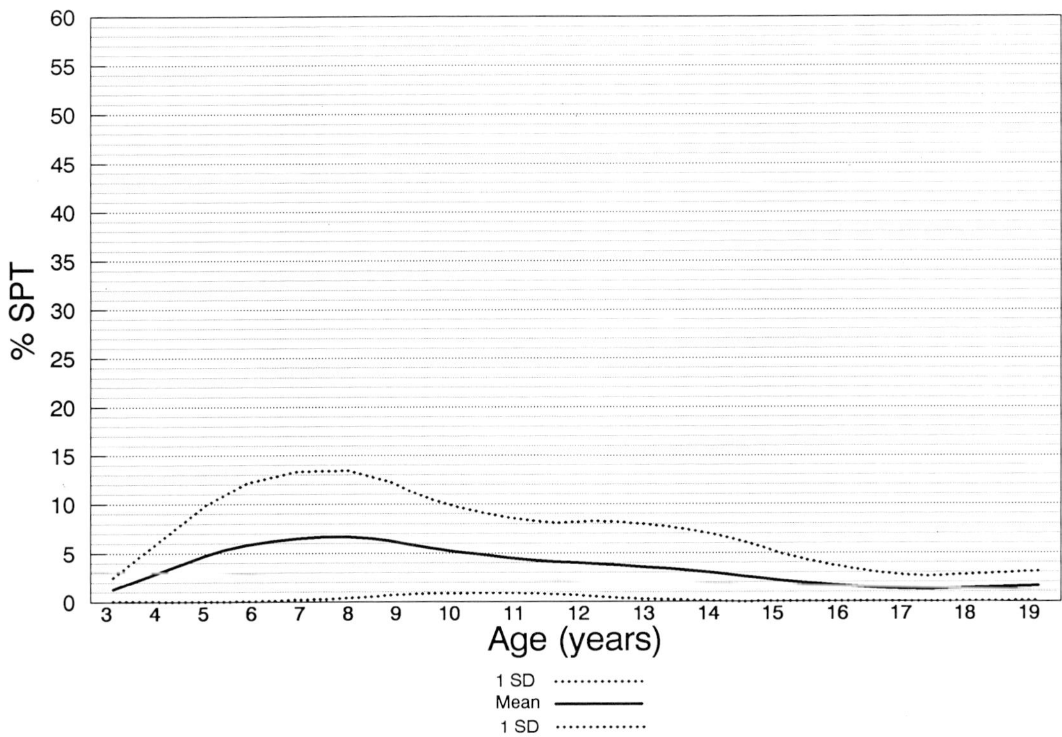

FIGURE A2–6. Polysomnographic variables: wake after sleep onset. (Data derived and modified from Williams RL, Karacan I, and Hursch CJ: Electroencephalogram (EEG) of human sleep. New York, Wiley, 1975, pp 35-45; and Cobel PA et al: EEG sleep of healthy children 6 to 12 years of age. In Guilleminault C [ed]: Sleep and its disorders in children. New York, Raven Press, 1987, pp 32-33, with permission.)

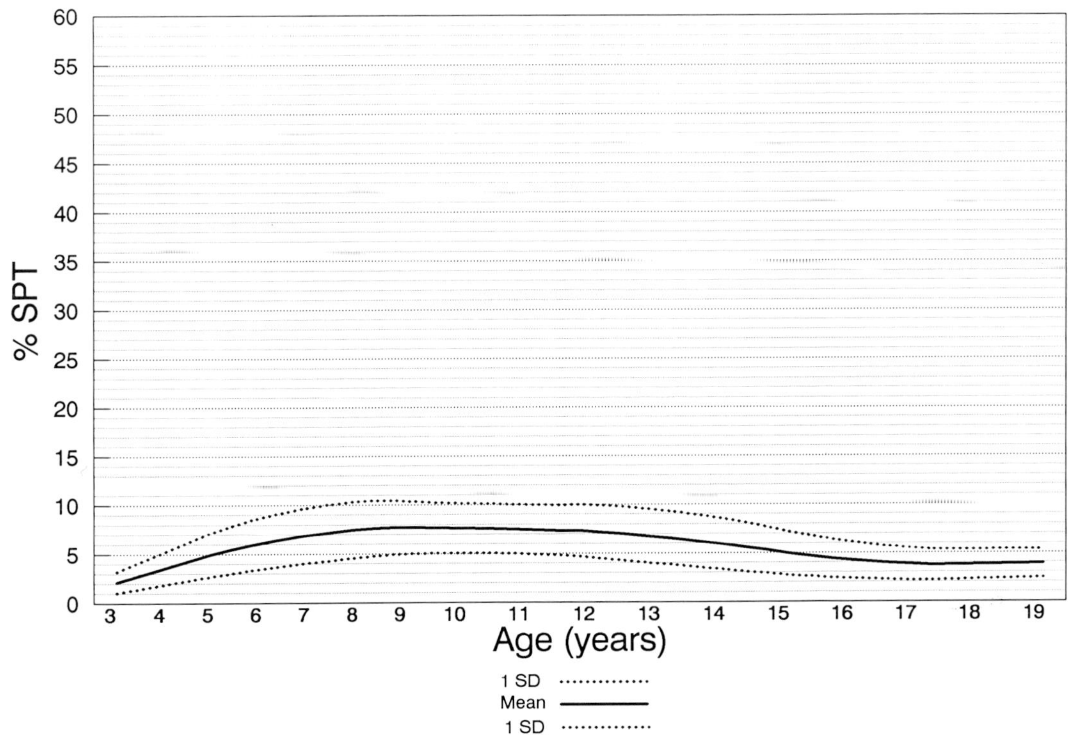

FIGURE A2–7. Polysomnographic variables: Stage 1 volume. (Data derived and modified from Williams RL, Karacan I, and Hursch CJ: Electroencephalogram (EEG) of human sleep. New York, Wiley, 1975, pp 35-45; and Cobel PA et al: EEG sleep of healthy children 6 to 12 years of age. In Guilleminault C [ed]: Sleep and its disorders in children. New York, Raven Press, 1987, pp 32-33, with permission.)

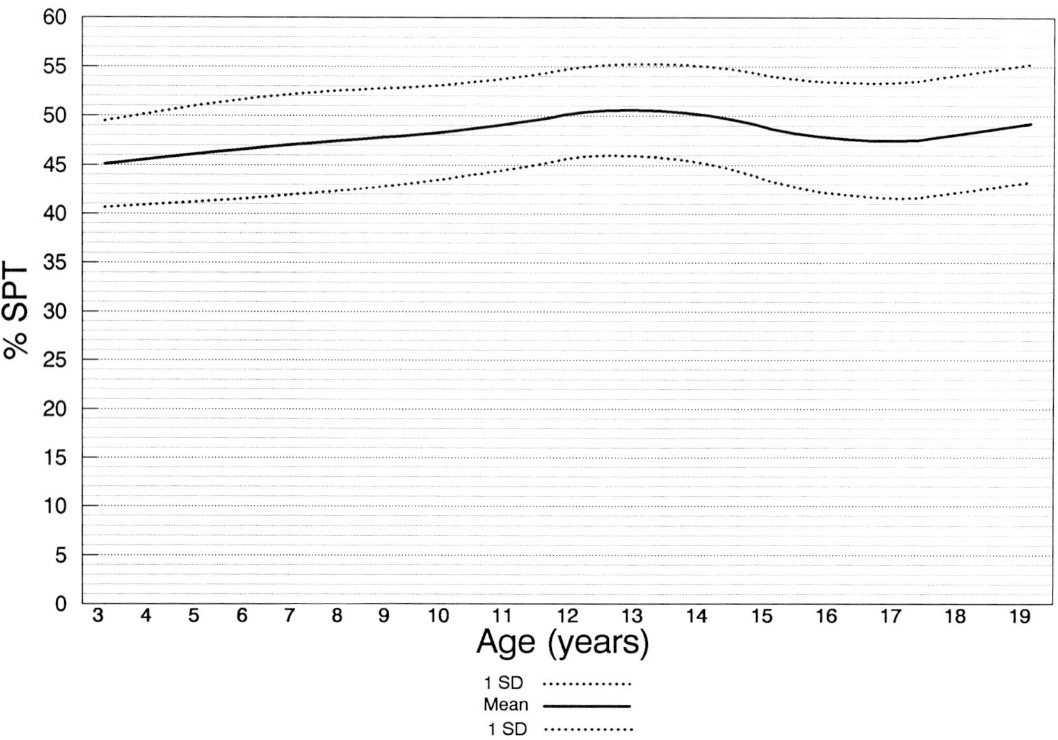

FIGURE A2–8. Polysomnographic variables: Stage 2 volume. (Data derived and modified from Williams RL, Karacan I, and Hursch CJ: Electroencephalogram (EEG) of human sleep. New York, Wiley, 1975, pp 35-45; and Cobel PA et al: EEG sleep of healthy children 6 to 12 years of age. In Guilleminault C [ed]: Sleep and its disorders in children. New York, Raven Press, 1987, pp 32-33, with permission.)

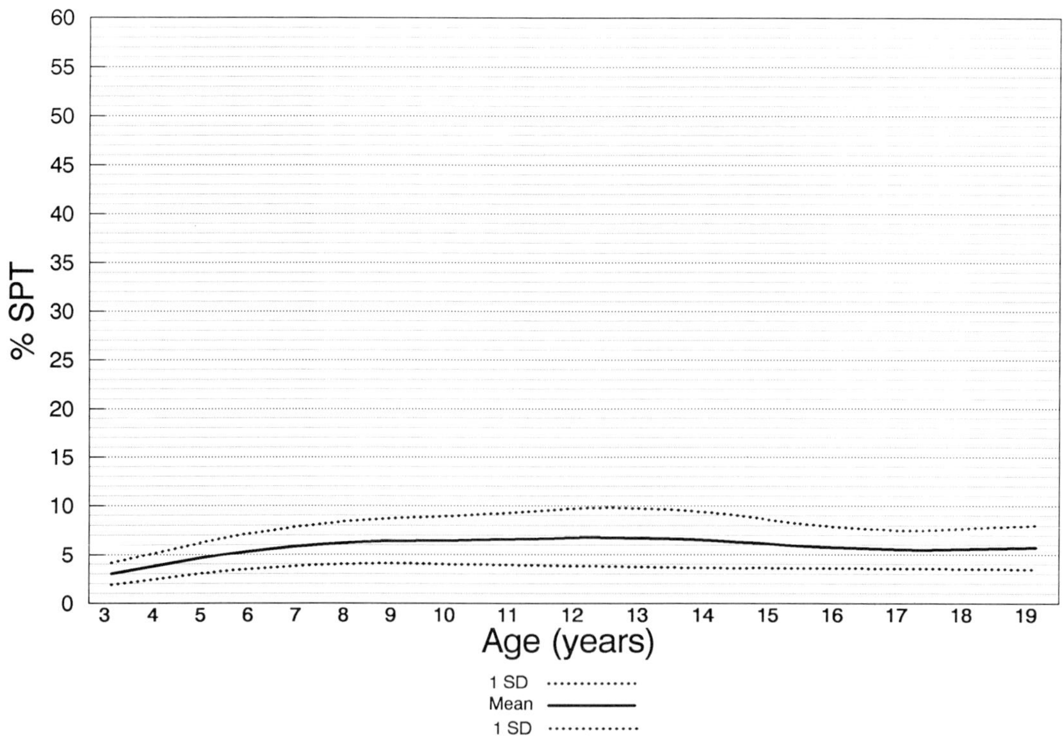

FIGURE A2–9. Polysomnographic variables: Stage 3 volume. (Data derived and modified from Williams RL, Karacan I, and Hursch CJ: Electroencephalogram (EEG) of human sleep. New York, Wiley, 1975, pp 35-45; and Cobel PA et al: EEG sleep of healthy children 6 to 12 years of age. In Guilleminault C [ed]: Sleep and its disorders in children. New York, Raven Press, 1987, pp 32-33, with permission.)

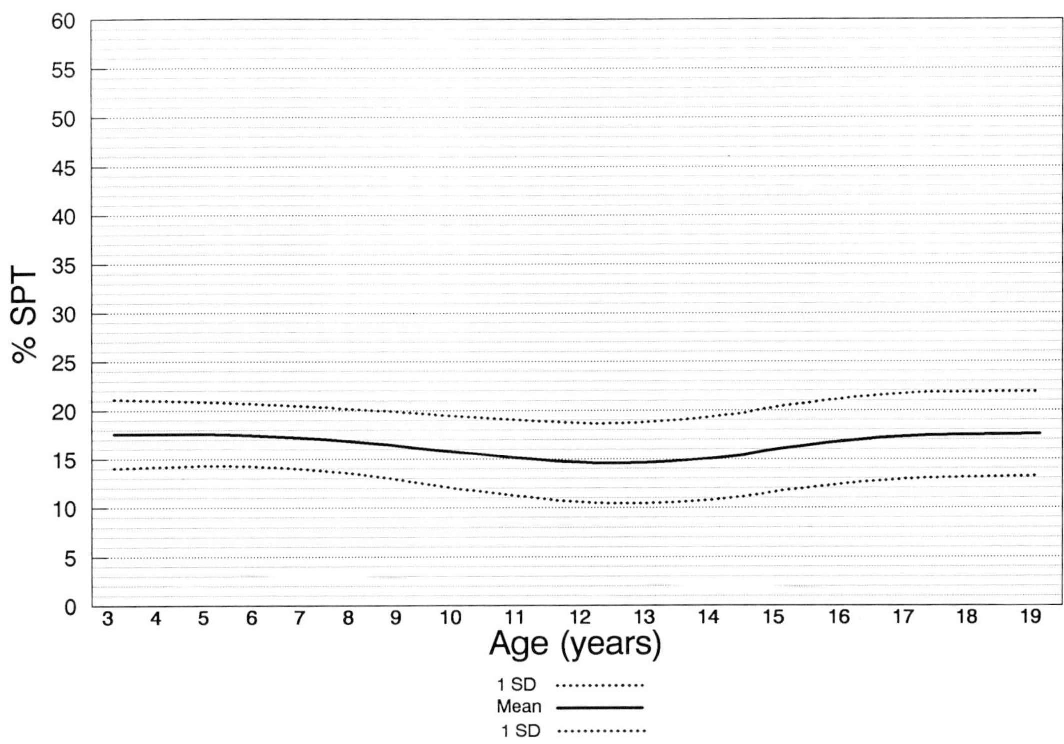

FIGURE A2–10. Polysomnographic variables: Stage 4 volume. (Data derived and modified from Williams RL, Karacan I, and Hursch CJ: Electroencephalogram (EEG) of human sleep. New York, Wiley, 1975, pp 35-45; and Cobel PA et al: EEG sleep of healthy children 6 to 12 years of age. In Guilleminault C [ed]: Sleep and its disorders in children. New York, Raven Press, 1987, pp 32-33, with permission.)

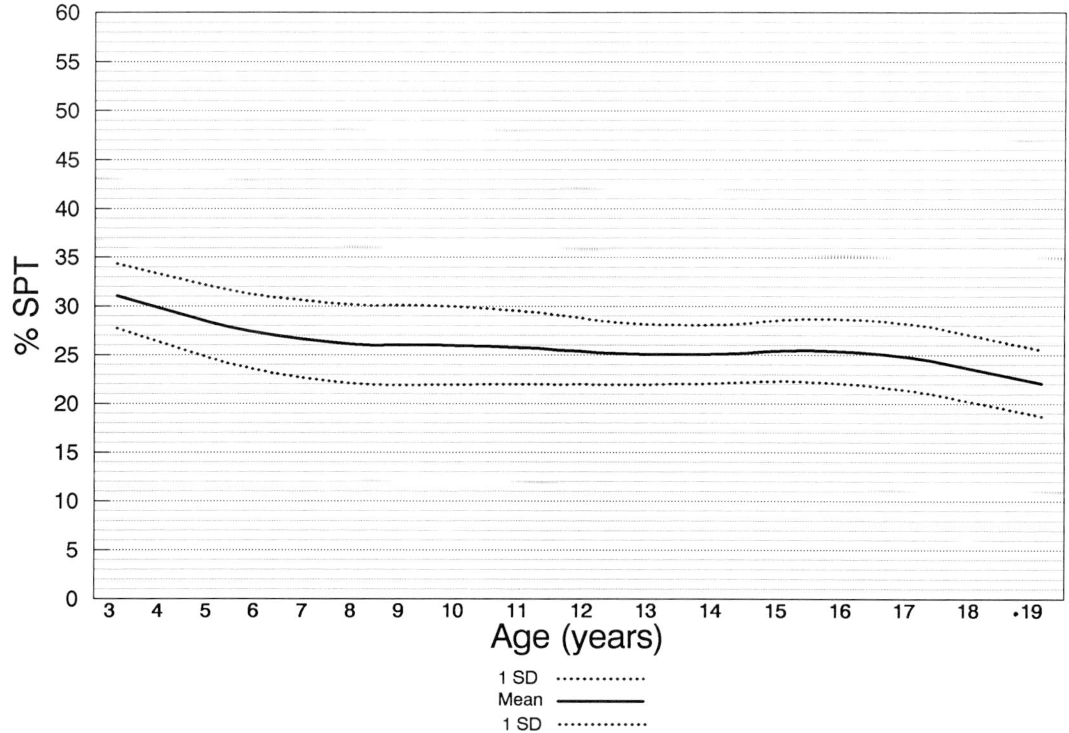

FIGURE A2–11. Polysomnographic variables: REM stage volume. (Data derived and modified from Williams RL, Karacan I, and Hursch CJ: Electroencephalogram (EEG) of human sleep. New York, Wiley, 1975, pp 35-45; and Cobel PA et al: EEG sleep of healthy children 6 to 12 years of age. In Guilleminault C [ed]: Sleep and its disorders in children. New York, Raven Press, 1987, pp 32-33, with permission.)

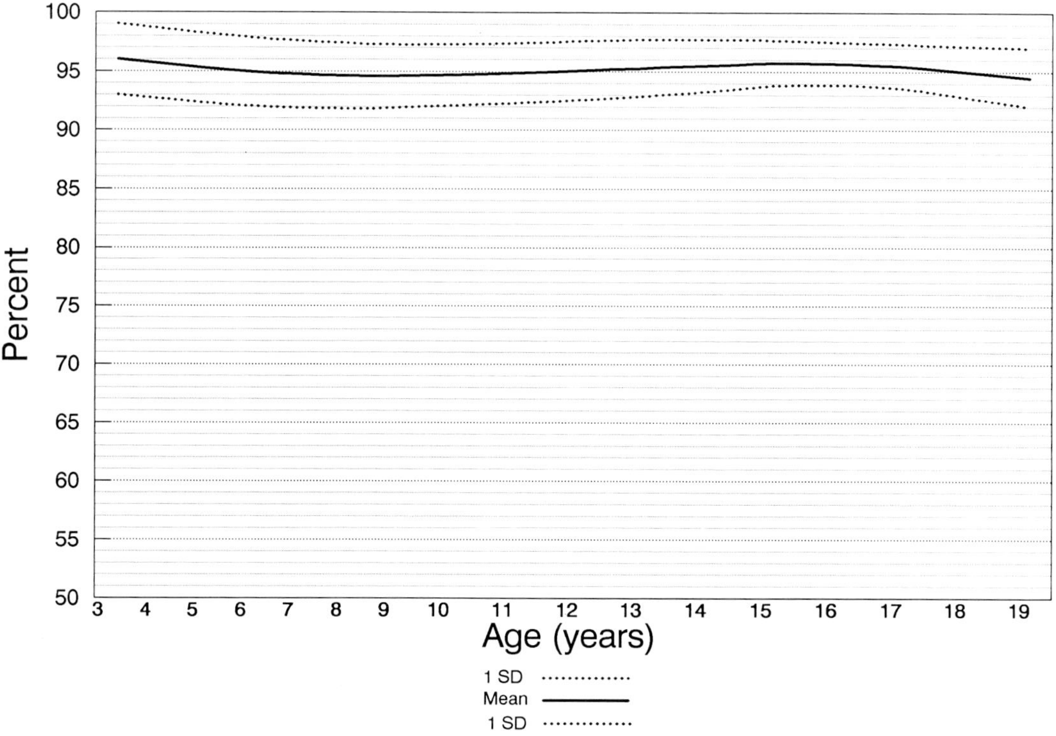

FIGURE A2–12. Polysomnographic variables: sleep efficiency. (Data derived and modified from Williams RL, Karacan I, and Hursch CJ: Electroencephalogram (EEG) of human sleep. New York, Wiley, 1975, pp 35-45; and Cobel PA et al: EEG sleep of healthy children 6 to 12 years of age. In Guilleminault C [ed]: Sleep and its disorders in children. New York, Raven Press, 1987, pp 32-33, with permission.)

APPENDIX 3

*Pediatric Sleep Medicine: Differential Diagnosis**

Appropriate recommendations for management of a child with sleep problems can be made only after an accurate diagnosis is established. In many cases the symptoms are vague and the parents seek medical advice only because the child's sleep problem is disrupting their sleep. Often difficulty in functioning during the day is the initial problem and the child's sleep is overlooked as a possible contributing or etiological factor. The practitioner may be faced with a dilemma of sorting out a confusing history. The cliché "If you never think of it, you'll never diagnose it" holds significance in pediatric sleep medicine.

The process of arriving at a diagnosis involves a complex series of inferences. Generating a hypothesis, testing the hypothesis by specific questioning and gaining information from physical examination, ordering the hypothesis set, and reordering the set according to the information acquired are the steps used by the clinician in solving clinical problems. The cornerstone of the process of reaching a diagnosis is adequacy and completeness of the hypothesis set. Too little information about sleep disorders and the sleep-wake cycle is taught in medical school and postgraduate training programs. This appendix is intended as a quick reference that a busy practitioner can use to develop appropriate hypotheses and subsequently a differential diagnosis that includes the various sleep disorders that may affect daytime and nighttime functioning. Clinical points that differentiate one clinical entity from another are listed and briefly described. Comprehensive descriptions of the various sleep disorders (and suggestions for management) are given elsewhere in this volume.

The classification and differential diagnosis given here have been modified from *The International Classification of Sleep Disorders: Diagnostic and Coding Manual*, published by the American Sleep Disorders Association in 1990. Descriptions of a number of the disorders have been revised so the practitioner can relate the diagnoses to clinical processes seen during childhood. Additional pediatric diagnoses have been proposed.

*Modified from Diagnostic Classification Steering Committee, Thorpy M (Chairman): International classification of sleep disorders: diagnostic and coding manual. Rochester, Minn, American Sleep Disorders Association, 1990, pp 331-336, with permission.

Much overlap exists. Many disorders that result in sleeplessness are also associated with excessive daytime sleepiness or may be classified as parasomnias. Descriptions of disorders are reiterated (although altered to relate to the primary presenting complaint) in the differential diagnosis to spare the reader from turning pages back and forth because of cross-referencing. Each diagnostic entity is covered more comprehensively elsewhere in the text. A number of sleep disorders listed have not been reported to occur during infancy, childhood, or adolescence but are included to ensure completeness and because they may be described in pediatric patients in the future.

DISORDERS OF INITIATING OR MAINTAINING SLEEP (D.I.M.S.)

The Insomnias

The insomnias are a heterogenous group of disorders that share the symptom of sleeplessness. Considerable overlap of symptoms may exist among disorders. The quality and quantity of the complaint and the presence or absence of associated symptoms may help the practitioner to differentiate among various conditions. Duplication is impossible to avoid, since a number of the sleep disorders may be manifested as sleeplessness, sleepiness, or both. This section focuses on the presenting complaint of an inability to initiate sleep or maintain sleep.

I. SLEEPLESSNESS ASSOCIATED WITH BEHAVIORAL PSYCHOPHYSIOLOGICAL CAUSES

Disorder	Clinical Presentation
Adjustment sleep disorder	This is a common complaint during childhood. Symptoms center on the child's inability to fall asleep at the routine bedtime or an unusually early morning waking. Onset of the problem is sudden and usually is related to a period of acute stress, anxiety, conflict, emotions, or environmental change. The inability to fall asleep is clearly different from the child's normal sleep pattern. The child or parent often identifies the stressor, such as viewing a frightening movie, parental conflict, or death in the family. Stressors may also include more pleasant or exciting events such as holidays, birthdays, or vacations. The problem usually remits when the stressor is removed or the child adapts to the stressful event.
Psychophysiological insomnia	This entity is rare during childhood and adolescence. Symptoms include an inability to fall asleep and decreased daytime functioning. The patient has profound inability to fall asleep at the desired time, although sleep onset may occur easily under soporific conditions during the day. Symptoms are chronic. The harder the patient tries to fall asleep, the more difficult sleep onset becomes. Often the patient has somatized tension, anxiety, and an intense preoccupation with the inability to fall asleep. This "conditioned" sleeplessness occurs primarily in the home environment; patients tend to sleep better in other environments.
Inadequate sleep hygiene	This is rare during childhood, since children seldom control their sleep patterns. It is more common in adolescence when this independence is obtained. Sleep onset is difficult, but the sleep complaint is variable and may be associated with irregular bedtimes and wake times. Bedtime may be disrupted by arousing activities (e.g., homework, exercise, parties, or other activities associated with high levels of concentration).

DISORDER	CLINICAL PRESENTATION
Inadequate sleep hygiene—cont'd	Patients may nap or sleep excessively several days per week. The sleep environment is often chaotic, disruptive, cluttered, and used for other activities (especially when homework, eating, watching television, or other arousing activities are done in the bed). Environmental temperature may be too hot or cold, or the bed may be uncomfortable and inconducive to sleep.
Limit-setting sleep disorder	This is often seen in childhood and may be associated with daytime manifestations of behavioral disorders or with dysfunctions of parenting. It is rare during infancy when the child sleeps in a crib. The typical complaint involves the child *refusing* to go to sleep at a time desired by the parents. Children frequently get out of bed and ask for a drink of water, to have another bedtime story read, or for some other favor that will stall bedtime. Some complain of fears associated with the sleeping environment. Symptoms of anxiety, however, are not intense, and daytime anxiety and fears are not reported. The parents give in to the child's protestations about sleep and rarely set limits. When limits are imposed, however, sleep onset is normal. Once sleep onset has occurred, quality and quantity of sleep are normal.
Sleep onset association disorder	This is common during childhood and generally affects children between the ages of 6 months and 3 years. Complaints of difficulty falling asleep at the beginning of the night are infrequent. Most complaints center on nocturnal wakings and an inability of the child to go back to sleep on his or her own after waking at night. Occasionally difficulties with sleep onset at bedtime are reported, but these are not as common as sleep maintenance problems. Sleep onset is *associated* with certain objects (e.g., a special blanket, pillow, or pacifier), being held in the parent's arms, rocking, nursing, or being carried. Children are often asleep when placed in the crib or bed. They have not learned to fall asleep in bed on their own. *Characteristic is the ability to fall back to sleep quickly once the associations are provided for the child.* Wakings are not as frequent as those in children receiving excessive fluids at night.
Excessive nocturnal fluids	This problem is common during infancy and early childhood. Parents complain that the child has frequent nighttime wakings, which sometimes are prolonged. Wakings may occur three to eight times per night, and sleep returns only after the ingestion of 4 to 8 ounces of fluid. The child may consume 12 to 32 ounces of fluid across the night. The amount of fluid ingested differentiates this disorder from sleep onset association disorder, since in the latter only small volumes of fluid are consumed and the problem is related more to associating the nipple and suckling with sleep than to consumption of fluids. The patient is usually fed just before bedtime. Wakings are also more frequent than with sleep onset association disorder. Diapers are often soaked in the morning, or frequent nighttime diaper changes are required.

II. SLEEPLESSNESS ASSOCIATED WITH PSYCHIATRIC DISORDERS

DISORDER	CLINICAL PRESENTATION
Psychoses	Many childhood psychoses are associated with sleeplessness or difficulty maintaining sleep. Disordered sleep is common in children with autism or childhood schizophrenia. Associated diurnal symptoms are typically present and are the reason treatment is sought. Sleep may be fragmented, and sleep-wake cycles significantly disorganized. Sleep efficiency is usually poor. Sleeplessness may alternate with excessive

Continued on following page

II. SLEEPLESSNESS ASSOCIATED WITH PSYCHIATRIC DISORDERS *Continued*

DISORDER	CLINICAL PRESENTATION
Psychoses—cont'd	sleepiness. Disordered sleep resulting from psychoses can be differentiated from an irregular sleep-wake schedule by the presence of daytime and functional symptoms in the former and their absence in the latter.
Mood disorders	Sleep problems secondary to mood disorders (e.g., depression) may occur in adolescents but are more common in young and middle-aged adults. Two patterns of insomnia are noted: (1) an inability to fall asleep at bedtime and (2) early morning awakening with an inability to go back to sleep. Daytime sleepiness and frequent napping may occur in milder mood disorders. Adolescents and young adult patients usually manifest a profound inability to fall asleep at night. Many patients complain about feeling tired during the day, and this may or may not be associated with true daytime sleepiness. Evaluation often indicates the presence of a mood disorder. The sleep complaint tends to increase in severity with the severity of the daytime symptoms and generally resolves with resolution of the mood disorder.
Anxiety disorder	Although anxiety disorder is seldom described in childhood, correlates exist. Children during middle childhood and adolescents may be affected. Sleep onset and sleep maintenance problems may be present. Anxiety and fears may be present during wakefulness, and the child or parent may be able to identify the stressor (e.g., parental separation, divorce, death in the family). Nightmares (anxiety dreams) often occur. Anxiety and fear seem to be generalized, with diurnal and nocturnal manifestations. Anxiety disorder can be differentiated from adjustment sleep disorder by the absence of a single precipitating event and by the presence of a more chronic course. Although anxiety and fears may be related to the sleeping environment, they do not center on anxiety about the inability to fall asleep, as occurs with psychophysiological insomnia in older patients.
Panic disorders	Panic disorders usually occur in young adults but may occur during middle childhood and adolescence. Sleep complaints center on an inability to fall asleep, sudden awakenings from sleep, and a profound inability to return to sleep after the awakening. The arousal is associated with intense fear, panic, and somatic symptoms of hyperarousal. Agoraphobia may be present. The patient may have an irrational fear of impending doom or of dying. Sleep terrors, on the other hand, are partial arousals from slow-wave sleep, are brief, and are not associated with sleep onset difficulties, agoraphobia, or daytime symptoms. Sleep returns quickly after a sleep terror episode, and the child does not remember the event. Nightmares tend to have a vivid, storylike quality, are specific rather than generalized, occur during early morning hours, and usually are associated with only mild autonomic arousal.
Alcohol misuse	Although alcoholism is rarely discussed in the context of pediatric sleep disorders, the increasing prevalence of alcohol misuse and abuse during middle childhood and adolescence demands its inclusion. Alcohol consumption has two major effects on sleep. First there is an increase in sleepiness, which lasts for several hours. This sleepiness is followed by an increase in wakefulness, which occurs 2 to 3 hours after sleep onset. Sleep becomes fragmented by frequent brief arousals and significant restlessness, and rebound increases in REM sleep may occur. Nightmares often occur. Disruption in sleep continuity and architecture often results in excessive sleepiness and poor performance during the day.

III. SLEEPLESSNESS ASSOCIATED WITH ENVIRONMENTAL FACTORS

Disorder	Clinical Presentation
Environmental sleep disorder	Children and adolescents are susceptible to sleep disruption from environmental factors. Complaints of sleeplessness (onset and maintenance insomnia) are common. An easily identifiable environmental stimulus (e.g., excessive noise, excessive heat or cold, movement of a bed partner, or crying of a younger sibling) that has a temporal relationship to the onset of the sleep complaint is often identified. Symptoms are related to the physical presence of the noxious stimulus, rather than a psychological or emotional reaction to the offending agent. Symptoms of sleeplessness resolve after removal of the disturbing environmental factors. Daytime symptoms may include excessive sleepiness resulting from nocturnal sleep deprivation, attention span problems, restlessness, poor school performance, lethargy, and malaise.
Food allergy insomnia	Onset is usually within the first 2 years of life and is often associated with the introduction of cow's milk protein into the diet. Allergies to other food products may cause a similar pattern of onset of the sleep disturbance. Sleep onset difficulties may be profound and associated with significant agitation and incessant crying. Arousals and awakenings from sleep are frequent and may be prolonged. Diurnal symptoms of irritability; skin lesions; wheezing, rhinorrhea, and other respiratory tract complaints; colicky abdominal pain and hematochezia; agitation; and lethargy may accompany the sleep complaints. Removal of the allergen results in resolution of the symptoms (diurnal symptoms tend to resolve before nocturnal symptoms). Food allergy may be differentiated from sleep-disordered respiration by the absence of snoring or respiratory pauses during sleep and by the involvement of other body systems. Nocturnal asthma, gastroesophageal reflux, and colic may be difficult to differentiate from food allergy, and significant laboratory testing may be necessary to eliminate these as causes of the sleep complaint (especially if allergic respiratory symptoms predominate).
Toxin-induced sleep disorder	Sleep disturbance secondary to heavy metal intoxication is fairly common during early childhood. Chronic lead intoxication is the most common cause. Even low-dose lead exposure and increased body lead burden can result in nocturnal (sleep-related) symptoms. Sleep onset and maintenance insomnia may be present and associated with generalized central nervous system excitation. This may alternate with significant central nervous system depression and signs of increased intracranial pressure or encephalopathy. Nausea, vomiting, diarrhea, or constipation may occur. The child may have a history of pica and accidental ingestion of other substances. Other organ systems may be affected. Laboratory testing may be necessary to differentiate this cause from other causes of childhood sleeplessness.

IV. SLEEPLESSNESS ASSOCIATED WITH DRUG DEPENDENCY

Disorder	Clinical Presentation
Hypnotic-dependent sleep disorder	Although dependence on hypnotic drugs is not typically considered a pediatric disorder, correlates may be identified in children and adolescents. Similar problems may result when children are inappropriately given hypnotic medication in the treatment of

Continued on following page

IV. SLEEPLESSNESS ASSOCIATED WITH DRUG DEPENDENCY *Continued*

Disorder	Clinical Presentation
Hypnotic-dependent sleep disorder—cont'd	sleeplessness. Even a few days of hypnotic drug use may result in rebound sleeplessness when the medication is discontinued. This may lead to reinstitution of the hypnotic drug. Long-term use results in the development of tolerance and the need for increased doses to obtain a clinical effect. Hypnotics may shorten sleep onset latency, but rarely do they improve sleep quality. Medications with long half-lives may result in carryover daytime symptoms of excessive sleepiness, lethargy, malaise, poor functioning, poor coordination, visual-motor problems, restlessness, and anxiety. Sudden cessation of hypnotics generally results in rapid return of severe sleepiness (to the premedication level). The sleep architecture gradually improves over 2 to 3 weeks, but the patient perceives that sleep is worse than before the hypnotics were begun.
Stimulant-dependent sleep disorder	Although stimulant dependence is more typically seen in adolescents and young adults, children inappropriately maintained on stimulant medication for hyperactivity or behavior problems may manifest similar symptoms. Sleep onset may be profoundly delayed, and there may be long periods of sleep suppression followed by periods of extreme somnolence. Anecdotal evidence indicates that disrupted sleep in children with attention deficit hyperactivity disorder is somewhat improved after administration of stimulant medication if bedtime is delayed long enough after the last dose (half-life dependent). Withdrawal from chronic abuse of stimulant medications during adolescence results in severe sleepiness.
Alcohol-dependent sleep disorder	This sleep disorder has not been described during childhood. Typical age of onset is during the fifth decade of life. The patient complains of chronic insomnia. Sleep onset is assisted by the repeated consumption of alcohol. Tolerance to the hypnotic effect occurs, necessitating consumption of greater quantities of alcohol. With long-term use of alcohol, sleep is significantly disrupted and fragmented by frequent arousals and awakenings. Sudden awakening from REM sleep may occur and is often accompanied by xerostomia and cephalalgia. Sometimes the patient uses other hypnotics (e.g., benzodiazepines) in conjunction with alcohol.

V. SLEEPLESSNESS ASSOCIATED WITH SLEEP-INDUCED RESPIRATORY IMPAIRMENT

Disorder	Clinical Presentation
Obstructive sleep apnea syndrome	Sleep onset difficulties are seldom present in childhood obstructive sleep apnea syndrome. Occasional or frequent nocturnal awakenings may occur. The parents may note snoring, brief respiratory pauses, and gasps. Snoring is characteristic but may be more subtle than the snoring of adults. Sleep-related enuresis is a common associated feature. As a result of nocturnal sleep fragmentation, varying degrees of daytime sleepiness may occur. Children tend to mask the sleepiness by becoming overstimulated and hyperactive. Daytime symptoms include hyperactivity, unrefreshing naps, attention span problems, fidgety behavior, motor restlessness, school difficulties, unusual aggressiveness, social withdrawal, pathological shyness, morning headaches, and dry mouth. Since hypertrophic tonsils and adenoids are the most common

Disorder	Clinical Presentation
Obstructive sleep apnea syndrome—cont'd	cause of obstructive sleep apnea in children, symptoms and signs referable to this primary underlying condition are often present and include adenoidal facies, adenoidal speech, dull expression, periorbital edema, mouth breathing, swallowing difficulties, and frequent episodes of otitis media. Chronic sleep-related airway obstruction may result in systemic hypertension, pulmonary hypertension, and cor pulmonale.
Central sleep apnea syndrome	Central sleep apnea syndrome in childhood is often asymptomatic, but when symptoms are present, sleep maintenance insomnia is the typical complaint. The nighttime sleep period is interrupted by several awakenings, during which the child may have a frightening feeling of choking or being unable to breathe. If awakenings do not occur, parents may notice episodes of pauses in respiratory effort. Daytime sleepiness and fatigue may result from nocturnal sleep disruption but are not as severe as in obstructive sleep apnea syndrome. If present, daytime symptoms may be mistaken for laziness or behavioral problems. Learning and memory difficulties may occur. During infancy, central sleep apnea syndrome may present as an Apparent Life Threatening Event (ALTE). Prolonged presence of central sleep apnea may result in systemic and pulmonary hypertension and cardiac arrhythmias.
Central alveolar hypoventilation syndrome	Sleep onset is usually normal. Sleep maintenance problems exist with manifestations of arousals to lighter stages of sleep and awakening from sleep. Sleep fragmentation may cause excessive daytime sleepiness. Central control of respiration is disturbed, and hypoventilation results in oxygen desaturation and arousal. An apparent life-threatening event (cyanosis, pallor, apnea, bradycardia) at sleep onset early in infancy may be the first manifestation. In some patients the syndrome does not appear until adolescence or young adulthood. Hypoxia and hypercapnia are common during childhood, but clinical signs may be subtle when evidence of respiratory distress is absent. Chemoreceptors are generally unresponsive to the hypoxia and hypercapnia. When hypoventilation in children occurs during both sleep and wakefulness, the inability to sustain spontaneous ventilation during wakefulness later in life may occur. Neurological disorders that affect the brainstem mechanisms for control of breathing may be identified.
Chronic obstructive pulmonary disease	Sleep disturbances are common and consist of difficulty in initiating sleep, as well as maintenance insomnia. There are frequent awakenings, coughing, shortness of breath, and respiratory distress. Medications often used in daytime management of chronic obstructive pulmonary disease (e.g., methylxanthines) may exacerbate the sleep complaints. Daytime sleepiness may result from nocturnal sleep disruption and architectural fragmentation. Sleep efficiency is reduced, and early morning wakings occur. Evidence of chronic underlying pulmonary disease (e.g., cystic fibrosis) is often present.
Sleep-related asthma	Frequent nocturnal wakings occur and are associated with respiratory distress, wheezing, and coughing. Excessive production of thick, tenacious mucus takes place. The severity of nighttime symptoms typically parallels the severity of daytime symptoms, although patients with mild diurnal manifestations can exhibit clinically significant nocturnal symptoms. Bronchodilator therapy often alleviates symptoms. However, bronchodilators (especially methylxanthine derivatives) may exacerbate nocturnal wakings and complaints of insomnia.
Altitude insomnia	Altitude insomnia may occur at any age. There is an acute onset (within 72 hours) of sleeplessness after travel to elevations higher than 4,000 m above sea level. Associated symptoms include headache, fatigue, and anorexia. Awakenings are often related to apneic events, and patients awaken with a perception of difficulty breathing. Underlying pulmonary disease and anemia may predispose individuals to insomnia from high altitudes. Symptoms often improve after acclimation to lower ambient oxygen tensions.

VI. SLEEPLESSNESS ASSOCIATED WITH MOVEMENT DISORDERS

Disorder	Clinical Presentation
Sleep starts	Sleep starts are usually benign and run an uneventful course. They are considered normal events. When severe or frequent, however, sleep starts may result in a sleep onset insomnia. A massive, brief, single contraction of the legs (and occasionally the arms and head) occurs at sleep onset and results in arousal. A conscious perception of falling or a visual dream or hypnogogic hallucination often occurs. If sleep onset is delayed significantly, sleep deprivation (and its resultant symptoms) can occur. Occasionally bruising from hitting a foot or hand on a fixed object (bedpost, nightstand) may occur. Subjective complaints are rare during childhood, although parents may notice and report concern about these major myoclonic movements.
Restless leg syndrome	The peak onset of restless leg syndrome is in middle age, and the disorder has rarely been reported in infancy and childhood. Patients complain of disturbing sensations in the legs. These may include aches, tingling, itching, or creeping sensations before sleep onset, resulting in an inability to keep the legs still and inhibiting sleep onset. Sensations occur anywhere in the legs or feet. In some cases the arms are involved. Symptoms may last for only a few minutes or may be prolonged for hours, significantly delaying sleep. Movement of the legs results in resolution of the perceptions, and cessation of leg movements causes return of the sensation and symptoms.
Periodic limb movement disorder	This disorder is rarely seen in childhood and is most prevalent during middle adulthood. Some clinical correlates may exist during childhood and adolescence. The patient's history may reveal frequent awakenings and unrefreshing sleep. Numerous partial arousals occur and significantly disrupt sleep architecture and continuity. There are repetitive and stereotypical movements of one or both legs. The arms may also be involved. Parents may express concern about these periodic jerking movements. More commonly, patients are unaware of the partial or brief arousals and complaints center on symptoms of excessive daytime sleepiness.
Nocturnal leg cramps	Although this disorder has not been described during infancy, children may be awakened at night by leg pains and cramps. The history may reveal occasional nighttime wakings or early morning arousal and difficulty returning to sleep. Both upper and lower leg musculature may be involved. Rubbing or massage of the affected area may relieve the discomfort. Nocturnal leg pains and cramps must be differentiated from those of clear organic origin, including but not limited to arthritis, arthralgia, metabolic disorders, dystonia, seizure disorders, peripheral neuropathies, and myelopathies.
Rhythmical movement disorders	Rhythmical movement disorders may occur at the onset of sleep or during sleep. A variety of manifestations occur. The history may reveal rhythmical head banging, head rolling, body rocking, or head rocking. The patient has paroxysms of stereotypical, repetitive movements of large muscle groups. Episodes occur at sleep onset, during light sleep, or during slow-wave sleep. Similar rhythmical behaviors may occur during daytime naps and during wakefulness. Onset of symptoms is typically during the first 2 years of life, and symptoms tend to resolve during middle childhood and adolescence. Occasionally symptoms persist. Episodes may occur almost nightly or less than once per week. Diurnal symptoms are unusual, and the affected children are normal neurologically, behaviorally, and psychologically. If symptoms are severe (especially in patients with head banging [jactatio capitis nocturna]), bruising and other physical injury may occur.

Disorder	Clinical Presentation
REM sleep behavior disorder	Sleep onset is typically normal. The history reveals sudden arousal, swinging of the arms, punching, leaping from bed, mumbling incoherently, and running from the bed. These behaviors appear to be consistent with dream enactment. A paradoxical increase in muscle tone (absence on normal skeletal muscle inhibition) takes place during REM sleep. Typical episodes occur at least 90 minutes after sleep onset or during the early morning hours when REM sleep predominates and REM sleep duration and intensity are greatest. Violent and frightening behaviors can occur, and injuries are frequent. Although this condition is typically described in elderly men, a number of cases in children have been reported. Underlying neurological abnormalities have been described in a large number of patients. Sleep continuity is significantly disrupted. Evidence of excessive limb twitching and body movements during sleep has been reported.
Nocturnal paroxysmal dystonia	The history consists of choreoathetotic or ballistic movements occurring before sleep onset, during sleep, or after an arousal from sleep. These paroxysmal movements are associated with dystonic posturing, especially of the hands. No daytime symptoms occur. Episodes may be brief (lasting less than 1 minute but recurring in frequent paroxysms throughout the night) or prolonged (lasting 1 hour or more). Episodes occur almost nightly. Vocalizations may be present. After paroxysms cease, the person is not disoriented and returns quickly to sleep. The symptoms must be differentiated from those of sleep-related seizures. Evidence that nocturnal paroxysmal dystonia is a manifestation of seizure activity has not been established.

VII. SLEEPLESSNESS ASSOCIATED WITH CIRCADIAN RHYTHM DISORDERS

Disorder	Clinical Presentation
Time zone change/jet lag syndrome	Children of all ages are susceptible. The severity of symptoms depends on the number of time zones traversed, as well as the individual's innate ability to delay or advance the sleep phase. Patients complain of an inability to fall asleep at the socially desired hour in the new time zone, difficulty in waking in the morning, and excessive sleepiness during the day. Adaptation of the sleep-wake cycle to the new time zone generally takes 2 to 3 days but may take considerably longer after travel from west to east, which requires a phase advance. Adaptation of other physiological rhythms may take considerably longer than the sleep-wake cycle. In most cases symptoms are self-limited, lasting less than 2 weeks. Persistence for a longer period may represent an inappropriate response to the symptoms or the presence of other sleep related disorders.
Shift work sleep disorder	Although children are not subjected to shift work, many parents are. To increase time spent with their children (or out of necessity to prepare for day care, night care, or other activities), parents may permit or force their children to follow unusual sleep-wake schedules. Sleep phase shifts, inability to fall asleep at desired times, and excessive daytime sleepiness may result. Complaints of insomnia, when they occur, usually focus on sleep maintenance problems, night wakings, or early morning arousals. More commonly, excessive sleepiness, performance deficits, and behavioral problems develop, especially when the child's social responsibilities are out of phase with the parents'. Sleep onset and maintenance problems may persist in children after the parents' shift rotates to a more appropriate time.

Continued on following page

VII. SLEEPLESSNESS ASSOCIATED WITH CIRCADIAN RHYTHM DISORDERS *Continued*

Disorder	Clinical Presentation
Delayed sleep phase syndrome	Delayed sleep phase syndrome is common during childhood. The most frequent complaints are bedtime struggles and sleep onset difficulties. Sleep onset may be delayed for hours beyond the parents' desired bedtime for the child. Older infants and toddlers still sleeping in a crib often cry and fuss for significant periods at bedtime. Older children often climb out of bed, protest, or make numerous requests to stall bedtime. Sleep onset generally occurs at the same time each night (although later than desired). Sleep is continuous, and nocturnal wakings are unusual. If the child has early morning responsibilities (e.g., school), he or she may seem impossible to arouse in the morning. When no responsibilities require early wake-up times (e.g., on weekends and vacations), the child sleeps into the late morning or early afternoon. Children with delayed sleep phase syndrome are generally most wide awake and alert in the late afternoon or evening. School work may be poorer in the morning than in the afternoon. The early portion of the week tends to be more difficult than the latter portion because of adaptation. Symptoms of sleep deprivation may appear. The child recovers somewhat on the weekends when he or she can sleep later into the day, only to show symptoms again during the school week. Symptoms may persist for months or years.
Advanced sleep phase syndrome	This is much less common than delayed sleep phase syndrome, and sleep complaints are few. If they are present, they center on morning waking at a time significantly earlier than desired. Sleep onset is usually not a problem but occurs early in the evening. Sleep is otherwise normal and uninterrupted. Unlike other disorders of sleep maintenance, early morning awakenings occur after otherwise normal amounts of undisturbed sleep. Daytime symptoms are notably absent, but children are incapable of staying awake at night. For parents of younger children this is usually not a problem, and sleep complaints are not brought to the attention of the health professional. Older children, who have social responsibilities in the evening, may have difficulty staying awake and concentrating on tasks such as homework. Typically, however, stimulating evening activities delay and entrain the sleep phase, synchronizing the sleep-wake cycle to more appropriate times.
Non-24-hour sleep-wake syndrome	Sleep complaints in this syndrome are variable and changing because of a continual 1- to 2-hour per day delay in the phase of the sleep-wake cycle. The pattern of the cycle is similar to that seen in the free-running state. Patients alternate from periods of extreme inability to sleep at night and severe sleepiness during the day, to a brief period in which no particular sleep-related complaints occur (i.e., when the sleep-wake cycle is in phase with the 24-hour light-dark cycle). At times wake periods may be prolonged (24 to 40 hours in length) and followed by prolonged sleep periods (14 to 24 hours in length). This sleep pattern is common in patients who are blind (congenital or acquired). It is less commonly associated with mental retardation or psychiatric disorders. Non-24-hour sleep-wake syndrome can be differentiated from sleep phase delay syndrome (which has many similar characteristics) by an inability to achieve a stable sleep-wake pattern during vacations from school.
Irregular sleep-wake pattern	Sleep and wake patterns are significantly variable, haphazard, and disorganized. No clear sleep-wake pattern can be discerned. Complaints may focus on sleeplessness, sleepiness, or both. Total sleep time over a 24-hour period is usually within age group norms, but the timing of long sleep periods and long wake periods is unpredictable. An inability

DISORDER	**CLINICAL PRESENTATION**
Irregular sleep-wake pattern—cont'd	to fall asleep may be the primary complaint, and the frequent daytime sleep episodes may be mistakenly related to the child's inability to sleep at night. Parents may complain that their child "never sleeps." Sleep patterns may resemble the ultradian pattern seen in infancy, although the total sleep time is much shorter and usually within normal limits for the patient's age. Cognitive and performance difficulties are common. Irregular sleep-wake pattern is most common in children with severe congenital or developmental central nervous system dysfunction. It may also be seen in otherwise normal children in the presence of severe familial dysfunction. In these cases the remainder of the child's day (including the timing of other classic zeitgebers) is also dysfunctional, disorganized, haphazard, and chaotic.

VIII. SLEEPLESSNESS ASSOCIATED WITH PARASOMNIAS

DISORDER	**CLINICAL PRESENTATION**
Confusional arousals	Confusional arousals are common during early childhood and decrease in frequency as middle childhood progresses. The typical history involves severe disorientation and confusion after an arousal from slow-wave sleep, during the first part of the night. Similar symptoms may occur after arousal from a daytime nap if it contains slow-wave sleep. During an episode speech is slow and mumbled, orientation to time and place is poor, and response to parents is slow and incoherent. Inappropriate and bizarre behaviors may occur. Forced awakenings also may precipitate events. Occasionally, unusual aggressiveness occurs and injury results. Restraint during a period of confusional arousal may increase the aggressiveness. Behaviors may last only a few minutes or may be prolonged for several hours. The individual generally forgets the event and shows normal waking behavior. Confusional arousals must be differentiated from complex partial seizure disorders.
Sleep terrors (pavor nocturnus)	A sudden, explosive arousal from slow-wave sleep occurs during the first half of the night. Episodes are heralded by a piercing cry or scream and are accompanied by severe autonomic discharges manifested by tachycardia, tachypnea, diaphoresis, pupillary dilatation, flushing, and increased muscle tone. Confusion and disorientation are severe, and parental attempts to comfort the child often worsen the symptoms. Vocalizations may occur, but they are mumbled and garbled. Enuresis is common. Episodes last only a few minutes, and the child rapidly returns to sleep. There is amnesia for the event. No significant daytime symptoms, neurological abnormalities, or psychological dysfunction is present. Occasionally the child falls or climbs from the bed and runs frantically around the house. If this occurs, injury is common.
Nightmares (anxiety dreams)	In contrast to sleep terrors, nightmares result in arousal from REM sleep during early morning hours (typically the last third of the sleep period, although they may occur during any REM sleep period). Nightmares are less intense than sleep terrors and are associated with significantly less autonomic arousal. Long dream mentation occurs and is frightening or anxiety laden. Verbal reports of the frightening dream are common and have a storylike quality. The dream content that causes fear and anxiety associated with nightmares may not be considered disturbing by others. Displacement from the bed is rare, injuries are infrequent, and children respond well to parental efforts to comfort them. Return to sleep may be significantly delayed.

Continued on following page

VIII. SLEEPLESSNESS ASSOCIATED WITH PARASOMNIAS *Continued*

Disorder	Clinical Presentation
Sleep hyperhidrosis	Symptoms include profuse diaphoresis during sleep, which may result in arousal or awakening because of the discomfort. Diurnal diaphoresis may or may not be present. Sleep sweats may occur during febrile illnesses or may be associated with autonomic nervous system dysfunction (e.g., familial dysautonomia). Sleep hyperhidrosis may be associated with other organically based disorders, such as seizure disorders, hyperthyroidism, head injury, hypothalamic lesions, diabetes insipidus, and cerebral palsy. Excessive sweating during sleep is also common in patients with obstructive sleep apnea syndrome.

IX. SLEEPLESSNESS ASSOCIATED WITH CENTRAL NERVOUS SYSTEM DISORDERS (NOT OTHERWISE CLASSIFIED)

Disorder	Clinical Presentation
Sleep-related epilepsy	Seizure disorders may be classified as diurnal, nocturnal, or random (occurring during sleep and wake). Sleep is an important activator of epileptogenesis. Generalized tonic-clonic, simple partial, and partial complex seizures, as well as partial benign focal epilepsy of childhood (Rolandic epilepsy), are particularly associated with sleep. Seizures during sleep may cause awakenings or unusual stereotypical movements noted by parents. Seizures may disrupt the continuity of sleep and result in daytime sleepiness. Sleep-related seizures may be accompanied by complex motoric activity, which must be differentiated from other paroxysmal sleep-related behaviors and rhythmical movement disorders (e.g., somnambulism, bruxism, and sleep terrors). Nocturnal sleep-related enuresis, hyperhidrosis, apnea, and injuries occurring during sleep may also be manifestations of sleep-related epilepsy. Often repetitive seizures during sleep are isolated to the sleep state, but many patients with a single nocturnal seizure develop daytime seizures. Sleep-related seizures may be generalized or focal and may be associated with automatisms and tongue biting. Postictal confusion is present if arousal from sleep occurs.
Fatal familial insomnia	This has not been described in children and has only recently been described in a few families. It typically occurs during the fifth or sixth decade of life and rarely during young adulthood. An initial complaint of difficulty falling asleep progresses within months to a complete lack of sleep. Spontaneous lapses from quiet wakefulness to sleep occur. Dissociated features of REM sleep and apparent dream enactment are seen. Autonomic dysfunction ensues, and death occurs within 2 years of the onset of symptoms.
Cerebral degenerative disorders	This classification refers to a heterogeneous group of disorders that share symptoms of slow progression, abnormal behaviors, involuntary movements, and motor system degeneration. Complaints of insomnia or excessive sleepiness or both can occur. Age of onset varies according to the primary underlying disease process, which may be torsion dystonia, spastic torticollis, Huntington's disease, dystonia musculorum deformans, hereditary progressive dystonia, hereditary ataxia, blepharospasm, or segmental dystonia and dyskinesia. Movements during sleep are common, and diurnal symptoms may be suggestive of the diagnosis. Diurnal symptoms of degenerative central nervous system abnormalities are often present.

X. SLEEPLESSNESS ASSOCIATED WITH NO OBJECTIVE SLEEP DISTURBANCE

DISORDER	CLINICAL PRESENTATION
Sleep state misperception	This disorder can occur at any age, but onset is most common in young adulthood. The complaint is an inability to sleep, but there is no objective evidence of disordered sleep. The patient may state that he or she cannot fall asleep, that sleep is fragmented or disrupted, or that complete sleeplessness is present. The history is convincing and honest. This complaint is generally impossible to differentiate from true sleeplessness on clinical grounds alone. Polysomnography reveals normal sleep onset latency and normal quantity and quality of sleep. Patients often report sleeplessness in the laboratory, despite objective evidence of normal sleep.
Sleep choking syndrome	Sleep choking syndrome is not known to occur in children. It is characterized by awakening from sleep with a sudden sensation of choking. Episodes occur frequently and often repetitively during a single night. Patients awaken suddenly with a feeling of an inability to breathe, are frightened and anxious, and rapidly become fully awake. Respiratory distress or stridor is not present, and other forms of sleep-related anxiety attacks or sleep-disordered respiration are not manifested. Tachycardia occurs on awakening, and there is often a fear of impending death. Once the patient is awake, fear and anxiety rapidly resolve.
Munchausen's syndrome by proxy	Munchausen's syndrome by proxy is a severe form of child abuse in which the caretaker (most often the mother) produces factitious symptoms in her child, necessitating multiple invasive and expensive tests. Histories are fabricated, signs are artificially produced by alteration of laboratory specimens or data, or actual illness is induced (e.g., by surreptitiously administering medication to the child). Commonly the patient has symptoms of a central nervous system disorder (e.g., seizures, incoordination, excessive sleepiness). Chronic sleeplessness may be the initial complaint. The sleeplessness may be fabricated or may be induced by the parent, who deliberately wakens the child during the night. Factitious reports of apnea and sleep-related cardiorespiratory arrest have been described. The patient usually has a history of a long series of medical evaluations, multiple medical complaints, and unsuccessful treatments. The child generally appears healthy, and no objective evidence of a sleep disorder or medical abnormality can be found to explain the symptoms. The mother seems less concerned about the child's illness than does the medical professional, mother and child appear to be overly emotionally involved, the symptoms occur only in the presence of the mother, and the mother seems knowledgeable about medical procedures and techniques. Severe maternal psychopathology is often present, and suicide attempts after disclosure of the diagnosis have been reported.

XI. SLEEPLESSNESS ASSOCIATED WITH IDIOPATHIC INSOMNIA

DISORDER	CLINICAL PRESENTATION
Idiopathic insomnia	Idiopathic insomnia begins in infancy or early childhood. There is a clear complaint of sleeplessness that is relentless, unchanging, and unresponsive to management. Sleeplessness does not vary through periods of good and poor emotional and behavioral adaptation. In

Continued on following page

XI. SLEEPLESSNESS ASSOCIATED WITH IDIOPATHIC INSOMNIA *Continued*

Disorder	Clinical Presentation
Idiopathic insomnia—cont'd	addition to the history of insomnia, daytime performance deficits are observed. Patients have decreased motivation, low levels of vigilance, poor concentration, and attention span difficulties. Children may have soft neurological findings, reading disability, or hyperactivity. Preoccupation with the inability to sleep, characteristic of psychophysiological insomnia, is absent. There may be a family history of insomnia, and symptoms are lifelong. The condition is often complicated by other sleep-related factors (such as long-term use of hypnotic drugs) and is diagnosed when the onset of the insomnia can be traced to infancy, before the introduction of other factors that may disrupt sleep. Other health-related problems are remarkably absent.

XII. OTHER CAUSES OF SLEEPLESSNESS

Disorder	Clinical Presentation
Infantile colic	Parental complaints center on crying, fussiness, and the infant's inability to fall asleep in the evening. These evening symptoms may last for hours. Characteristically onset of the disorder occurs at 2 to 3 weeks of age. Children are otherwise healthy but experience paroxysms of inconsolable irritability that last for more than 3 hours per day, occur at least 3 days per week, and persist for at least 3 weeks. Violent screaming and relatively uninhibited motor activity occur during a paroxysm, and infants have been described as hypertonic during episodes. The infant may grimace and appear to be in pain. Attacks typically occur in the late afternoon or evening (5 PM to midnight) but may occur from 7 PM to 2 AM. Rarely are episodes randomly distributed throughout the day. Occasionally the history reveals brief, irregular daytime sleep episodes. Symptoms resolve spontaneously in almost all infants by 4 months of age. Complaints of sleeplessness persisting beyond 4 months of age are usually a result of parental mismanagement of the sleep problem during the colicky period, and other causes for sleeplessness should be sought.
Sleep-related gastroesophageal reflux	Although most commonly described in adults over 40 years of age, sleep-related gastroesophageal reflux can occur in infants, and childhood correlates may exist. Infants awaken frequently at night and often appear to be in pain. Symptoms may be easily confused with colic. Older children may complain of abdominal pain, substernal chest pain, or tightness in the chest. Nocturnal wheezing or laryngospasm can occur if there is reflux into the pharynx, and infants may have apneic episodes or an apparent life-threatening event. Daytime symptoms of gastroesophageal reflux may be present, and a history of frequent spitting up or regurgitation may be elicited. In severe forms esophagitis and signs of failure to thrive may be prominent.
Pain syndromes	Any cause of acute or chronic pain may result in a complaint of sleeplessness. Acute illness such as otitis media may result in a profound sleep onset or maintenance insomnia. Associated features of local or systemic infection may be present. Persistence of the sleep problem after resolution of the acute infection is usually the result of parental mismanagement, and other causes for the sleep disruption should be sought. Chronic pain from disorders such as juvenile rheumatoid arthritis may cause profound and prolonged sleep disruption.

DISORDER	CLINICAL PRESENTATION
Pain syndromes—cont'd	Sleep tends to be nonrefreshing, and wakings may be associated with pain or stiffness. Teething pain, posttraumatic pain, myalgia, cephalalgia, orthopedic disorders, or any other disease associated with chronic pain may disrupt nocturnal sleep. Daytime symptoms of sleep disruption may be present, and diurnal signs and symptoms of the underlying disease process may establish the diagnosis.
Short sleeper	A short sleeper habitually sleeps substantially less (less than 75%) than the norm for his or her age group. Parents may complain that their child has a very short nocturnal sleep period. Symptoms usually begin during adolescence but may appear earlier. Short sleepers sleep continuously at night. Sleep onset is not delayed, although the time of sleep onset may be later than expected, and early morning wakings occur. Patients are unable to sleep longer, despite opportunities or attempts. Sleep is *refreshing*. Diurnal symptoms are absent, and the individual functions well during the day. Complications occur when attempts are made to extend sleep artificially with medications.
Menstrual-associated sleep disorder	A sleep onset or maintenance insomnia that is temporally related to the premenstrual stage (typically 1 week before the onset of menses) may be the chief complaint. Symptoms generally recur for at least 3 consecutive months. Sleep efficiency is reduced, sleep is fragmented, and frequent awakenings occur during the symptomatic phase. At all other times sleep is normal and there are no sleep-related complaints.
Pregnancy-associated sleep disorder	This sleep disorder can occur in pregnant women of any age. Insomnia generally begins toward the end of the second trimester and is characterized by frequent nocturnal awakenings. Sleep onset is delayed, and waking after sleep onset increases as term approaches. Sleeplessness can be profound and may be related to an inability to assume a comfortable sleeping position, back pain, fetal movements, small functional bladder capacity, and urinary frequency. Sleeplessness may persist after delivery, and child care activities may prolong the sleepless periods. Symptoms gradually subside.
Terrifying hypnogogic hallucinations	Frightening dreams are common during early and middle childhood but are usually associated with REM sleep. Frightening dreams at sleep onset may be terrifying to the child, have a hallucinatory quality, and may be associated with other sensory misperceptions, vague thoughts, and illusions. Mumbling, screaming, and body movements may occur. Fear or anxiety-laden awakening is common. As with nightmares, autonomic activation may be present but is significantly milder than that seen with sleep terrors. The sleeping environment may be involved in the dream mentation.
Sleep-related abnormal swallowing syndrome	This entity is rare in infants and children, but clinical correlates may exist, especially in infants and children with esophageal incoordination or central nervous system disturbances that interfere with the gag reflex and swallowing of pooled secretions. Sleep is restless and interrupted. The person awakens suddenly with coughing, gagging, and choking. These episodes tend to follow periods of gurgling sounds during sleep. Significant apnea is not present, although aspiration of pooled hypopharyngeal secretions may occur. Awakenings are typically of short duration, and return to sleep is rapid.
Sleep-related laryngospasm	This is most often described in middle age, but correlates may exist in childhood. A sudden awakening from sleep occurs and is accompanied by respiratory difficulties, an intense feeling of choking, and profound stridor. Episodes are brief and resolve spontaneously after a few minutes. Patients may panic during the episode because they feel unable to breathe. During childhood this condition is easily differentiated from the awakening and stridor associated with supraglottitis by the absence of fever or cyanosis and by the spontaneous resolution of symptoms.

Continued on following page

XII. OTHER CAUSES OF SLEEPLESSNESS *Continued*

Disorder	Clinical Presentation
Sleep-related laryngospasm—cont'd	Differentiating sleep-related laryngospasm from spasmodic croup may be difficult, and spasmodic croup may be a childhood variant of this sleep disorder.

DISORDERS OF EXCESSIVE SOMNOLENCE (D.O.E.S.)

Disorders of excessive somnolence are a heterogeneous group of sleep abnormalities of both functional and organic origin. Symptoms include undesirable sleeping during waking hours, unavoidable sleep episodes (sleep attacks), excessive tendency to sleep, increased total sleep time in a 24-hour period, or problems achieving full arousal on awakening. Numerous cognitive and performance problems may result. Significant overlap among the disorders exists, and a number of the disorders may be manifest as sleepiness, sleeplessness, or both. Duplication of diagnoses and their description is unavoidable; the descriptions are modified to focus on the disorder when the presenting complaint is excessive sleepiness.

Symptoms of excessive sleepiness in children are highly variable and less clear than those of sleeplessness. Extreme degrees of hypersomnolence are usually obvious. Children are noted to fall asleep at inappropriate times (e.g., at the dinner table, during birthday parties, while opening presents at Christmas). However, most sleepy children manifest behaviors that are not typically associated with sleepiness and may be mistaken for symptoms of other disorders or behavioral problems. These symptoms may include, but are not limited to, the following:

Hyperactivity	Attention span problems
Poor concentration	Easy distractibility
School failure	Unusual aggressiveness
Pathological shyness	Motor restlessness
Fidgety behaviors	Rapid mood swings
Napping in school	Decreased appetite
Impulsiveness	Cognitive deficits
Performance deficits	Reading disability

These signs and symptoms are associated with many childhood disorders. Evaluation should be considered incomplete if possible disorders of excessive somnolence are not comprehensively sought and assessed.

I. SLEEPINESS ASSOCIATED WITH BEHAVIORAL AND PSYCHOPHYSIOLOGICAL DISORDERS

Disorder	Clinical Presentation
Inadequate sleep hygiene	Sleep complaints associated with inadequate sleep hygiene are variable. Daytime sleepiness often appears during adolescence when youngsters become more independent and assume greater responsibility for determining the timing of sleep, caring for the sleep environment, and scheduling other nighttime and daytime activities. Irregular bedtimes and wake times emerge. Bedtime may be delayed by arousing or stimulating activities (e.g., homework, exercise, parties). Because of extreme variability in sleep schedules, patients may spend excessive time sleeping and may nap several times per week in attempts to

DISORDER	CLINICAL PRESENTATION
Inadequate sleep hygiene—cont'd	recover. The sleeping environment may not be conducive to sleep. It may be cluttered and used for other activities (especially doing homework in bed, eating in bed, and watching television in bed). The room may be too hot or too cold. The bed may be disheveled and uncomfortable.
Insufficient sleep syndrome	The typical complaint is of excessive sleepiness, but prepubertal children may also have difficulty initiating sleep. There is a *voluntary* restriction of total sleep time, and the habitual sleep episode is considerably shorter than age-related norms. When given the opportunity to lengthen the sleep episode, the patient typically has no problem initiating or maintaining sleep or sleeping for a longer period. In fact, sleep periods tend to be longer on weekends and holidays, and patients awaken spontaneously. Secondary symptoms include concentration problems, attention span difficulties, low levels of vigilance, easy distractibility, restlessness, irritability, poor coordination, malaise, and myalgias. These symptoms may become the focal point of the presenting complaint. The disparity between the need for sleep and the amount of sleep actually obtained is significant. Findings of the physical examination are unremarkable, and usually no physical basis for the excessive sleepiness is found.
Limit-setting sleep disorder	Limit-setting sleep disorder is common during childhood and may be associated with other manifestations of behavioral disorders or disorders of parenting. Excessive sleepiness is the result of the parents' inability to set limits on bedtime, which leads to a decrease in nocturnal sleep. Parents state that their child refuses to go to sleep at a time the parents have established. The child frequently gets out of bed, asks for another drink of water or a bedtime story, or finds some other excuse to stall bedtime. The parents give in to the child's demands and rarely set limits on the child's behavior. When limits are set and enforced, sleep onset is normal, the sleep period time returns to the age-related norm, quality and quantity of sleep become normal, and symptoms of excessive daytime sleepiness resolve.

II. SLEEPINESS ASSOCIATED WITH PSYCHIATRIC DISORDERS

DISORDER	CLINICAL PRESENTATION
Mood disorders	Sleep problems from mood disorders are only occasionally seen in prepubertal children. Adolescents may manifest sleep abnormalities secondary to depression, but this problem is most commonly seen during the third and fifth decades of life. Daytime sleepiness and frequent napping may be present in milder forms of the disorder. Many patients complain about feeling tired during the day, and this may or may not be associated with true or manifest daytime sleepiness. Inability to fall asleep at bedtime and early morning awakenings with an inability to fall back to sleep are common associated complaints. Daytime evaluation often reveals the mood disorder, and the sleep complaints tend to increase in severity with the severity of the behavioral symptoms. Sleep problems usually improve or resolve with improvement or resolution of the mood disorder.
Psychoses	Daytime and functional symptoms are usually the focus of the parents' complaints. Many childhood psychoses are associated with sleep-related symptoms (e.g., childhood autism, childhood schizophrenia). Nocturnal sleep may be fragmented, and the sleep-wake cycle profoundly disorganized. Excessive daytime sleepiness may be manifested as any of

Continued on following page

II. SLEEPINESS ASSOCIATED WITH PSYCHIATRIC DISORDERS *Continued*

DISORDER	CLINICAL PRESENTATION
Psychoses—cont'd	the typical childhood symptoms or may be associated with frequent or prolonged daytime sleep periods. Daytime sleepiness may alternate with nocturnal sleeplessness. Sleep efficiency is typically poor.
Alcoholism	Although alcoholism is rarely discussed in the context of pediatric sleep disorders, the increasing prevalence of alcohol abuse and misuse during middle to late childhood and adolescence demands its inclusion. Daytime sleepiness is a common complaint and may lead the parents to bring their child to the health professional for evaluation. Excessive daytime somnolence results from severe nocturnal sleep fragmentation caused by frequent brief arousals. Although awakenings may not occur, sleep may appear restless. Alcohol consumption has two major effects on sleep. First, there is an increase in sleepiness lasting for several hours. REM suppression occurs during the early part of the evening, and REM rebound takes place during the latter portion of the sleep period (after the alcohol has been metabolized). Nightmares are common. Increased sleepiness is followed by an increase in wakefulness 2 to 3 hours after sleep onset. This disruption in the architecture and continuity of sleep may be responsible for the daytime symptoms of excessive sleepiness.

III. SLEEPINESS ASSOCIATED WITH ENVIRONMENTAL FACTORS

DISORDER	CLINICAL PRESENTATION
Environmental sleep disorder	Symptoms of excessive daytime sleepiness (e.g., attention span problems, poor school performance, lethargy, malaise) may be the initial factors that bring the child to the attention of the health care professional. The parents may not recognize the influence of environmental factors in disrupting the child's nocturnal sleep. Children and adolescents of any age are susceptible to sleep fragmentation and disruption from environmental factors. If pursued, environmental stimuli are often easily identified (e.g., excessive noise from living near a highway or airport, excessive heat or cold, movements of a bed partner when co-sleeping, crying of a younger sibling). Sleeplessness at night may also be reported. There is a temporal relationship between the onset of the sleepiness (and other sleep-related complaints) and the presence of the environmental factors. Symptoms are related to the physical existence of the noxious environmental stimulus, rather than a psychological or emotional reaction to it. Symptoms resolve after removal of the disturbing factor(s).
Toxin-induced sleep disorder	Sleep disturbances secondary to heavy metal intoxication are fairly common during early childhood. Chronic lead intoxication is the most common heavy metal intoxication during childhood (although other heavy metal poisonings and toxins can precipitate similar symptoms). The associated sleep abnormalities are not well described in the literature. Because of the subtle nature of the signs and symptoms, as well as the frequent absence of diurnal symptoms, abnormal sleep may be the first sign of intoxication. Even low-dose exposure and increased body lead burden can result in sleep-related complaints. Significant central nervous system depression and daytime sleepiness may occur. There may be a history of pica or accidental ingestion of other substances. Sleepiness may alternate with sleeplessness (because of

DISORDER	CLINICAL PRESENTATION
Toxin-induced sleep disorder—cont'd	generalized central nervous system excitation). Diurnal signs and symptoms of increased intracranial pressure or encephalopathy may occur. Nausea, vomiting, diarrhea, or constipation may be present. Laboratory testing may be necessary to differentiate this cause of sleepiness from others.

IV. SLEEPINESS ASSOCIATED WITH DRUG DEPENDENCY

DISORDER	CLINICAL PRESENTATION
Hypnotic-dependent sleep disorder	Although hypnotic dependence is not considered a pediatric disorder, correlates may be identified during childhood and similar problems may develop when children are inappropriately given hypnotic medication in the treatment of sleeplessness. Daytime sleepiness typically occurs after the ingestion of hypnotics that have long half-lives. Carryover daytime symptoms of excessive sleepiness, lethargy, malaise, poor functioning, poor coordination, visual-motor problems, motor restlessness, and anxiety often occur. Hypnotics decrease sleep onset latency, but rarely do they improve sleep. Even a few days of hypnotic use may result in rebound sleeplessness when the medication is discontinued. The sleeplessness may lead to reinstitution of the medication. Long-term use often results in the development of tolerance, and patients require increased doses to obtain a clinical effect. The chance for carryover sleepiness increases with increasing doses.
Stimulant-dependent sleep disorder	This is typically seen during adolescence and young adulthood. However, children inappropriately maintained on stimulant medication for hyperactivity or behavior problems may manifest similar symptoms. The presenting complaint may focus on extreme degrees of daytime sleepiness, cognitive deficits, and performance problems. These often follow long periods of sleep suppression by the stimulant medication. Withdrawal after long-term use, abuse, or misuse of stimulant drugs during adolescence often results in profound symptoms of daytime sleepiness.

V. SLEEPINESS ASSOCIATED WITH SLEEP-INDUCED RESPIRATORY IMPAIRMENT

DISORDER	CLINICAL PRESENTATION
Obstructive sleep apnea syndrome	Because obstructive apneas greatly disrupt nocturnal sleep, they frequently cause extreme daytime sleepiness. Sleepiness is a significantly more common complaint than sleeplessness, especially during childhood. Sleepiness is often manifested as paradoxical symptoms of hyperactivity and overstimulation. Unrefreshing naps, attention span problems, fidgety behavior, motor restlessness, school performance difficulties, unusual aggressiveness, social withdrawal, pathological shyness, morning headaches, and dry mouth may be present. Sleep-related enuresis is common. Nocturnal sleep may be interrupted by occasional or frequent awakenings. Snoring, brief respiratory pauses, and gasping may be noted during sleep. Snoring is characteristic, although it may be more subtle than that of adults. Since hypertrophic tonsils and adenoids are the most common cause of

Continued on following page

V. SLEEPLESSNESS ASSOCIATED WITH SLEEP-INDUCED RESPIRATORY IMPAIRMENT *Continued*

Disorder	Clinical Presentation
Obstructive sleep apnea syndrome—cont'd	cause of obstructive sleep apnea in children, symptoms and signs referable to this primary underlying condition are often present and include adenoidal facies, adenoidal speech, dull expression, periorbital edema, mouth breathing, swallowing difficulties, and frequent episodes of otitis media. Chronic sleep-related airway obstruction may result in systemic hypertension, pulmonary hypertension, and cor pulmonale.
Central sleep apnea syndrome	Central sleep apnea syndrome is often asymptomatic. Excessive daytime sleepiness and fatigue may result from nocturnal sleep disruption and may be the presenting complaint (if awakenings do not occur from the apneic events). In the absence of nocturnal awakenings, daytime symptoms may be mistaken for laziness or behavioral problems. Learning and memory deficits may occur. Often patients also complain of a sleep maintenance insomnia. The sleep period is interrupted by several awakenings, which may be accompanied by a frightening feeling of choking or being unable to breathe. Prolonged, untreated central sleep apnea may result in systemic and pulmonary hypertension and cardiac arrhythmias. During infancy, central sleep apnea syndrome may present as an Apparent Life Threatening Event.
Central alveolar hypoventilation syndrome	Excessive daytime sleepiness may be the presenting complaint when this form of sleep-disordered respiration results in nocturnal arousal to lighter sleep stages without frank awakenings. Sleep onset is usually normal. During sleep, central control of respiration is disturbed and hypoventilation occurs. The hypoventilation results in oxygen desaturation and arousal. The syndrome may appear early in infancy with an apparent life-threatening event (which may include cyanosis, pallor, apnea, and bradycardia). In other patients it first appears during adolescence or young adulthood. Hypoxia and hypercapnia are common in children with this disorder, but clinical signs may be subtle when respiratory distress is absent. Chemoreceptors are generally unresponsive to the hypoxia and hypercapnia. When hypoventilation occurs during both sleep and wakefulness, the inability to sustain spontaneous ventilation during wakefulness may appear later in life. Neurological disorders that affect the brainstem mechanisms for control of breathing are identified in some patients.
Sleep-related neurogenic tachypnea	This is a rare disorder characterized by sustained tachypnea (an increase in respiratory rate of more than 20% above baseline waking level). The tachypnea begins at sleep onset, persists throughout the sleep period, and resolves spontaneously immediately on awakening. Excessive daytime sleepiness is the usual presenting complaint, but diurnal symptoms may be related to significant underlying central nervous system (especially brainstem and medulla) pathology. Brainstem medullary dysfunction, pseudotumor cerebri, explosive nocturnal arousals, intense nightmares, and other sleep-related respiratory signs and symptoms have been reported. Hypoxia and hypercapnia are notably absent.

VI. SLEEPINESS ASSOCIATED WITH MOVEMENT DISORDERS

Disorder	Clinical Presentation
Periodic limb movement disorder	Periodic limb movement disorders are rare during childhood, although some clinical correlates may exist. These disorders are most prevalent in middle adulthood. The most common presenting complaint is excessive daytime sleepiness, and associated symptoms are often present. Often the periodic limb movements are not perceived to disrupt sleep. The mode of presentation is extremely variable. Sleep is described as unrefreshing. Frequent arousals to lighter stages of sleep occur (in the absence of frank awakenings). When co-sleeping, the bed partner may notice paroxysms of leg (or arm) jerks and movements. There are repetitive and stereotypical movements of one or both legs and sometimes the arms. Parents observing their child sleeping may notice these periodic jerking movements. Significant disruption of sleep architecture and continuity occurs, although patients themselves are unaware of these movements and partial arousals.

VII. SLEEPINESS ASSOCIATED WITH DISORDERS OF CIRCADIAN RHYTHM

Disorder	Clinical Presentation
Long sleeper	A long sleeper habitually sleeps substantially more during a 24-hour period than the conventional amount of sleep obtained by individuals in the same age group (see Fig. A2–3, Appendix 2). Onset of symptoms usually occurs during childhood. When patients are allowed to sleep their habitual amount of time, sleep is continuous and sleep efficiency and timing are normal (although sleep is longer than expected). Frequently there are no sleep complaints. Some patients (or parents) may complain of hypersomnia. Associated symptoms of excessive daytime sleepiness (e.g., daytime napping, performance deficits, hyperactivity, cognitive difficulties) are notably absent unless sleep is restricted because of social obligations (e.g., school, homework). The history reveals that the pattern of long sleep requirement is stable and long standing.
Time zone change/jet lag syndrome	Children of all ages are susceptible. Symptom severity and presenting complaints depend on the number of time zones traversed and the individual's ability to delay or advance the sleep phase. Patients complain of severe daytime sleepiness, a profound inability to fall asleep at the socially desired time, and difficulty waking in the morning. Adaptation of the sleep-wake cycle to the new time zone generally takes 2 to 3 days but may take considerably longer after eastward travel. Adaptation of other physiological functions to the new time zone may take much longer. In most cases symptoms are self-limited, lasting no more than 2 weeks. Symptoms persisting for a longer period may represent the presence of other sleep disorders.
Shift work sleep disorder	Although children do not participate in shift work, disordered sleep from parental shift work is common. Parents may force unusual sleep-wake schedules on their children to increase time spent with the children or out of necessity to prepare for day care, night care, or other activities. Excessive daytime sleepiness, performance problems, hyperactivity, persistent napping, behavioral abnormalities, and phase shifts may occur. The child may have a history of inability to fall asleep at parentally enforced times. Symptoms generally appear when the

Continued on following page

VII. SLEEPINESS ASSOCIATED WITH DISORDERS OF CIRCADIAN RHYTHM *Continued*

DISORDER	CLINICAL PRESENTATION
Shift work sleep disorder—cont'd	child's social responsibilities are out of phase with the parents' work schedule. Disrupted sleep may persist in children even after the parents' shift rotates to a more appropriate time.
Delayed sleep phase syndrome	Delayed sleep phase syndrome is common during childhood. Although the most frequent presenting complaints center on difficulties falling asleep, bedtime struggles, and other sleep onset problems, excessive daytime sleepiness, performance problems, and related symptoms are also common. Sleep onset may be delayed for hours beyond the scheduled bedtime. Older infants and young toddlers still sleeping in a crib may cry and fuss for significant periods at bedtime. Older children may climb out of bed with many requests or protestations. Sleep onset generally occurs at the *inherent physiological time* each night. Once sleep occurs, it is continuous and rarely broken by awakenings. A child with no social obligations sleeps into late morning or early afternoon hours, and this may be acceptable to the parents. If, however, there are early morning responsibilities (e.g., school), parents frequently report that the child is extremely difficult to waken, disoriented on awakening, sluggish, lethargic, cranky, aggressive, and unable to perform required tasks. Symptoms of excessive sleepiness are generally restricted to the morning hours. Parents typically report the child to be most awake and alert in the late afternoon or evening. Morning school work may be significantly poorer than that accomplished in the afternoon. Symptoms are more apparent early in the week than later. Symptoms of sleep deprivation are present, but the child recovers somewhat on weekends, only to show symptoms again when the school week begins. Symptoms may persist for months or years.
Advanced sleep phase syndrome	Advanced sleep phase syndrome is much less common than delayed sleep phase syndrome. Excessive daytime sleepiness is typically not a complaint of children with advanced sleep phase syndrome. It becomes a concern of parents when the child has significant nighttime responsibilities or obligations. In these situations the history usually reveals the child's inability to remain awake in the early evening hours. If forced to remain awake, the child becomes cranky and irritable. Often it is impossible to keep the child awake. A younger child may fall asleep under inappropriate circumstances or in unusual places (e.g., curled up on the floor). More often the sleep complaint centers on morning wakings at a time significantly earlier than desired. Sleep is otherwise normal and uninterrupted. For parents of younger children, sleep phase advance syndrome is usually not a problem; the parents welcome the time alone in the early evening when the child is sleeping. After middle childhood and during adolescence, stimulating evening activities tend to entrain the sleep phase to a later time, better synchronizing the sleep-wake cycle to the light-dark cycle.
Non-24-hour sleep-wake syndrome	Sleep complaints are variable and tend to change from week to week because of a continual 1- to 2-hour per day delay in the phase of the sleep-wake cycle. The cycle pattern is similar to that seen in a free-running state. The patient appears to lack entrainment to the 24-hour day, and the circadian pacemaker cycles at its inherent periodicity. Patients alternate from periods of profound daytime sleepiness and an inability to sleep at night to a brief period when there are no particular sleep-related complaints. This occurs when the sleep-wake cycle comes into phase with the 24-hour light-dark cycle. In some cases symptoms of hypersomnia are present and the child sleeps for prolonged periods (up to 24 continuous hours). This is often preceded by a surprisingly

Disorder	Clinical Presentation
Non-24-hour sleep-wake syndrome—cont'd	prolonged period of wake (24 to 40 hours). This sleep abnormality is often seen in patients who have congenital or acquired blindness. It is less commonly associated with psychiatric disorders and mental retardation. Non-24-hour sleep-wake syndrome shares some features with the sleep phase delay syndrome. Patients with sleep phase delay syndrome, however, are able to achieve a stable sleep-wake pattern during vacations from school, whereas children with non-24-hour sleep-wake pattern cannot.
Irregular sleep-wake pattern	Complaints may focus on excessive daytime sleepiness, frequent naps, long daytime sleep periods, sleeplessness at night, or a combination of symptoms. Sleep-wake cycles may resemble the ultradian pattern seen during infancy. Distribution of sleep and wake throughout the 24-hour day is haphazard, disorganized, and variable. At times no clear sleep-wake pattern can be discerned. The total sleep time over a 24-hour period, however, is usually within age group norms. The longest sleep periods and longest wake periods are temporally unpredictable. Cognitive and performance difficulties are common. Non-24-hour sleep-wake pattern occurs most commonly in children with severe developmental or congenital central nervous system dysfunction. It may also occur in otherwise normal children in the presence of severe familial dysfunction. In these cases the remainder of the child's day (including the timing of other classic zeitgebers such as meals) is also dysfunctional, disorganized, haphazard, and chaotic.

VIII. SLEEPINESS ASSOCIATED WITH THE CENTRAL NERVOUS SYSTEM (NOT OTHERWISE CLASSIFIED)

Disorder	Clinical Presentation
Narcolepsy	Excessive daytime sleepiness is the most common complaint in narcolepsy. Daytime naps are frequent, brief (usually 10 to 20 minutes), and surprisingly *refreshing*. A period of refractory alertness occurs after the daytime nap. Daytime sleepiness tends to follow an ultradian pattern. The short nap is followed by 2 to 4 hours of alertness, which in turn is followed by a period of extreme sleepiness. Sudden and irresistible "sleep attacks" occur at undesirable times (e.g., in the classroom or while talking, eating, or opening presents at a birthday party). In addition to the excessive daytime sleepiness, cataplexy is characteristic and unique to narcolepsy. Weakness, wobbling, a "draining feeling," head nodding, or frank collapse to the ground is precipitated by emotions (especially laughing, crying, or being startled). Cataplexy may be the symptom that brings the patient to the attention of the health professional. Hypnogogic hallucinations (unusual and frightening dreams or illusions that occur at sleep onset) and sleep paralysis (an inability to move or speak at sleep onset or offset) complete the tetrad of symptoms. Any combination of symptoms may be present, but almost all patients manifest excessive daytime sleepiness or exhibit constant drowsiness during waking hours. Automatic behaviors, memory lapses, sleep drunkenness, and inappropriate behaviors are auxiliary symptoms. Nocturnal sleep fragmentation and frequent nocturnal arousals and awakenings occur in most patients.
Idiopathic hypersomnia	The onset of idiopathic hypersomnia usually takes place during adolescence, but the diagnosis is often delayed for years. Patients complain of persistent and profound daytime sleepiness, as well as long periods of drowsiness. Daytime naps are common and may be

Continued on following page

VIII. SLEEPINESS ASSOCIATED WITH THE CENTRAL NERVOUS SYSTEM (NOT OTHERWISE CLASSIFIED) *Continued*

Disorder	Clinical Presentation
Idiopathic hypersomnia—cont'd	differentiated from narcoleptic naps by their length (typically 1 to 2 hours). Brief naps may also occur, but they are characteristically *unrefreshing*. Nocturnal sleep may be normal in length or prolonged. Sleep is continuous (not disrupted by frequent arousals and awakenings as in narcolepsy), and awakening in the morning is relatively easy. Confusion and disorientation (sleep drunkenness) may occur on awakening from nocturnal sleep or from naps. Sleep attacks may also occur, but cataplexy is notably absent. Associated symptoms include migrainous cephalalgia, syncope, orthostatic hypotension, and Raynaud-type phenomena. Syncope and orthostatic symptoms may be confused with cataplexy. They may be easily differentiated by the maintenance of consciousness during cataplectic attacks and the absence of tachycardia and blood pressure changes. Also, in contrast to narcolepsy, naps of patients with idiopathic hypersomnia do not contain REM sleep. Despite these differences, polysomnography and the Multiple Sleep Latency Test are often necessary to differentiate idiopathic hypersomnia from narcolepsy in some patients.
Posttraumatic hypersomnia	Typical complaints focus on excessive daytime sleepiness and frequent daytime sleep episodes. Nocturnal sleep may or may not be prolonged. A history of head trauma is obtained. The posttrauma sleep pattern and daytime sleepiness are considerably different from the patient's habitual sleep pattern before the trauma. Headaches, fatigue, decrease in attention span, inability to concentrate, and memory difficulties may be associated symptoms. Posttraumatic narcolepsy may also occur.
Recurrent hypersomnia (Kleine-Levin syndrome)	Symptoms include recurrent periods of hypersomnia and excessive daytime sleepiness separated by asymptomatic periods lasting weeks or months. The hypersomnolent phases may or may not be associated with binge eating and hypersexuality. Onset is typically during middle adolescence. Patients may sleep for prolonged periods (18 to 20 hours) during hypersomnolent periods. Episodes may last a few days to a few weeks, spontaneously resolve, and may recur 2 to 12 times per year. Social impairment during attacks is severe.
Subwakefulness syndrome	Complaints center on a subjective feeling of daytime sleepiness. Daytime naps and sleep attacks do not occur. Persistent drowsiness may result in decreased attention span, poor concentration, memory deficits, and poor performance. Clear objective evidence of a sleep disorder is absent. Polysomnography reveals sleep that is normal in quality and quantity. The Multiple Sleep Latency Test results are also normal. Twenty-four-hour monitoring may reveal waxing and waning of Stage 1 sleep intruding into the waking state.
Fragmentary myoclonus	Symptoms of fragmentary myoclonus are unusual during childhood or adolescence, although clinical correlates may exist. Fragmentary myoclonus is characterized by brief (75 to 150 msec) jerks and twitches that involve the legs, arms, and facial muscles and are asynchronous and asymmetrical. Episodes may last from less than 10 minutes to several hours. These twitches and episodes are usually benign and asymptomatic, but when periods of twitching are prolonged, sleep fragmentation may occur and daytime sleepiness may result. Fragmentary myoclonus can be differentiated from periodic limb movement disorders by the length of the twitch (0.5 to 5 seconds with periodic limb movements) and the lack of clustering and clear periodicity (which occur in fragmentary myoclonus).

DISORDER	CLINICAL PRESENTATION
Sleeping sickness	This is a rare, protozoal disease caused by *Trypanosoma brucei* and transmitted through the bite of a tsetse fly. Extreme degrees of hypersomnolence and fragmented nocturnal sleep occur in the middle to late stages of the disease. The acute phase is characterized by remitting fever, generalized lymphadenopathy, and severe cephalalgia. Edema of the hands, feet, and periorbital region is common. A circinate rash may be present. Encephalopathy results in hypersomnolence, vacant facial expression, ptosis, slow speech, confusion, disorientation, and seizures. Coma and death occur in persons with untreated disease.

IX. OTHER CAUSES OF EXCESSIVE SLEEPINESS

DISORDER	CLINICAL PRESENTATION
Menstrual-associated sleep disorder	This is a recurrent hypersomnia that is temporally related to menstruation. Onset of symptoms may occur during adolescence. Hypersomnolence and daytime sleepiness begin approximately 1 week before onset of menses. Intermenstrual intervals are generally asymptomatic, and sleep is normal during these times. Nocturnal sleep during symptomatic episodes tends to be fragmented by frequent awakenings, and sleep efficiency is reduced.
Pregnancy-associated sleep disorder	This sleep disorder can occur in pregnant women of any age. Excessive daytime sleepiness generally begins toward the end of the second trimester. Fragmentation of nocturnal sleep is often the presenting complaint. Nocturnal sleeplessness can be profound and is often related to an inability to assume a comfortable sleeping position as term approaches.
Munchausen's syndrome by proxy	This is a severe form of child abuse in which the patient's caretaker (usually the mother) produces factitious symptoms and illnesses in the child. Often multiple invasive and expensive medical tests are performed. Histories are fabricated, or actual signs are artificially produced. A majority of patients have symptoms related to central nervous system disorders (e.g., seizures, incoordination), and excessive sleepiness and other sleep-related complaints (e.g., apnea, cardiorespiratory arrest) are often present. The parent may fabricate the sleepiness or may induce it by frequent intentional wakings. There is usually a history of a long series of medical evaluations, multiple medical complaints, "doctor shopping," and unsuccessful diagnostic and treatment regimens. The child generally appears to be healthy, symptoms tend to occur only in the mother's presence, and no objective evidence of a sleep disorder or medical abnormality can be found. The mother may seem less concerned about the child's illness than is the medical professional, mother and child appear to be overly emotionally involved, and the mother seems to be quite knowledgeable about medical procedures and techniques.

SLEEP DISORDERS WITH PRESENTING SYMPTOMS OTHER THAN SLEEPLESSNESS OR SLEEPINESS

As previously noted, many sleep disorders in childhood can present symptoms of sleeplessness, sleepiness, or both. At times, however, the presenting signs and symptoms are not referable to either decreased or excessive sleep. Again, significant duplication and overlap exist. In this section, entities that are manifested most commonly as disorders of initiating or maintaining sleep or as disorders of excessive somnolence are only briefly mentioned and the differences pointed out. Sleep disorders with major presenting manifestations unrelated to sleepiness or sleeplessness are described in greater detail.

I. SLEEP DISORDERS ASSOCIATED WITH BEHAVIORAL OR PSYCHOPHYSIOLOGICAL DISORDERS

Disorder	Clinical Presentation
Nocturnal eating/drinking syndrome	This syndrome is characterized by frequent nocturnal wakings. Digestive and endocrine rhythms are affected, and the child's eating and drinking pattern remains at a more infantile level (e.g., feeding every 3 to 4 hours). The child cannot return to sleep without eating or drinking significant amounts, and the sleep-wake pattern is therefore disrupted.

II. SLEEP DISORDERS ASSOCIATED WITH PSYCHIATRIC DISORDERS

Disorder	Clinical Presentation
Panic disorders	Periods of intense fear and somatic symptoms (e.g., dizziness, dyspnea, palpitations, diaphoresis, trembling) occur unexpectedly and without apparent cause. Agoraphobia is common. Panic attacks can be associated with sudden awakening from sleep. They are differentiated from sleep terrors by their occurrence during daytime waking hours (as well as during sleep episodes), absence of heralding scream that occurs out of slow-wave sleep, and presence of agoraphobia. Nightmares are differentiated from panic disorders by their distribution, dream cognition, and clustering during early morning hours.

III. SLEEP DISORDERS ASSOCIATED WITH SLEEP-INDUCED RESPIRATORY IMPAIRMENT

Disorder	Clinical Presentation
Primary snoring	Primary snoring refers to loud, sonorous, rhonchous, upper airway (pharyngeal) breathing sounds. *Apnea, hypopnea, and hypoventilation are notably absent.* Family members or bed partners usually complain of being kept awake by the noisy breathing. At times the patient is aware of the snoring at sleep onset or after a brief awakening. Excessive sleepiness or sleeplessness are not present.
Obstructive sleep apnea syndrome/upper airway resistance syndrome	Correlates of obstructive sleep apnea syndrome may be seen during childhood without clear nocturnal waking, insomnia, or excessive daytime sleepiness. Daytime symptoms of hyperactivity, attention span problems, motor restlessness, performance problems, and behavioral abnormalities may be the presenting complaints. Sleep is fragmented and disrupted by an increase in the respiratory resistive load.
Central sleep apnea syndrome	Infants with central sleep apnea syndrome may be brought to the physician for assessment after an apparent life-threatening event. Parents

Disorder	Clinical Presentation
Central sleep apnea syndrome—cont'd	may seek medical attention because of observed respiratory pauses during sleep. If this respiratory abnormality is of long standing, systemic hypertension, pulmonary hypertension, and cardiac arrhythmias may be the presenting symptoms. In older children and young adults, cognitive difficulties, memory impairment, and depression may occur.
Congenital central hypoventilation syndrome	Congenital central hypoventilation syndrome most often is present at birth. Spontaneous breathing does not occur, resuscitation is required, and the infant cannot be weaned from mechanical ventilatory support. Congenital central hypoventilation syndrome may also occur in an otherwise normal child as an apparent life-threatening event. The infant or child may not breathe spontaneously, or respiratory efforts may be erratic and cease at sleep onset. Progressive pulmonary hypertension, cor pulmonale, and cerebral hypoxic encephalopathy can occur. Patients may require diaphragmatic pacing.
Sleep-related asthma	Diurnal symptoms of asthma may be present. Symptoms related to performance deficits during the day may persist even after adequate control of symptoms during the daytime hours.
Sleep-related neurogenic tachypnea	This is not generally described in children. Parents or caretakers may notice an increase in respiratory rate at sleep onset and the persistence of tachypnea during sleep. The respiratory rate is normal during waking hours. Excessive daytime sleepiness is the most common complaint.

IV. SLEEP DISORDERS ASSOCIATED WITH MOVEMENT DISORDERS

Disorder	Clinical Presentation
Sleep starts	Parents may be concerned about major, massive jerking movement of a leg, arm, or entire body at the time of sleep onset. Complaints of excessive daytime sleepiness or excessive somnolence are usually absent. Sleep starts are most often considered normal phenomena.
Somnambulism (sleep walking)	Symptoms of somnambulism range from simple sitting up in bed to frantic running. Most often the history reveals episodes of quiet walking around the house and the performance of complex and sometimes bizarre behavior. Enuresis is common, and the child may urinate in unusual places around the house. Sleep walking can occur at any age after the child learns to walk. Other parasomnic symptoms may have been present at an earlier age. Children may leave the house, and injury is common (especially when the sleep walking is agitated). Episodes may occur as frequently as several times per week or may be rare and take place only when precipitating factors are present (e.g., fever, sleep restriction, some medications, bladder distention). Sleep walking may also be associated with obstructive sleep apnea syndrome. Children awakened from a somnambulistic episode often appear confused, disoriented, and frightened. At times choreoathetotic movements may be seen. Somniloquy can occur during sleep walking, but the speech is often mumbled and incoherent.
Sleep terrors	Sleep terrors are characterized by a sudden, abrupt partial arousal from slow-wave sleep during the early part of the sleep period. They are heralded by a terrifying scream. Severe crying, shouting, and agitation occur. Intense autonomic discharges result in pupillary dilatation, tachycardia, tachypnea, diaphoresis, and tremors. Parental intervention in attempts to comfort the child only makes the symptoms worse. Displacement from the bed is common, and injuries may occur. Episodes are brief and resolve spontaneously. The child rapidly falls

Continued on following page

IV. SLEEP DISORDERS ASSOCIATED WITH MOVEMENT DISORDERS *Continued*

Disorder	Clinical Presentation
Sleep terrors—cont'd	back to sleep and does not recall the event. Parents observing a sleep terror also become frightened and may seek medical attention for the child. The parents may describe the episode as a bad nightmare, but usually the physician can easily differentiate sleep terrors from nightmares.
Sleep bruxism	Loud, unpleasant sounds are generated by the child forcibly grinding and clenching the teeth. The sound is unmistakeable and disturbs parents and siblings more than the patient. Since abnormal wear to the crowns of the teeth, periodontal damage, and jaw pain may occur, the dentist may be the first to identify the presence of bruxism.
Periodic limb movement disorders	These disorders are rarely described during childhood, but clinical correlates may exist. Parents may observe repetitive and stereotypical movements of one or both legs. Arms may also be involved. Clusters of movements appear, and each movement lasts 0.5 to 5 seconds. Episodes occur infrequently or may be prolonged during NREM sleep. They generally do not occur during REM sleep.
Sleep paralysis	Children, adolescents, and adults can be affected. Although sleep paralysis is one symptom of the classic tetrad of narcolepsy, it may occur in an isolated or a familial (X-linked dominant) form. Symptoms of the isolated form of this disorder typically occur at sleep offset. Although awake and alert, the patient cannot move the arms, legs, trunk, and head. There may be a sensation of an inability to breathe. Ocular and respiratory movements remain intact, however. Attacks usually last only a few minutes and end spontaneously. Episodes can occasionally be aborted by the patient rapidly moving the eyes. Familial sleep paralysis (and the sleep paralysis of narcolepsy) tends to occur at sleep onset and follows a more chronic course.
Nocturnal leg cramps	This disorder is not described during infancy. Children and young adolescents may awaken at night or complain of leg pains and cramps at the time of sleep offset. No organic disorder can be found to account for the symptoms. Rubbing or massage of the affected limb may relieve the discomfort.
REM sleep behavior disorder	Sudden partial arousal from REM sleep occurs with apparent dream enactment. Punching, swinging, leaping from the bed, running around the room, and loud vocalizations often occur. Injuries are common, especially when displacement from the bed occurs.
Nocturnal paroxysmal dystonia	Paroxysms of choreoathetoid or ballistic movements of the extremities and dystonic posturing (especially of the hands and arms) are noted during sleep. Episodes may be brief or may last for hours. No daytime symptoms are noted, and the disorder may occur in otherwise normal individuals.
Rhythmical movement disorders	Complaints of rhythmical head banging, head rolling, body rocking, or body rolling are characteristic. These movement disorders are common during infancy and childhood and tend to resolve spontaneously as the child matures. The behaviors can also occur during wakefulness but tend to cluster around times of sleep onset and persist into light stages of sleep.

V. SLEEP DISORDERS ASSOCIATED WITH PARASOMNIAS (NOT OTHERWISE CLASSIFIED)

Disorder	Clinical Presentation
Nightmares	Nightmares are anxiety dreams that occur during REM sleep, most often during the early morning hours. Although there is some autonomic discharge, it is not as intense as that seen during a sleep terror. The child typically responds well to parental comforting and often reports the storylike imagery associated with the nightmare.
Somniloquy (sleep talking)	Somniloquy is generally benign and is characterized by clear speech, vocalizations, moans, or other utterances. Episodes may occur spontaneously or may be precipitated by talking to the sleeper. Sleep talking may be annoying to other family members and is often associated with other parasomnias.
Sleep enuresis	Sleep enuresis is bed wetting after the age of 5 years. Primary sleep-related enuresis consists of continuous bed wetting without a period of at least 3 consecutive months of dry nights. It may occur nightly or be intermittent. Arousal generally does not occur, and the child is unaware of the episode. Urological, medical, and psychiatric findings are normal. Secondary enuresis is present when bed wetting recurs after 3 consecutive months of dry nights. Significant embarrassment occurs, and enuretic children often have poor self-esteem.
Sleep-related painful erections	These generally are not described in prepubertal children (although they do manifest REM-related penile tumescence). Adolescent and adult males may complain of painful erections during sleep. Daytime genitourinary functioning is normal, and erections during wakefulness are not painful. There is no associated sexual dysfunction.

VI. SLEEP DISORDERS ASSOCIATED WITH THE CENTRAL NERVOUS SYSTEM (NOT OTHERWISE CLASSIFIED)

Disorder	Clinical Presentation
Sleep-related epilepsy	In this disorder a sudden, paroxysmal discharge of seizure activity occurs during sleep. Sleep is an important factor facilitating seizure activity. Sleep-related seizures may or may not be associated with motor manifestations (focal movements, generalized tonic-clonic movements, automatisms) or autonomic manifestations (including tachycardia, diaphoresis, enuresis, and respiratory difficulties). Occasionally, sleep-related epilepsy is the cause of an apparent life-threatening event.
Electrical status epilepticus of sleep	Continuous spike and slow-wave activity occurs during NREM sleep. Underlying epilepsy is usually present and discovered well before the sleep related electrical status epilepticus is diagnosed. Epilepsies are typically generalized or partial tonic-clonic, with absence seizures. Similar motor manifestations during sleep are rare, despite the severe abnormality of cerebral electrical activity. The disorder is rare but is most often seen in childhood in the setting of mild to moderate mental retardation or known CNS congenital abnormalities. The onset is typically between 4 and 14 years of age.
Fragmentary myoclonus	Parents may notice twitching and jerking of the arms, legs, or facial muscles. The movements are brief and not clustered. They are typically benign and are infrequently associated with diurnal symptoms.

VII. OTHER SLEEP DISORDERS WHICH MAY NOT INCLUDE SLEEPINESS OR SLEEPLESSNESS

Disorder	Clinical Presentation
Other	Sleep-related gastroesophageal reflux, sleep-related sinus arrest, sleep-related abnormal swallowing syndrome, sleep-related laryngospasm, sleep choking syndrome, and terrifying hypnogogic hallucinations may also present symptoms unrelated to sleepiness or sleeplessness. Most have not been reported during childhood (although clinical correlates might exist) or are extremely rare in children. The reader is referred to these topics elsewhere in the text for full descriptions.

APPENDIX 4

Differential Diagnosis Based on Polysomnographic Variables*

The following are general descriptions of polysomnographic characteristics identified in each diagnostic category. Significant overlap exists. For each diagnosis, polysomnographic data may vary. Definitive diagnosis requires evaluation of both polysomnographic information and clinical manifestations.

DISORDERS OF INITIATING AND MAINTAINING SLEEP

Diagnosis	Polysomnographic Characteristics
Adjustment sleep disorder	*Latencies:* Sleep onset latency is prolonged. REM latency is normal. *Architecture:* The number and duration of wakings after sleep onset are increased. Sleep efficiency is reduced. Premature waking occurs. Total sleep time may be slightly prolonged. Stage volumes are relatively normal. *EMG:* Normal. *EEG:* Normal. *Respiration:* Normal. *Comments:* An MSLT may demonstrate a reduced mean sleep onset latency.
Psychophysiological insomnia	*Latencies:* Sleep onset latency is increased. REM latency is normal. *Architecture:* Waking after sleep onset is increased, and sleep efficiency is decreased. Stage 1 volume is increased, and slow-wave sleep is decreased.

Continued on following page

*Modified from Diagnostic Classification Steering Committee, Thorpy M (Chairman): International classification of sleep disorders: diagnostic and coding manual. Rochester, Minn: American Sleep Disorders Association, 1990, pp 331-336, with permission.

DISORDERS OF INITIATING AND MAINTAINING SLEEP *Continued*

Diagnosis	Polysomnographic Characteristics
Psychophysiological insomnia—cont'd	*EMG:* Increased muscle tone may be noted. *EEG:* Normal. Alpha intrusions into NREM sleep may occur. *Respiration:* Normal. *Comments:* A reversed first night effect may be seen; that is, patients often sleep better in the laboratory than at home.
Inadequate sleep hygiene	*Latencies:* Sleep onset latency is variable: it may be prolonged or shortened. REM latency is normal. *Architecture:* All stages of sleep are present. The progression of stages across the sleep period is normal. Architecture is fragmented by frequent arousals, and sleep efficiency is decreased. There may be early morning spontaneous waking. *EMG:* Normal. *EEG:* Normal. *Respiration:* Normal. *Comments:* The MSLT may show a decreased mean sleep onset latency. Patients may sleep better in the laboratory when principles of sleep hygiene are enforced. A sleep log or wrist actigraphy may be helpful in diagnosis.
Limit-setting sleep disorder	*Latencies:* Sleep onset latency is normal if limits are set in the laboratory. REM latency is normal. *Architecture:* All sleep stages are seen, and stage volumes are normal. The progression of stages across the sleep period is normal. *EMG:* Normal. *EEG:* Normal. *Respiration:* Normal. *Comments:* Quantity and quality of sleep are normal when limits are enforced. A sleep log may be helpful in diagnosis.
Sleep onset association disorder	*Latencies:* Sleep onset latency is increased if sleep onset associations are absent. It is within normal limits when associations are present. REM latency is normal. *Architecture:* If sleep onset associations are absent, the number and length of wakings after sleep onset are increased. Stage volumes and progression are normal. *EMG:* Normal. *EEG:*Normal. *Respiration:* Normal. *Comments:* Sleep is quantitatively and qualitatively normal if the sleep onset associations are present. Abnormalities appear only when the associations are absent.
Excessive nocturnal fluids	*Latencies:* Sleep onset latency is normal. REM latency is normal. *Architecture:* All sleep stages are present and normal in volume, and there is a normal progression across the sleep period. Architecture is disrupted and fragmented by frequent awakenings. *EMG:* Normal. *EEG:* Normal. *Respiration:* Normal. *Comments:* The sleep period is normal except for frequent nocturnal wakings to eat or drink.
Psychoses	*Latencies:* Sleep onset latency is prolonged. REM latency is normal or decreased. *Architecture:* Abnormalities depend on the type and severity of the psychosis. Total sleep time may be decreased. Architecture is fragmented, and there is an increase in waking after sleep onset. Slow-wave sleep volume is decreased. Time spent in REM sleep may be increased, normal, or decreased. REM density is increased.

DIAGNOSIS	POLYSOMNOGRAPHIC CHARACTERISTICS
Psychoses—cont'd	*EMG:* Normal. *EEG:* Normal. However, there may be increased activity in the beta frequency (especially over the frontal regions). *Respiration:* Normal. *Comments:* A reversed first night effect may occur. Patients may sleep better in the laboratory on the first night than the characteristic sleep at home.
Mood disorders	*Latencies:* Sleep onset latency is prolonged. REM latency is significantly decreased (less than 50% of normal). *Architecture:* REM volume is increased, and slow-wave sleep volume is decreased. Architecture is fragmented, and the number of wakings after sleep onset is increased. Sleep efficiency is decreased. After a long, intense first REM period, REM episodes tend to decrease in length and intensity across the sleep period. Slow-wave sleep episodes tend to cluster later in the sleep period. *EMG:* Normal. *EEG:* Normal. *Respiration:* Normal. *Comments:* MSLT findings may be normal, or a decrease in the mean sleep onset latency may occur.
Anxiety disorders	*Latencies:* Sleep onset latency is prolonged. REM latency is relatively normal. *Architecture:* Slow-wave sleep volume is decreased, and volumes of Stages 1 and 2 are increased. Increase in the frequency and duration of nocturnal waking is seen, and there is a mild decrease in sleep efficiency. *EMG:* Normal. *EEG:* Normal. *Respiration:* Normal. *Comments:* The MSLT reveals a normal or increased mean sleep onset latency.
Panic disorders	*Latencies:* Sleep onset latency is prolonged. REM latency is relatively normal. *Architecture:* Stage volumes and progression are normal. Abrupt awakenings out of Stage 2 or Stage 3 NREM sleep result in a decrease in sleep efficiency. Occasionally the awakenings are noted at sleep onset. Movement time is increased. *EMG:* Normal. *EEG:* Normal. *Respiration:* Normal (although the respiratory rate may increase during the period of panic). *Comments:* The MSLT reveals a normal sleep onset latency.
Alcoholism	*Latencies:* Sleep onset latency is significantly decreased. REM latency is significantly prolonged. *Architecture:* Total sleep time is decreased. Sleep is highly fragmented. Slow-wave sleep is increased during the first half of the night. REM sleep, arousals, and wakes are increased during the second half of the night. A significant decrease in slow-wave sleep is noted during short-term abstinence. *EMG:* Normal. *EEG:* Normal. However, alpha intrusions and an alpha-delta pattern can be seen. *Respiration:* Normal. However, obstructive and central apneas may be exacerbated by alcohol consumption. *Comments:* The MSLT consistently shows excessive sleepiness with a mean sleep onset latency of less than 10 minutes.

Continued on following page

DISORDERS OF INITIATING AND MAINTAINING SLEEP *Continued*

Diagnosis	Polysomnographic Characteristics
Environmental sleep disorder	*Latencies:* Sleep onset latency may be normal or shortened in the laboratory, compared with the increased latency at home. REM latency is normal. *Architecture:* All stages of sleep are seen, and the progression of stages across the sleep period is normal. Total sleep time in the laboratory tends to be longer than at home. Sleep efficiency is normal. *EMG:* Normal. *EEG:* Normal. *Respiration:* Normal. *Comments:* The MSLT frequently reveals a mean sleep onset latency of less than 10 minutes.
Food allergy insomnia	*Latencies:* Sleep onset latency is normal. REM latency is normal. *Architecture:* All stages are seen, and the progression is normal. The frequent arousals and awakenings, which occur in any sleep stage, result in decreased sleep efficiency. *EMG:* Normal. *EEG:* Normal. *Respiration:* Normal. If the patient has associated allergic respiratory symptoms, respiratory changes (e.g., increased respiratory resistive load, coughing, wheezing) may be noted. *Comments:* The MSLT may reveal a shortened sleep onset latency.
Toxin-induced sleep disorder	*Latencies:* Little information about polysomnographic variables is available. Sleep onset latency is usually variable (i.e., may be prolonged, normal, or shortened). REM latency may also be variable and dependent on the presence of an encephalopathic process. *Architecture:* There may be decreased sleep efficiency, frequent arousals and awakenings, and an early morning wake time. *EMG:* Normal? *EEG:* May be normal or may reveal encephalopathic changes (e.g., diffuse slowing, paroxysmal epileptiform discharges). *Respiration:* May be normal. *Comments:* The MSLT may show a short mean sleep onset latency.
Hypnotic-dependent sleep disorder	*Latencies:* Sleep onset latency may be normal while the patient is receiving medication but prolonged when the hypnotic is not taken. REM latency is prolonged. *Architecture:* There are decreases in Stages 1, 3, and 4 NREM sleep. REM sleep is also decreased in volume. The percentage of Stage 2 is increased. There are frequent stage changes and architectural fragmentation of NREM and REM sleep. *EMG:* Normal. *EEG:* Decreases in the number of K-complexes and delta wave activity are noted. Pseudospindles with a frequency of 14 to 18 Hz are present, and alpha and beta activity is increased. *Respiration:* Normal. *Comments:* The number and quality of REM sleep eye movements are significantly decreased.
Stimulant-dependent sleep disorder	*Latencies:* Sleep onset latency is increased, and REM latency is prolonged. On withdrawal from the stimulant medication, a significant decrease in the sleep onset latency and a decrease in REM latency are noted. *Architecture:* Total sleep time is decreased, and time awake after sleep onset is increased. REM volume is decreased. Withdrawal from the medication increases total sleep time, and a significant REM rebound occurs (REM latency is decreased and REM volume is increased).

Diagnosis	Polysomnographic Characteristics
Stimulant-dependent sleep disorder—cont'd	*EMG:* Normal. *EEG:* Normal. *Respiration:* Normal. *Comments:* After withdrawal of the stimulant medication, the MSLT may be suggestive of narcolepsy. A significantly reduced mean sleep onset latency (often less than 7 minutes) may be seen.
Alcohol-dependent sleep disorder	*Latencies:* Sleep onset latency is increased. REM latency is increased. *Architecture:* Slow-wave sleep is increased. Arousals and wakings occur frequently, and stage transitions are common during the second half of the sleep period. REM activity is increased, but REM sleep becomes fragmented. *EMG:* Normal. *EEG:* Normal. *Respiration:* Normal, but obstructive and central apneas may become exacerbated. *Comments:* The MSLT has variable findings and may show an increased or decreased mean sleep onset latency.
Obstructive sleep apnea syndrome	*Latencies:* Sleep onset latency is increased if apneas occur at the time of sleep onset. REM latency may be prolonged, or REM sleep may be absent. *Architecture:* Arousals or state changes at each apneic event usually occurs. Slow-wave sleep and REM sleep may be decreased or absent. Stage 1 and 2 sleep volume is increased. *EMG:* Snore artifact is often noted on chin muscle EMG. *EEG:* Normal. *Respiration:* Obstructive apneas lasting longer than 10 seconds occur frequently (more than five apneas per hour of sleep). Oxygen desaturation, arousal to a light sleep stage, and frequent awakening are associated findings. ECG changes are commonly associated with the respiratory events. *Comments:* Bradyarrhythmias and tachyarrhythmias are commonly associated with apneic events. The MSLT often reveals a mean sleep onset latency of less than 10 minutes. Sleep onset REM periods may be present if there is significant sleep deprivation and may be confused with narcolepsy. An all-night polysomnogram *before* the MSLT is mandatory for a correct diagnosis.
Central sleep apnea syndrome	*Latencies:* Sleep onset latency is variable. It may be prolonged if the apneas occur at sleep onset, or it may be short if there has been significant sleep disruption. REM latency may be normal or variable. *Architecture:* Architectural disruptions and fragmentation may be significant. Frequent arousals and stage changes after an apneic event are common. *EMG:* Normal. *EEG:* Normal. *Respiration:* Frequent central apneas lasting more than 10 seconds (20 seconds in infancy) occur. They may be brief or prolonged to 30 seconds or longer. Often rebound hyperventilation follows the central apneic event. Oxygen desaturation is variable but is usually less significant than the desaturation occurring with obstructive events. *Comments:* Excessive sleepiness is often noted on the MSLT. Mean sleep onset latency may be less than 10 minutes but is usually not as profoundly decreased as in obstructive sleep apnea syndrome. Bradyarrhythmias and tachyarrhythmias may be noted on the ECG.
Central alveolar hypoventilation syndrome	*Latencies:* Sleep onset latency is prolonged if decreased ventilatory effort results in arousal at sleep onset. The sleep onset latency is often short because of architectural disruption. *Architecture:* An increase in the frequency of body movements and frequent awakenings fragment and disrupt architecture.

Continued on following page

DISORDERS OF INITIATING AND MAINTAINING SLEEP *Continued*

DIAGNOSIS	POLYSOMNOGRAPHIC CHARACTERISTICS
Central alveolar hypoventilation syndrome—cont'd	*EMG:* Normal. *EEG:* Normal. *Respiration:* Episodes of decreased tidal volume occur and last for several minutes. There is significant decrease in oxygen saturation, which is lowest during REM sleep. Obstructive sleep apneas may be present. There is often an associated increase in arterial carbon dioxide concentration. *Comments:* The MSLT often reveals excessive sleepiness with mean sleep onset latencies of less than 10 minutes.
Chronic obstructive pulmonary disease	*Latencies:* Sleep onset latency is prolonged. REM latency is variable. *Architecture:* Architecture is disrupted by frequent arousals, stage changes, and awakenings. Total sleep time, slow-wave sleep, and REM volume are decreased. *EMG:* Normal. *EEG:* Normal. *Respiration:* Because shortness of breath may occur when the patient is recumbent, it may be necessary to conduct the polysomnography with the patient in the sitting position. Coughing and expectoration of pooled secretions occur frequently. Oxygen desaturation that is independent of apneas or hypopneas is noted. *Comments:* Cardiac arrhythmias may occur independent of obstructive or central respiratory events. The MSLT frequently reveals a decrease in the mean sleep onset latency characteristic of excessive daytime sleepiness.
Sleep-related asthma	*Latencies:* Sleep onset latency is variable. It may be prolonged if respiratory difficulties prevent sleep onset or shortened if the architecture is significantly disrupted. REM latency is relatively normal. *Architecture:* All stages of sleep are present in relatively normal volumes. Stages occur in a normal progression across the sleep period. Waking after sleep onset is increased. These awakenings may be prolonged during a sleep-related asthma attack. *EMG:* Normal; may be increased during a period of bronchospasm. *EEG:* Normal. *Respiration:* Bronchoconstriction and wheezing occur, most often during Stage 2 NREM sleep. They typically do not occur during slow-wave sleep or early in the sleep period. *Comments:* The MSLT may show evidence of excessive daytime sleepiness. Daytime symptoms of asthma are often present.
Altitude insomnia	*Latencies:* Sleep onset latency is prolonged. REM latency is normal. *Architecture:* There is a significant decrease in sleep efficiency and a decrease in total sleep time. Body movements are increased. REM volume is typically decreased. *EMG:* Normal. *EEG:* Normal. *Respiration:* Periodic breathing occurs. Central apneas appear. Often an alternation between hypopnea and hyperpnea is associated with periodic fluctuations in hemoglobin oxygen saturation. *Comments:* Arterial oxygen and carbon dioxide tensions are decreased. Variable degrees of compensated respiratory alkalosis can be identified.
Sleep starts	*Latencies:* Sleep onset latency may be prolonged following a hypnic myoclonic jerk. REM latency is normal. *Architecture:* Stage volumes are normal. Sleep starts may be identified at sleep onset and early in Stage 1 sleep. The myoclonic jerk may prolong sleep onset. There is typically no other disruption or fragmentation of sleep architecture.

DIAGNOSIS	POLYSOMNOGRAPHIC CHARACTERISTICS
Sleep starts—cont'd	*EMG:* Brief high-amplitude potentials are noted at sleep onset. These may be single or successive. *EEG:* Normal. High-voltage, negative vertex sharp waves may be seen at the time of the myoclonic jerk. *Respiration:* Normal. *Comments:* A brief period of tachycardia may be present after the myoclonic jerk.
Restless leg syndrome	*Latencies:* Sleep onset latency is prolonged. REM latency is normal. *Architecture:* Stage volumes are typically normal. The progression of stages across the sleep period is normal. Periods of awakening during the night may be prolonged because of frequent, sometimes continuous, leg movements (of which the patient seems to be partially aware) during the waking state, and sleep efficiency may be decreased. The leg movements may be quite complex. *EMG:* Sustained tonic EMG may be identified in the anterior tibialis tracing of the EMG. The sustained tone and muscle movements may alternate from one leg to the other before sleep onset. *EEG:* No paroxysmal, focal, or epileptiform activity is present during the movements. *Respiration:* Normal. *Comments:* The anterior tibialis muscle sustained tone may persist into Stage 1 sleep.
Periodic limb movement disorder	*Latencies:* Sleep onset latency is normal or shortened. REM latency is normal. *Architecture:* Progression of stages is typically normal, but significant fragmentation and disruption of the architecture result from arousals and awakenings secondary to leg movements. *EMG:* Episodes of repetitive contractions lasting 0.5 to 5 seconds (mean 1.5 to 2.5 seconds) are seen in one or both legs. The typical interval between movements is 20 to 40 seconds. Movements with intervals of less than 5 seconds or greater than 90 seconds are not counted in the episode. *EEG:* Normal. K-complexes often occur in association with the leg movements. *Respiration:* Normal. *Comments:* Periodic movements are notably absent during REM sleep. They begin in Stage 1, become maximum in Stage 2, and tend to decrease in slow-wave sleep. A mild increase in heart rate and blood pressure is seen. This movement disorder may also affect the musculature of the arms.
Nocturnal leg cramps	*Latencies:* Sleep onset latency and REM latency are typically normal. *Architecture:* Stage volumes and progression of stages across the sleep period are usually normal. Awakenings occur and may be prolonged. Early morning waking may also be noted. Sleep efficiency may be decreased. *EMG:* EMG activity is increased in the affected leg. The increase in muscle activity with nocturnal leg cramps may be sustained and does not reveal any periodicity. *EEG:* Normal. *Respiration:* Normal. *Comments:* Painful sensations may be alleviated by rubbing or massage.
Rhythmical movement disorders	*Latencies:* Sleep onset latency is normal to prolonged. REM latency is normal. *Architecture:* Stage volumes and progression of stages tend to be normal. Rhythmical movements of the body or head are noted during wakefulness (immediately before sleep onset), may persist into light NREM Stage 1 sleep, or may be noted during slow-wave sleep.

Continued on following page

DISORDERS OF INITIATING AND MAINTAINING SLEEP *Continued*

Diagnosis	Polysomnographic Characteristics
Rhythmical movement disorders—cont'd	*EMG:* Increase in EMG activity is noted during movements. Otherwise, the EMG shows no abnormalities. *EEG:* Normal. No focal, paroxysmal, or epileptiform activity is noted. *Respiration:* Normal. *Comments:* Similar rhythmical behaviors may be noted during normal waking hours.
REM sleep behavior disorder	*Latencies:* Sleep onset latency is normal. REM latency is normal. *Architecture:* Stage volumes and progression tend to be normal. An abrupt arousal out of REM sleep occurs. REM eye movement density is increased. *EMG:* Chin muscle potential is increased. There is a *paradoxical* increase in chin muscle tone during REM sleep. Excessive phasic twitching is also present. *EEG:* Normal. No focal, paroxysmal, or epileptiform activity is noted. *Respiration:* Normal. *Comments:* Excessive body jerking and limb movement take place throughout sleep. Complex violent behaviors often result in displacement from the bed and injury to self and sometimes to others.
Nocturnal paroxysmal dystonia	*Latencies:* Sleep onset latency is normal or prolonged. REM latency is normal. *Architecture:* All stages of sleep are seen, and the progression of stages across the sleep period is usually normal. Arousal, movement, and dystonic posturing are noted during an event. Episodes typically occur in Stage 2 but may also occur in slow-wave sleep. *EMG:* Chin muscle tone is increased during the event. *EEG:* Arousal rhythm often precedes the event by a few seconds. Questionable epileptiform activity has been occasionally noted in some patients. *Respiration:* Normal. *Comments:* MSLT findings are usually normal.
Short sleeper	*Latencies:* Sleep onset latency is often shortened. REM latency is normal. *Architecture:* Arousals from sleep are much less frequent than in normal sleepers. Stage 2 NREM sleep is decreased. Absolute volume of slow-wave sleep is normal for the patient's age. *EMG:* Normal. *EEG:* Normal. *Respiration:* Normal. *Comments:* A patient with a history of a chronically short sleep period who reveals an increase in slow-wave sleep is most likely rebounding from sleep deprivation and cannot be classified as a short sleeper (even in the absence of daytime symptoms). Short sleepers have a normal MSLT mean sleep onset latency. A patient with chronic sleep deprivation shows a shortened sleep onset latency on the MSLT.
Time zone change/jet lag syndrome	*Latencies:* Sleep onset latency is variable but is often increased if the polysomnography is done in the new time zone (and at the socially acceptable time of sleep) within a day or two of travel. REM latency is generally normal. *Architecture:* An increase in Stage 1 volume and a variable decrease in slow-wave sleep occur. An increase in the number of arousals is noted. Sleep efficiency is decreased. *EMG:* Normal. *EEG:* Normal. *Respiration:* Normal.

Diagnosis	Polysomnographic Characteristics
Time zone change/jet lag syndrome—cont'd	*Comments:* This disorder occurs mainly when two or more time zones are traversed. The sleep-wake rhythm is disordered for the first few days after east-to-west travel. This may persist for longer periods after west-to-east travel. The MSLT during the day in the new time zone reveals excessive daytime sleepiness. Sleep studies done during the patient's normal inherent sleep period produce normal findings.
Shift work sleep disorder	*Latencies:* Little is known about the effect of parents' shift work on children. If there is no sleep-wake schedule disruption, sleep onset latency and REM latency are normal. Parents experience an increase in sleep onset latency, and their REM latency is normal or variable. *Architecture:* Parents' total sleep time is reduced. Their sleep is fragmented and there is an increase in the number of arousals and waking after sleep onset. *EMG:* Normal. *EEG:* Normal. *Respiration:* Normal. *Comments:* Sleep disruption from parents' shift work is variable, and little is known of this disorder. There may be a loss of chronobiological rhythmicity. This disorder is usually diagnosed on the basis of the history, and sleep studies are generally not necessary. Polysomnography, if performed, should be conducted during the shifted sleep period. The MSLT should be conducted during the shifted wake period.
Delayed sleep phase syndrome	*Latencies:* Sleep onset latency is increased. A mild to moderate decrease in REM latency can be seen. *Architecture:* Stage volumes are usually normal, and there is a normal progression of stages across the sleep period. Sleep efficiency is lower than normal for the patient's age. Arousals and awakenings are infrequent (less than those seen in normal control subjects of the same age). *EMG:* Normal. *EEG:* Normal. *Respiration:* Normal. *Comments:* The patient has difficulty wakening at a socially desired time in the morning. The MSLT may reveal a decreased sleep onset latency during morning naps and a normal latency during afternoon naps. A sleep log or wrist actigraphy may be necessary for diagnosis.
Advanced sleep phase syndrome	*Latencies:* On the first night of study the sleep onset and REM latencies are normal. On the second night of study the sleep onset latency may be decreased. *Architecture:* Stage volumes and progression are normal for the patient's age. An early morning spontaneous wake-up time is usually noted. *EMG:* Normal. *EEG:* Normal. *Respiration:* Normal. *Comments:* Two consecutive nights of polysomnography separated by an MSLT should be performed. The first night's polysomnography should be performed during the patient's habitual sleep period. The second night is performed during the desired sleep period. The intervening MSLT usually shows no abnormalities.
Non-24-hour sleep-wake syndrome	*Latencies:* There is a progressive 1- to 2-hour prolongation of the sleep onset latency on successive days. The REM latency may be concomitantly delayed. *Architecture:* There is a progressive decrease in the total sleep time on successive days. Otherwise, the architecture is relatively normal. *EMG:* Normal. *EEG:* Brain-damaged or mentally retarded patients may have significantly lower than normal spindle activity and number of K-complexes.

Continued on following page

DISORDERS OF INITIATING AND MAINTAINING SLEEP *Continued*

DIAGNOSIS	POLYSOMNOGRAPHIC CHARACTERISTICS
Non-24-hour sleep-wake syndrome—cont'd	*Respiration:* Normal. *Comments:* Little polysomnographic information is available. Twenty-four-hour temperature monitoring reveals a progressive delay in the nadir by 1 to 2 hours on successive days. Wrist actigraphy may be helpful in diagnosis.
Irregular sleep-wake pattern	*Latencies:* Sleep onset latency and REM latency are variable. *Architecture:* Architecture may be disrupted by frequent, prolonged wakings. Architectural changes are variable. The volume of slow-wave sleep may be decreased. *EMG:* Normal. *EEG:* The number of spindles and K-complexes is often decreased. *Respiration:* Normal. *Comments:* Few data are available. There is a loss of the normal sleep-wake pattern on 24-hour monitoring. Wrist actigraphy for several days or maintenance of a sleep log can often assist in the diagnosis.
Confusional arousals	*Latencies:* Sleep onset latency is normal. REM latency is normal. *Architecture:* Stage volumes are normal for age, and there is a normal progression of stages across the sleep period. An abrupt arousal from slow-wave sleep during the first third of the sleep period may be noted. *EMG:* Activity of the chin muscle (as well as other monitored muscles) increases during arousal. *EEG:* Delta and Stage 1 theta activity is present during the arousal. Often, poorly reactive alpha waves and repeated microsleep periods are seen. *Respiration:* Normal. The respiratory rate may be increased during the arousal. *Comments:* Confusional arousals are rare during naps or other NREM stages.
Sleep terrors	*Latencies:* Sleep onset latency is normal. REM latency is normal. *Architecture:* Stage volumes are normal, and there is a normal progression of stages across the sleep period. A sudden, abrupt partial arousal from slow-wave sleep occurs during the first third of the sleep period. Partial arousals without major motor manifestations are commonly present. *EMG:* Chin muscle tone is increased during the arousal. *EEG:* Normal. The EEG tracing is often obscured by muscle artifact during the arousal. No focal, paroxysmal, or epileptiform activity is present. *Respiration:* Tachypnea is often present during the arousal. *Comments:* The sleep terror is heralded by a sudden piercing scream. Intense autonomic discharge is present during the partial arousal. Tachycardia is typically present.
Nightmares	*Latencies:* Sleep onset latency is normal. REM latency is normal. *Architecture:* Stage volumes and progression are normal. The patient abruptly awakens from REM sleep and remains awake longer than 10 minutes. REM density tends to be increased. *EMG:* Normal. *EEG:* Normal. *Respiration:* Normal. *Comments:* A variable increase in heart rate and respiratory rate takes place. Although some autonomic discharge occurs, it is significantly less intense than that seen in sleep terrors. Patients often report a vivid, frightening dream.

Diagnosis	Polysomnographic Characteristics
Sleep hyperhidrosis	*Latencies:* Sleep onset and REM latencies are normal. *Architecture:* Architecture is most likely normal, although wakings caused by discomfort may be noted. *EMG:* Most likely normal. *EEG:* Most likely normal. *Respiration:* Most likely normal. *Comments:* Significant polysomnographic data have not been reported. The preceding characteristics are speculative.
Sleep-related epilepsy	*Latencies:* Sleep onset latency and REM latency may be variable. *Architecture:* Architecture may be normal or variably disrupted by seizure activity. *EMG:* Potentials are normal to increased during ictal events. *EEG:* Characteristics vary depending on the underlying process. NREM sleep is an important activator of seizure activity. Interictal sleep EEG in generalized epilepsies often reveals bilateral synchronous spikes and slow waves, multiple spike and slow-wave complexes, or focal unilateral spikes. Partial epilepsies may exhibit spikes and sharp transients in a localized distribution. Benign focal epilepsy of childhood (Rolandic epilepsy) may reveal high-amplitude negative sharp waves that have a centrotemporal distribution or may be multifocal. A stereotypical morphology of these sharp waves may be noted. *Respiration:* Normal to variable during seizure activity (especially if there are motor components). *Comments:* EEG abnormalities can occur in any stage of sleep. A full-montage EEG is recommended when evaluating patients for sleep-related seizures. Videopolysomnography is essential to correlate motor activity with EEG abnormalities.
Fatal familial insomnia	*Latencies:* Sleep onset latency is prolonged. REM latency may be normal initially but is often variable. *Architecture:* As the disorder advances, sleep architecture becomes progressively destroyed. There is a significant decrease in or complete absence of slow-wave sleep. Stage 1 sleep alternates with EEG desynchronization. REM bursts occur, and periods of skeletal muscle atonia intrude. *EMG:* A variable decrease in muscle tone accompanies the REM intrusions. Irregular myoclonic movements and tremors may be seen. *EEG:* In the late stages the EEG becomes unreactive and progressively flattens until death ensues. *Respiration:* Quite variable. *Comments:* The disorder has not been described in childhood. It appears uniformly progressive and fatal in adults.
Cerebral degenerative disorders	*Latencies:* Sleep onset latency is prolonged. REM latency is variable. *Architecture:* Significant decreases in slow-wave sleep and REM sleep are noted. Architectural fragmentation is common, and the number of arousals and awakenings is increased. *EMG:* Tonic and phasic limb contractions are noted. Chin muscle tone may be increased during REM sleep. *EEG:* EEG changes often depend on the type of cerebral degenerative disorder encountered. There may be generalized low amplitude of the waveforms, poor spindle formation, and seizure activity. *Respiration:* Respiratory irregularities are common. Obstructive and central apneas and hypopneas may be present. *Comments:* REM volume is often decreased, and REM sleep eye movements may be of poor quality. The polysomnographic presentation depends on the underlying disease or disorder.

Continued on following page

DISORDERS OF INITIATING AND MAINTAINING SLEEP *Continued*

Diagnosis	Polysomnographic Characteristics
Sleep state misperception	*Latencies:* Sleep onset latency is normal. REM latency is normal. *Architecture:* All stages of sleep are seen. There is a normal progression of stages across the sleep period. All stage volumes are within normal limits. *EMG:* Normal. *EEG:* Normal. No focal, paroxysmal, or epileptiform activity is noted. *Respiration:* Normal. *Comments:* Patients often report that they did not sleep or did not sleep well in the laboratory, despite objective evidence of normal sleep.
Sleep choking syndrome	*Latencies:* Sleep onset latency and REM latency are normal. *Architecture:* Sleep architecture is normal. Stage volumes and progression are normal. *EMG:* Normal. *EEG:* No abnormalities are noted. *Respiration:* Characteristically normal. No obstructive, central, or mixed apneas or hypopneas are noted. Oxygen saturation remains within normal limits. *Comments:* Sleep choking episodes generally do not occur in the laboratory. Polysomnography is performed to rule out other cardiorespiratory causes for the patient's symptoms.
Munchausen's syndrome by proxy	*Latencies:* Sleep onset latency is normal. REM latency is normal. *Architecture:* Sleep architecture is normal. Stage volumes and progression across the sleep period are within normal limits for the patient's age. *EMG:* Normal. *EEG:* Normal. *Respiration:* Normal. *Comments:* Polysomnographic characteristics of Munchausen's syndrome by proxy have only been described anecdotally in the literature. Since the complaints are factitious, all objective polysomnographic variables are usually normal. Objective signs may occur if the parents intentionally wake the child and deprive him or her of sleep. In this case the MSLT may show abnormalities and all-night polysomnography may reveal objective evidence of rebound from sleep deprivation. Munchausen's syndrome by proxy is a very severe form of child abuse. Although the complaints often center on sleepiness, sleeplessness, or cardiorespiratory problems during sleep, no abnormalities that explain the symptoms can be found on polysomnography. Videopolysomnography is helpful.
Idiopathic insomnia	*Latencies:* Sleep onset latency is prolonged. REM latency is shortened. *Architecture:* Sleep efficiency is decreased. The number and duration of awakenings after sleep onset are increased. Long REM periods that are devoid of eye movements may be noted. *EMG:* Normal. *EEG:* Poorly formed spindles may be seen. *Respiration:* Normal. *Comments:* The number of body movements noted is decreased. A reversed first night effect may be present (i.e., the patients sleep better on the first night in the laboratory than on subsequent nights).
Sleep-related gastroesophageal reflux	*Latencies:* Sleep onset latency is normal or prolonged. REM latency is normal. *Architecture:* Stage volumes and progression are normal. Architecture is disrupted by an increased number of arousals and awakenings. *EMG:* Normal. *EEG:* Normal.

Diagnosis	Polysomnographic Characteristics
Sleep-related gastroesophageal reflux—cont'd	*Respiration:* Normal. However, central or obstructive apneas may occur if there is reflux into the pharynx. Respiration may become labored if gastric contents are aspirated. *Comments:* Concurrent esophageal monitoring of pH shows a decrease in pH during periods of reflux.
Pain syndromes	*Latencies:* Sleep onset latency is prolonged. REM latency is generally normal. *Architecture:* All stages of sleep are present unless awakenings disrupt the continuity of sleep. The progression of stages across the sleep period is generally normal. *EMG:* Periodic limb movements may be noted. Chin muscle EMG shows no abnormalities. *EEG:* Alpha intrusions into NREM sleep and an alpha-delta sleep pattern may be noted. *Respiration:* Normal. *Comments:* Mean sleep onset latency on the MSLT may be significantly decreased.
Menstrual-associated sleep disorder	*Latencies:* During symptomatic phases, sleep onset latency is prolonged. REM latency may be normal. *Architecture:* Stage volumes tend to be within normal limits, but there are frequent stage transitions and an abnormal progression of stages across the sleep period. Prolonged awakenings occur, and sleep efficiency is decreased. Intermenstrual architecture is normal. *EMG:* Normal. *EEG:* Normal. *Respiration:* Normal. *Comments:* Findings of intermenstrual sleep studies are within normal limits.
Pregnancy-associated sleep disorder	*Latencies:* Sleep onset latency is prolonged during the second and third trimesters. REM latency is normal. *Architecture:* Total sleep time is increased during the first trimester. Awakenings after sleep onset increase dramatically during the second and third trimesters. Slow-wave sleep declines as term approaches. *EMG:* Normal. *EEG:* Normal. *Respiration:* Normal. *Comments:* The MSLT typically reveals a mean sleep onset latency of less than 10 minutes. After delivery of the infant, REM volume decreases. It then returns to normal levels over a 2-week period. Slow-wave sleep volume also returns to normal levels after delivery.
Terrifying hypnogogic hallucinations	*Latencies:* A prolongation of sleep onset latency may be noted. REM latency may be extremely short, and sleep onset REM periods may occur. *Architecture:* Stage volumes are generally within normal limits for age. Progression of stages may be abnormal because of the presence of a sleep-onset REM period. *EMG:* Normal. *EEG:* Normal. *Respiration:* Normal. *Comments:* Few data regarding the polysomnographic variables are available.
Sleep-related abnormal swallowing syndrome	*Latencies:* Sleep onset latency may be normal, prolonged, or shortened. REM latency is generally normal. *Architecture:* There are frequent brief awakenings lasting 5 to 10 minutes. Slow-wave sleep may be profoundly decreased or entirely absent. *EMG:* Normal. *EEG:* Normal.

Continued on following page

DISORDERS OF INITIATING AND MAINTAINING SLEEP *Continued*

Diagnosis	Polysomnographic Characteristics
Sleep-related abnormal swallowing syndrome—cont'd	*Respiration:* Brief apneas may be associated with pooling of secretions in the pharynx. *Comments:* Polysomnography is generally performed to rule out other causes for the symptoms (e.g., obstructive sleep apnea syndrome, central sleep apnea syndrome).
Sleep-related laryngospasm	*Latencies:* Sleep onset latency is variable. REM latency is generally normal. *Architecture:* Sleep stages and progression are normal. Awakenings occur with the onset of symptoms. *EMG:* Normal. *EEG:* Normal. *Respiration:* Normal. Obstructive apneas and other cardiorespiratory abnormalities are notably absent. *Comments:* Two consecutive nights of polysomnography are recommended. Sleep-related laryngospasm is often difficult to document in the laboratory.
Infantile colic	*Latencies:* Sleep onset latency may be significantly prolonged by intense crying episodes during the colicky period at night. At the end of the colicky episode the infant falls asleep. REM latency may be normal for age. *Architecture:* During evening episodes periods of quiet sleep are often missed. Colicky crying spells have been postulated to occur during undifferentiated or indeterminate sleep states. After 3 to 4 months of age, colic and unexplained crying disappear and the architecture returns to age-related normal limits. *EMG:* Periods of hypertonicity or uninhibited motor activity can be seen during colicky crying spells. *EEG:* Normal. *Respiration:* Normal. *Comments:* Irregular sleep or sleep-wake patterns and frequent wakings after 3 to 4 months of age are most likely due to parental mismanagement of the child's sleep patterns during the colicky period.

DISORDERS OF EXCESSIVE SLEEPINESS

Diagnosis	Polysomnographic Characteristics
Inadequate sleep hygiene	*MSLT:* Mean sleep onset latency is shortened (usually less than 10 minutes). Typically, no sleep onset REM periods are noted unless sleep deprivation is profound. *Nocturnal polysomnography:* Sleep onset latency may be short or prolonged. Architecture is fragmented by frequent arousals and an early morning spontaneous awakening. Sleep efficiency is decreased. *EMG:* Normal. *EEG:* No abnormalities are noted. *Respiration:* Normal. No apneas nor hypopneas are present. *Comments:* Sleep logs may be helpful in diagnosis. Patients often sleep better in the sleep laboratory than in the home environment.
Insufficient sleep syndrome	*MSLT:* The test may show extreme degrees of daytime sleepiness. Mean sleep onset latencies often range between 5 and 8 minutes. Episodes of sleep onset occur in most naps throughout the day. Stage 1 is achieved

DIAGNOSIS	POLYSOMNOGRAPHIC CHARACTERISTICS
Insufficient sleep syndrome—cont'd	in approximately 99% of the naps, and Stage 2 in greater than 80%. If sleep deprivation is severe, a sleep onset REM period may appear, especially in the first (early morning) nap, but usually *less than 2* sleep onset REM periods are seen across a five-nap study. *Nocturnal polysomnography:* Sleep onset latency is shortened. REM latency may be short or normal. There are a high sleep efficiency and an increased total sleep time. Sleep architecture and distribution and progression of stages are normal. *EMG:* Normal. *EEG:* Normal. *Respiration:* Normal. *Comments:* Patients often sleep longer in the laboratory than at home.
Limit-setting sleep disorder	*MSLT:* Mean sleep onset latency is shortened when limits are not set. Mean latencies are within normal age ranges when limits are placed on the child's sleep. No sleep onset REM periods are present. *Nocturnal polysomnography:* Normal in quantity and quality when limits are set. Sleep onset latency may be prolonged when limits are not set. *EMG:* Normal. *EEG:* Normal. *Respiration:* Normal. *Comments:* A sleep log may be of assistance in arriving at a diagnosis.
Mood disorders	*MSLT:* Mean sleep onset latency is reduced. Sleep onset REM periods are not present, despite the shortened REM latency noted in the nocturnal polysomnogram. *Nocturnal polysomnography:* Sleep onset latency is prolonged, and REM latency is reduced. Sleep efficiency is decreased because of an increase in the number of wakings after sleep onset. Slow-wave sleep is reduced in volume and is shifted to a period later in the night. The first REM period is often long and intense. REM periods tend to decrease in length and intensity as the sleep period progresses. *EMG:* Normal. *EEG:* Normal. *Respiration:* Normal. *Comments:* Results of testing may vary with the type and severity of the mood disorder.
Psychoses	*MSLT:* Results may vary significantly. Excessive sleepiness may be manifest during times of significant nocturnal sleep disruption. *Nocturnal polysomnography:* Variable. Sleep onset latency may be shortened. Sleep efficiency and slow-wave sleep are decreased, and Stages 1 and 2 NREM sleep and the frequency and duration of waking after sleep onset are increased. REM volume may be variable, and REM density is increased. *EMG:* Normal. *EEG:* Most often normal. *Respiration:* Normal. *Comments:* A polyphasic sleep pattern may be seen. Symptoms may be significantly variable, with periods of insomnia alternating with periods of hypersomnia. Specific polysomnographic findings depend on whether the patient is chronically ill or is experiencing an acute exacerbation of the illness. At times polysomnographic findings are quite normal.
Alcoholism	*MSLT:* Mean sleep onset latency is characteristic of excessive sleepiness (i.e., less than 10 minutes). Sleep onset REM periods are not present. *Nocturnal polysomnography:* There is a decrease in total sleep time, and the architecture is fragmented. Slow-wave sleep is increased during the first half of the sleep period and REM sleep and wake are increased during the second half of the recording. A significant decrease in slow-wave sleep is seen during short-term abstinence.

Continued on following page

DISORDERS OF EXCESSIVE SLEEPINESS *Continued*

Diagnosis	Polysomnographic Characteristics
Alcoholism—cont'd	*EMG:* Normal. *EEG:* An alpha-delta pattern may be present. *Respiration:* Typically normal, but alcohol may exacerbate obstructive and central apneas. *Comments:* Sleep onset latency may be decreased on nocturnal polysomnography, and the REM latency is often prolonged.
Environmental sleep disorder	*MSLT:* Characteristic of excessive sleepiness. Mean sleep onset latency is less than 10 minutes. Sleep onsets occur in most naps. Sleep onset REM periods are usually not present; however, if the degree of nocturnal sleep disruption and restriction caused by environmental factors are significant, an occasional sleep onset REM period may be seen on a five-nap study. *Nocturnal polysomnography:* Total sleep time tends to be longer in the laboratory than at home (since the disturbing environmental factors are absent). Sleep efficiency is normal to increased. Architecture is generally normal. *EMG:* Normal. *EEG:* Normal. *Respiration:* Normal. *Comments:* Patients tend to sleep better in the laboratory than at home.
Toxin-induced sleep disorder	*MSLT:* Little information is available regarding polysomnographic variables in this disorder. The MSLT might reveal a short mean sleep onset latency, indicative of excessive sleepiness. *Nocturnal polysomnography:* Sleep onset latency on nocturnal studies may be prolonged. Sleep efficiency may be decreased, and frequent awakenings may occur after sleep onset. Early morning spontaneous waking is present. *EMG:* Normal. *EEG:* May be normal or may reveal changes indicative of encephalopathy (e.g., diffuse slowing, seizure activity). *Respiration:* Normal. *Comments:* Since little is known about the changes that occur with this disorder, the preceding findings should be considered speculative and extrapolations from clinical data.
Hypnotic-dependent sleep disorder	*MSLT:* Demonstrated evidence of excessive sleepiness with chronic long-acting hypnotic use. Sleep onset latency is generally less than 10 minutes when hynotic medications are discontinued suddenly. *Nocturnal polysomnography:* Nocturnal sleep latency may be normal while the patient is receiving medication, but it is significantly prolonged when the medication is discontinued. Stage 1, REM, and slow-wave sleep is diminished, Stage 2 is increased, there are frequent stage changes, and sleep architecture is fragmented. *EMG:* Normal. *EEG:* Decreases in K-complexes and delta wave activity are seen. Pseudospindles at a frequency of 14 to 18 Hz are present, and alpha and beta activity may be increased. *Respiration:* Normal. *Comments:* REM sleep eye movements may be decreased. A urine drug screen may be helpful in diagnosis.
Stimulant-dependent sleep disorder	*MSLT:* On withdrawal of stimulant medication, a severe decrease in the mean sleep onset latency occurs. The MSLT may be suggestive of narcolepsy. *Nocturnal polysomnography:* Medication causes an increase in the sleep onset and REM latencies. Total sleep time is decreased. REM volume is decreased, and there is an increase in waking after sleep onset. This

Diagnosis	Polysomnographic Characteristics
Stimulant-dependent sleep disorder—cont'd	architecture is dramatically reversed after discontinuation of the drug. Sleep onset and REM latencies are shortened, total sleep time increases, and a significant rebound in REM sleep time occurs. *EMG:* Normal. *EEG:* Normal. *Respiration:* Normal. *Comments:* A urine drug screen before polysomnography may be helpful in diagnosis.
Obstructive sleep apnea syndrome	*MSLT:* Mean sleep onset latency is significantly short (less than 10 minutes). Sleep onset occurs in most, if not all, naps in a five-nap study. If nocturnal sleep disruption is profound, the mean sleep onset latency may be less than 5 minutes and sleep onset REM periods may occur. Differentiation between obstructive sleep apnea syndrome and narcolepsy based only on MSLT may be difficult. Nocturnal polysomnography before the MSLT is required for accurate diagnosis. *Nocturnal polysomnography:* Sleep onset latency is severely shortened, and many patients fall asleep during the setup procedure or are asleep at the time of lights out. Frequent arousals and stage changes result from the respiratory events. Slow-wave sleep and REM sleep may be severely reduced or absent. Stage 1 and 2 sleep is increased. Sleep efficiency is poor. *EMG:* Significant snore artifact is often present on the chin muscle EMG. *EEG:* Normal. *Respiration:* Obstructive apneas lasting 10 seconds or longer occur at a frequency of five or more apneas per hour. Oxygen desaturation and arousal are associated with the respiratory events. Paradoxical breathing can be demonstrated during obstructive events. *Comments:* Bradyarrhythmias, tachyarrhythmias, and other ECG changes are commonly associated with apneic events.
Central sleep apnea syndrome	*MSLT:* Mean sleep onset latency is typically less than 10 minutes. No sleep onset REM periods are present. *Nocturnal polysomnography:* Sleep onset latency may be shortened or prolonged. Frequent arousals and stage changes are noted. *EMG:* Normal. *EEG:* Normal. *Respiration:* Central apneas longer than 10 seconds (20 seconds in infants) occur. Rebound hyperventilation may follow the apneas. Oxygen desaturation occurs but tends to be less severe than that seen with obstructive apneas. *Comments:* Bradyarrhythmias and tachyarrhythmias may be seen on ECG.
Central alveolar hypoventilation syndrome	*MSLT:* Excessive sleepiness is demonstrated with a mean sleep onset latency of less than 10 minutes. Sleep onset REM periods are absent. *Nocturnal polysomnography:* Architecture is significantly disrupted by frequent awakenings. Movement time is increased. *EMG:* Normal. *EEG:* Normal. *Respiration:* Episodes of decreased tidal volume for several minutes occur. Decrease in oxygen saturation is present and becomes worse during REM sleep. Obstructive apneas may be present. *Comments:* Carbon dioxide tension may be increased.
Sleep-related neurogenic tachypnea	*MSLT:* Objective evidence of excessive sleepiness is present. The mean sleep onset latency is less than 10 minutes. Sleep onset REM periods are absent. *Nocturnal polysomnography:* Sleep onset latency is shortened, and sleep architecture is fragmented. Sleep efficiency is low. *EMG:* Normal.

Continued on following page

DISORDERS OF EXCESSIVE SLEEPINESS *Continued*

DIAGNOSIS	POLYSOMNOGRAPHIC CHARACTERISTICS
Sleep-related neurogenic tachypnea—cont'd	*EEG:* Normal. *Respiration:* The respiratory rate is increased 20% to 180% above waking rates. The tachypnea begins at sleep onset, and the rate immediately returns to normal on awakening. *Comments:* This disorder has not been described during childhood, but clinical correlates might exist.
Periodic limb movement disorders	*MSLT:* Excessive sleepiness is present, and mean sleep onset latency is less than 10 minutes. Sleep onset REM periods do not occur. *Nocturnal polysomnography:* Sleep onset latency is shortened, and architecture is disrupted by frequent arousals, awakenings, and movements. Movements begin in Stage 1 sleep, reach a maximum during Stage 2 sleep, and diminish during slow-wave sleep. *EMG:* Clusters of repetitive contractions lasting 0.5 to 5 seconds occur in one or both legs (arms may also be involved). Intervals are typically 20 to 40 seconds. *EEG:* K-complexes frequently occur with each muscle contraction. *Respiration:* Normal. *Comments:* Periodic limb movements disappear during REM sleep. There may be associated increases in heart rate and blood pressure during clusters of limb movements.
Long sleeper	*MSLT:* Mean sleep onset latency is normal (greater than 10 to 15 minutes). Sleep onsets are infrequent across a five-nap study but are most likely to occur during the midafternoon nap. *Nocturnal polysomnography:* Sleep onset latency and REM latency are normal. The progression of stages across the sleep period is normal. Slow-wave sleep volume is consistent with age-appropriate norms. REM sleep volume and Stage 2 volume are often greater than age-related norms. *EMG:* Normal. *EEG:* Normal. *Respiration:* Normal. *Comments:* Long sleepers are at one end of a normal continuum of total sleep time. Patients may show symptoms if and when they attempt to decrease their total sleep time to a level consistent with societal age-related norms.
Time zone change/jet lag syndrome	*MSLT:* Excessive sleepiness may be documented if the MSLT is done during daytime hours in the new time zone (and during the period when the patient is symptomatic, i.e., within the first few days after travel). *Nocturnal polysomnography:* Nocturnal sleep onset is prolonged. Sleep efficiency may be decreased. A variable decrease in slow-wave sleep volume and an increase in Stage 1 volume are observed. The sleep period is disrupted by frequent arousals. *EMG:* Normal. *EEG:* Normal. *Respiration:* Normal. *Comments:* Sleep-wake rhythm is lost for the first few days after travel. Other physiological rhythms may take longer to entrain to the new time zone.
Shift work sleep disorder	*MSLT:* Few data are available regarding the result of parental shift work on children. If sleep disruption or restriction occurs, mean sleep onset latency may be shortened and sleep may occur during several or all of the nap studies. Sleep onset REM periods are absent. *Nocturnal polysomnography:* Findings are variable. Parents show a decrease in total sleep time, fragmentation of architecture, and increase in the frequency of arousals and awakenings.

DIAGNOSIS	POLYSOMNOGRAPHIC CHARACTERISTICS
Shift work sleep disorder—cont'd	*EMG:* Normal. *EEG:* Normal. *Respiration:* Normal. *Comments:* This is usually diagnosed on the basis of the history. A sleep log may greatly assist in the diagnosis. A loss of chronobiological rhythmicity may occur.
Delayed sleep phase syndrome	*MSLT:* Sleep onset latencies are variable, and the average across a five-nap test may be considered normal. However, sleep onset latency may be significantly reduced during morning naps and normal during afternoon naps. Sleep onset REM periods are absent. *Nocturnal polysomnography:* Sleep onset latency may be prolonged for hours. Sleep efficiency is decreased for age. The sleep period is relatively free of arousals, and other than the long sleep onset latency, the architecture is normal. *EMG:* Normal. *EEG:* Normal. *Respiration:* Normal. *Comments:* Patients may be difficult to wake in the morning. Wrist actigraphy or a sleep log may greatly assist in diagnosis.
Advanced sleep phase syndrome	*MSLT:* Mean sleep onset latency is usually normal (greater than 10 minutes). No sleep onset REM periods are seen. *Nocturnal polysomnography:* Polysomnography should be performed on two consecutive nights separated by an MSLT. On the first night the study should begin at the patient's habitual sleep time. Sleep onset latency should be normal. Quantity and quality of sleep and sleep architecture are normal. The second night, conducted at the socially desired time, reveals a reduced sleep onset latency and a prolonged early morning wake. *EMG:* Normal. *EEG:* Normal. *Respiration:* Normal. *Comments:* Wrist actigraphy or a sleep log may be required for diagnosis.
Non-24-hour sleep-wake syndrome	*MSLT:* Little information is available. Mean sleep onset latency may be prolonged or profoundly shortened when the patient's chronophysiological sleep period is out of phase with the timing of the MSLT. When the sleep period and the test are in phase, the findings may be normal. *Nocturnal polysomnography:* A progressive decrease in the total sleep time occurs on successive days. A progressive increase in the sleep onset latency also takes place. Otherwise, the architecture may be relatively normal. *EMG:* Normal. *EEG:* Spindle formation and the number of K-complexes may be abnormally low in brain-damaged or mentally retarded patients. *Respiration:* Normal. *Comments:* Twenty-four-hour temperature monitoring shows progressive delay in the nadir by 1 to 2 hours on successive days. Many patients have congenital or acquired blindness.
Irregular sleep-wake pattern	*MSLT:* Few data are available. MSLT results may be significantly variable. Sleep onset latency may be normal or prolonged for some naps and significantly short for others. *Nocturnal polysomnography:* Architecture is quite variable. Total sleep time may be significantly decreased. *EMG:* Normal. *EEG:* Normal. *Respiration:* Normal.

Continued on following page

DISORDERS OF EXCESSIVE SLEEPINESS *Continued*

DIAGNOSIS	POLYSOMNOGRAPHIC CHARACTERISTICS
Irregular sleep-wake pattern—cont'd	*Comments:* Twenty-four-hour monitoring shows loss of a normal sleep-wake pattern. Wrist actigraphy or a sleep log may be required for diagnosis.
Narcolepsy	*MSLT:* Mean sleep onset latency is typically less than 7 minutes (and often less than 5 minutes) on a five-nap study. Frequent microsleeps may be seen during MSLT naps. Two or more sleep onset REM periods (REM occurring less than 15 minutes after sleep onset) are characteristic of narcolepsy. *Nocturnal polysomnography:* Sleep onset latency is significantly short. Sleep is frequently (but not universally) entered through REM sleep. REM latency is significantly short and generally occurs less than 15 minutes after sleep onset. Although the remainder of the architecture is relatively normal, sleep is fragmented by frequent arousals and awakenings. Stage 1 sleep may be somewhat increased. *EMG:* Normal. Decreased chin muscle tone is noted during the sleep onset REM period. *EEG:* Normal. *Respiration:* Normal. *Comments:* Although a profoundly short mean sleep onset latency and two or more sleep onset REM periods are characteristic, this pattern is not pathognomonic. Historical evidence of cataplexy (with or without sleep paralysis or hypnogogic hallucinations) virtually establishes the diagnosis.
Idiopathic hypersomnia	*MSLT:* Mean sleep onset latency is less than 10 minutes (most often between 7 and 9 minutes). An average of less than two sleep onset REM periods have been noted. Microsleeps may be noted on MSLT naps. *Nocturnal polysomnography:* Sleep onset latency is short. REM latency is normal. Total sleep time is slightly increased. Slow-wave sleep volume is normal to slightly increased. *EMG:* Normal. *EEG:* Normal. *Respiration:* Normal. *Comments:* Polysomnography is conducted to rule out other causes of excessive sleepiness. Clinical symptoms may not correlate with the severity of sleepiness seen on the MSLT.
Posttraumatic hypersomnia	*MSLT:* Objective measures of sleepiness are documented. Mean sleep onset latency is less than 10 minutes. In general, no sleep onset REM periods are noted. *Nocturnal polysomnography:* Sleep onset latency may be normal or decreased. Stage volumes are normal, and stages occur in a normal progression across the sleep period. *EMG:* Normal. *EEG:* May be normal or may show evidence of posttraumatic abnormalities (e.g., epileptiform activity). *Respiration:* Normal. *Comments:* Posttraumatic narcolepsy has been reported. In these patients the shortened sleep onset latency may be accompanied by two or more sleep onset REM periods and clinical evidence of cataplexy, hypnogogic hallucinations, or sleep paralysis.
Recurrent hypersomnia	MSLT: Mean sleep onset latency is less than 10 minutes. In general, no sleep onset REM periods are noted. Occasionally, less than two sleep onset REM periods may be seen. *Nocturnal polysomnography:* Sleep onset latency is decreased. REM latency is also shortened. Sleep efficiency tends to be increased, and

DIAGNOSIS	POLYSOMNOGRAPHIC CHARACTERISTICS
Recurrent hypersomnia—cont'd	slow-wave sleep volume is decreased. Progression of stages across the sleep period is normal. *EMG:* Normal. *EEG:* During episodes of hypersonmia there is often generalized low-voltage slow-wave activity or a diffuse alpha pattern. *Respiration:* Normal. *Comments:* Recurrent hypersomnia is also known as Kleine-Levin syndrome. Between hypersomnolent episodes, polysomnographic findings may be normal.
Subwakefulness syndrome	*MSLT:* Stage 1 sleep onset is seen in most MSLT naps (occasionally Stage 2 is noted). A pattern of persistent drowsiness during wakefulness may be observed. Mean sleep onset latency is less than 10 minutes but greater than 5 minutes. *Nocturnal polysomnography:* Sleep onset latency is shortened. REM latency is generally normal. Stage volumes are typically within normal limits, and progression of stages across the sleep period is normal. *EMG:* Normal. *EEG:* A slow and diffuse alpha pattern, Stage 1 drowsiness, or occasionally Stage 2 patterns are seen on a continuous daytime polysomnographic recording. These patterns wax and wane. Frequent microsleeps may be seen. *Respiration:* Normal. *Comments:* Subwakefulness syndrome is a very rare disorder. Sleepiness may be mild and is not frequent or irresistible. REM sleep does not occur during daytime sleep episodes.
Fragmentary myoclonus	*MSLT:* Mean sleep onset latency is less than 10 minutes. Sleep onset REM periods generally do not occur. *Nocturnal polysomnography:* Sleep onset latency is short. REM latency is normal. Architecture is typically normal, although fragmented by myoclonic jerks. *EMG:* Asymmetrical, asynchronous potentials lasting 75 to 150 msec are noted in the muscles of the arms, legs, and face. Amplitude of the potentials ranges from 50 to 300 μV or greater. Myoclonic potentials are seen in Stage 2, slow-wave sleep, and REM sleep. *EEG:* K-complexes are often seen in association with muscle potentials. *Respiration:* Normal. *Comments:* This disorder is not typically described in childhood. The most common age of onset is during adulthood.
Sleeping sickness	*MSLT:* Data are limited, but extreme daytime sleepiness may be demonstrated on the MSLT. *Nocturnal polysomnography:* Sleep onset latency is decreased. REM sleep may be normal. Slow-wave sleep is decreased or absent. *EMG:* Potentials are increased during microarousals. *EEG:* Vertex sharp transients, K-complexes, spindles, and theta activity are decreased. EEG activity becomes homogeneous, and sleep stages cannot be distinguished. Low-amplitude beta, alpha, or theta rhythms lasting 3 to 7 seconds may be noted. Epileptiform discharges may occur. *Respiration:* A transient increase in the respiratory rate may take place during microarousals. *Comments:* Untreated sleeping sickness is fatal.
Menstrual-associated sleep disorder	*MSLT:* During the premenstrual period, evidence of excessive sleepiness may be noted on the MSLT. Mean sleep onset latencies may be less than 10 minutes. *Nocturnal polysomnography:* Sleep onset latency may be increased or decreased when symptoms are present. There are frequent stage transitions, prolonged awakenings, and decreased sleep efficiency. The

Continued on following page

DISORDERS OF EXCESSIVE SLEEPINESS *Continued*

Diagnosis	Polysomnographic Characteristics
Menstrual-associated sleep disorder—cont'd	progression of stages across the sleep period is abnormal. During the intermenstrual period, polysomnographic findings are normal. *EMG:* Normal. *EEG:* Normal. *Respiration:* Normal. *Comments:* Intermenstrual periods are symptom free. Symptoms may be excessive sleepiness or excessive sleeplessness.
Pregnancy-associated sleep disorder	*MSTL:* Mean sleep onset latency is less than 10 minutes. No sleep onset REM periods occur. *Nocturnal polysomnography:* Sleep onset latency is increased during the second and third trimesters. Awakenings after sleep onset are increased in the second and third trimesters. During the first trimester the total sleep time may be increased. Slow-wave sleep volume is decreased near term. The postdelivery period is characterized by a decrease in REM sleep and a return of slow-wave sleep volume. REM sleep gradually returns to normal prepregnancy levels. *EMG:* Normal. *EEG:* Normal. *Respiration:* Normal. *Comments:* Excessive daytime sleepiness and sleep disruption may be due to an inability to assume a comfortable sleeping position.
Munchausen's syndrome by proxy	*MSLT:* Mean sleep onset latency is normal. No sleep onset REM periods are present. *Nocturnal polysomnography:* Stage volumes, stage progression, and sleep architecture are normal. *EMG:* Normal. *EEG:* Normal. *Respiration:* Normal. *Comments:* Sleep study findings are surprisingly normal despite the dramatic nature of the history.

OTHER SLEEP DISORDERS

Diagnosis	Polysomnographic Characteristics
Primary snoring	*Latencies:* Sleep onset latency is normal. REM latency is normal. *Architecture:* Stage volumes are normal, as is progression of stages across the sleep period. Sleep efficiency is normal. *EMG:* Snore artifact is often noted in the chin muscle EMG. *EEG:* Normal. No focal, paroxysmal, or epileptiform activity is noted. *Respiration:* Normal. No apneas, hypopneas, hypoventilation, oxygen desaturation, or paradoxical respiration is noted. *Comments:* Patients may be aware of the snoring at sleep onset or after an arousal. No daytime symptoms are observed.
Congenital central hypoventilation syndrome	*Latencies:* Sleep onset latency may be decreased. REM latency may be variable for the patient's age (the syndrome occurs at an age when sleep onset is through active sleep). *Architecture:* Sleep is disrupted and fragmented because of ventilatory instability. *EMG:* Normal. *EEG:* May be normal. Evidence of hypoxic encephalopathy (e.g., diffuse slowing, seizure activity) may be present.

Diagnosis	Polysomnographic Characteristics
Congenital central hypoventilation syndrome—cont'd	*Respiration:* Ventilatory effort ceases at sleep onset. In most patients the syndrome is diagnosed at birth and mechanical ventilation is required. Weaning the patient from the ventilator is difficult or impossible. Hypoxia and hypercapnia are present. *Comments:* This condition is often diagnosed at birth. It may first be noted during infancy as an apparent life-threatening event. Artificial ventilatory assistance is required.
Sleep-related increased respiratory resistive load	*Latencies:* Sleep onset latency is decreased. REM latency is usually normal. *Architecture:* Architecture is disrupted by frequent brief arousals and stage changes. Stage volumes are generally within normal limits, and progression of stages across the sleep period is normal. *EMG:* Chin muscle EMG may be increased during periods of increased respiratory resistive load. Intercostal EMG may show increased accessory muscle activity. *EEG:* Normal. *Respiration:* Paradoxical respiration is present and may persist for long periods. Variable decreases in oxygen saturation occur. No clear apneas or hypopneas are noted. *Comments:* Significant daytime symptoms may be present, and the MSLT may reveal excessive daytime sleepiness or microsleeps. Esophageal manometry shows increased intrathoracic pressure during periods of increased airway resistance. Symptoms and sleep disruption are more closely related to architectural fragmentation than to oxygen desaturation.
Sleep walking	*Latencies:* Sleep onset latency is normal. REM latency is normal for the patient's age. *Architecture:* All stages of sleep are seen, and stage volumes are within age-related norms. The progression of stages across the sleep period is normal. A sudden partial arousal from slow-wave sleep is noted. This generally occurs during the first third of the night, after the first or second episode of slow-wave sleep. *EMG:* Muscle tone is increased during the period of walking. *EEG:* Normal. No focal, paroxysmal, or epileptiform activity is noted during the sleep walking event. *Respiration:* Normal. *Comments:* Increased body movement and partial arousals during slow-wave sleep are noted (even in the absence of sleep walking).
Sleep terrors	*Latencies:* Sleep onset latency is normal. REM latency is normal for the patient's age. *Architecture:* Stage volumes and the progression of stages across the sleep period are normal. Sleep efficiency is normal. An abrupt, sudden arousal from slow-wave sleep occurs during the first third of the sleep period. The arousal is brief, and the patient rapidly returns to sleep after the episode. *EMG:* Potentials are increased during the terror. *EEG:* Normal. No focal, paroxysmal, or epileptiform activity is associated with the event. *Respiration:* Normal. The respiratory rate is often increased during the terror, reflecting the intense autonomic discharge. *Comments:* Intense autonomic discharges are noted. Displacement from the bed is common, and injuries are frequent. Partial arousals are more common during slow-wave sleep, even in the absence of major motor manifestations or a full-blown sleep terror episode.
Sleep bruxism	*Latencies:* Sleep onset and REM latencies are normal. *Architecture:* Stage volumes and progression of stages across the sleep period are normal. Paroxysms of bruxism are seen most often during Stage 2 sleep; however, they may occur in any stage (as well as during

Continued on following page

OTHER SLEEP DISORDERS *Continued*

DIAGNOSIS	POLYSOMNOGRAPHIC CHARACTERISTICS
Sleep bruxism—cont'd	wakefulness). Bruxism may also occur during REM sleep. *EMG:* Paroxysms of rhythmical masseter and temporalis muscle activity are observed. *EEG:* Normal. There is no evidence of seizure activity during periods of bruxism. If paroxysmal, focal, or epileptiform activity is present, sleep-related seizures are a more likely cause of the observed muscle activity. *Respiration:* Normal. *Comments:* Two consecutive nights of polysomnography may be necessary to confirm the diagnosis.
Sleep paralysis	*Latencies:* In the isolated and familial form of this disorder, sleep onset latency and REM latency are normal. Patients with sleep paralysis occurring with narcolepsy have a shortened sleep onset latency, and their REM periods occur within 15 minutes of sleep onset (although *not all* sleep onsets in narcoleptic patients are through REM sleep). *Architecture:* Stage volumes and progression are normal. Sleep efficiency is normal. *EMG:* During periods of sleep paralysis, skeletal muscle tone is profoundly decreased. *EEG:* Normal. Waking rhythm or a light Stage 1 pattern may be noted during periods of sleep paralysis. *Respiration:* Normal. However, patients often complain of a sensation of being unable to breathe. Clear apneas and hypopneas are absent. *Comments:* Extraocular and respiratory musculature remains intact during events. Blink artifact may be noted. The MSLT findings are normal unless the sleep paralysis is associated with narcolepsy.
REM sleep behavior disorder	*Latencies:* Sleep onset latency is normal. REM latency is normal. *Architecture:* Stage volumes and progression are normal. REM sleep is interrupted by sudden violent movements. An increase in REM density is noted. *EMG:* A paradoxical increase in muscle tone is noted during REM sleep. An increase in phasic twitching is also present. *EEG:* Normal. *Respiration:* Normal. *Comments:* Excessive body movements and jerking are seen. Complex behaviors and vocalizations occur during REM sleep.
Nocturnal paroxysmal dystonia	*Latencies:* Sleep onset latency and REM latency are normal. *Architecture:* Stage volumes are usually within age-related normal limits. Progression of stages across the sleep period also is normal. Choreoathetotic and dystonic body movements occur during Stage 2 and slow-wave sleep. They may also appear at sleep onset. *EMG:* Skeletal muscle tone is increased during the events. *EEG:* Arousal rhythm precedes the event by a few seconds. Abnormal EEG activity has been described in some patients, but it is questionable whether it is epileptiform. *Respiration:* Normal. *Comments:* Symptoms of dystonia are seldom present during normal waking hours.
Nightmares	*Latencies:* Sleep onset and latencies are normal. *Architecture:* Stage volumes and progression are normal. Abrupt awakening from REM sleep is noted, and patients generally remain awake for 10 minutes or longer. REM density may be increased. *EMG:* Normal. *EEG:* Normal. *Respiration:* Normal.

Diagnosis	Polysomnographic Characteristics
Nightmares—cont'd	*Comments:* Mild autonomic discharges are present, but they are significantly less intense than those seen with sleep terrors.
Sleep talking	*Latencies:* Sleep onset latency and REM latency are normal. *Architecture:* All stages of sleep are present, and the progression of stages across the sleep period is normal. *EMG:* Normal. Chin muscle tone may be increased during the episode of talking. *EEG:* Normal. *Respiration:* Normal. However, sleep talking may occur in patients with obstructive sleep apnea syndrome. *Comments:* Somniloquy occurs in all sleep stages. Dream mentation may be present and can be identified in 79% of REM, 46% of Stage 2, and 21% of slow-wave sleep episodes.
Sleep enuresis	*Latencies:* Sleep onset latency and REM latency are normal. *Architecture:* Stage volumes and progression across the sleep period are normal. *EMG:* Normal. *EEG:* Normal. Questionable high-amplitude delta activity may be seen before the episode of bed wetting. *Respiration:* With primary (functional) sleep enuresis, respiration is normal. Enuresis may be a component of obstructive sleep apnea syndrome. *Comments:* Sleep enuresis can occur during any stage of sleep. It may be associated with obstructive sleep apnea syndrome, epilepsy, or other parasomnias.
Sleep-related painful erections	*Latencies:* Sleep onset latency is normal. REM latency is normal. *Architecture:* Stage volumes and progression across the sleep period are normal. The patient awakens from REM sleep during periods of penile tumescence. *EMG:* Normal. *EEG:* Normal. *Respiration:* Normal. *Comments:* The patient awakens because of a painful sensation during normal penile tumescence. Interestingly, no sexual dysfunction is noted and erections during waking hours are normal and painless.
Sleep-related epilepsy	*Latencies:* Sleep onset and REM latencies may be variable. *Architecture:* Sleep stages and progression may be normal or disrupted by seizure activity. *EMG:* Generally normal. Potentials may be increased if motor manifestations are present during epileptic activity. *EEG:* Exact EEG manifestations depend on the underlying process. Most sleep-related seizures occur during NREM sleep (particularly Stage 2). An interictal sleep EEG may reveal significantly heterogeneous abnormalities, such as focal unilateral spikes, bilateral synchronous spike and slow-wave discharges, multiple spikes and slow waves, sharp transients in a localized distribution, and high-amplitude negative sharp waves with stereotypical morphology. *Respiration:* Normal. Breathing may be variable during ictal periods. *Comments:* The interictal EEG may not show abnormalities.
Electrical status epilepticus of sleep	*Latencies:* Sleep onset latency is normal. REM latency may be normal or variable in length. *Architecture:* Sleep stage volumes are normal and cycle in a normal pattern. *EMG:* Normal. *EEG:* Before sleep onset the EEG may reveal spikes or other interictal phenomena or may be normal. At sleep onset, bilateral, diffuse, 2 to 2.5 Hz spike and wave activity appears, is virtually continuous, and

Continued on following page

OTHER SLEEP DISORDERS *Continued*

DIAGNOSIS	POLYSOMNOGRAPHIC CHARACTERISTICS
Electrical status epilepticus of sleep—cont'd	occupies 85% to 100% of NREM sleep. This abnormal activity decreases or disappears with REM desynchronization. Infrequent paroxysmal bursts of diffuse spike and slow-wave or focal (predominantly frontal) discharges may be present. *Respiration:* Normal. *Comments:* Spindle activity, K-complexes, and vertex sharp transients are often difficult to distinguish from the abnormal background activity.

GLOSSARY

Every medical discipline has a vocabulary that, although similar to those of other disciplines, is specific, unique, and often confusing to the reader. Terminology used in this text follows that presented in *The International Classification of Sleep Disorders: Diagnostic and Coding Manual* (American Sleep Disorders Association, 1990, pp. 337-351). It is modified and included with permission from the American Sleep Disorders Association.

actigraph: A small biomedical instrument, typically worn on the wrist, that measures and records body movement. It can be used to define sleep-wake cycles clearly (and objectively), based on documentation of body movement during the waking state and lack of movement during sleep periods. It is extremely useful in the diagnosis of chronophysiological disorders.

active sleep: A term used in pediatric sleep medicine and phylogenetic literature to describe a sleep state considered to be equivalent to REM sleep. It is used to describe REM sleep in infants less than 3 months of age. In the scoring of active sleep, EEG criteria are supplemented by other physiological parameters, such as respiratory pattern, heart rate, body movements, eye movements, and chin muscle tone.

alpha activity: Relatively low-amplitude (less than 50 μV) EEG waveforms with a frequency of 8 to 13 Hz.

alpha-delta sleep: Alpha activity occurring during slow-wave sleep. Relatively low-amplitude, 8 to 13 Hz waveforms are superimposed upon slow (less than 4 Hz) delta waves.

alpha intrusions: Brief superimposition of alpha activity onto the characteristic EEG morphology of any stage of sleep.

alpha rhythm: EEG rhythm with a frequency of 8 to 13 Hz, characteristic of relaxed wakefulness in most individuals 4 years of age and older. Its frequency is relatively stable for each individual. The amplitude is variable (right hemisphere slightly greater than the left), but typically below 50 μV. The rhythm is most prominent over the parietooccipital cortex when the eyes are closed. Visual input and other arousing stimuli typically block it. The frequency range is variable: it is slower and more diffuse during drowsiness, and it is slower in children than in young and middle-aged adults.

apnea: Cessation of airflow lasting at least 10 seconds (central apneas lasting at least 20 seconds in infants). Apneas may be obstructive, central, or mixed (having characteristics of both obstructive and central apneas).

apnea-hypopnea index: The total number of obstructive, central, and mixed apneas and hypopneas per hour of sleep.

apnea index: The total number of obstructive, central, and mixed apneas per hour of sleep.

arise time: The time that an individual gets out of bed after the final wake of the major sleep period. It should be clearly differentiated from the final wake time.

arousal: A sudden change from any NREM sleep stage to a "lighter" stage of sleep or from REM sleep toward wakefulness. Wakefulness is a possible final outcome but is not invariable. Increased muscle tone, heart rate, and body movement may accompany an arousal.

arousal disorder: A parasomnia thought to be due to an abnormality in the arousal mechanism. Conflicting, simultaneous, asynchronous activity of the central arousal and sleep mechanism may be involved. Somnambulism, sleep terrors, and confusional arousals are examples of arousal disorders.

awakening: Return to the polysomnographically defined awake state from any stage of sleep. It is characterized by return of alpha and beta EEG activity, increase in EMG tone, and presence of voluntary eye movements and eye blinks and is paralleled by a reasonably alert state and awareness of the environment.

baseline: The normal state of an individual (or of a particular variable) before an intervention or experimental manipulation.

bedtime: The time of day when an individual begins to attempt to fall asleep (distinguished from the time the individual gets into bed).

beta activity: EEG waveforms with a frequency greater than 13 Hz.

beta rhythm: EEG rhythm in the range of 13 to 35 Hz. When beta rhythm is the predominant frequency, it is usually associated with an alert or vigilant state and is accompanied by high EMG tone. The amplitude is of relatively low voltage (less than 30 μV). Beta rhythm may also be drug induced.

biorhythm: Colloquial term used to describe a biological rhythm. See Chronobiology.

cataplexy: A sudden decrease in skeletal muscle tone and loss of deep tendon reflexes resulting in muscle weakness, paralysis, or postural collapse. Precipitating factors are usually associated with emotions (e.g., laughter, anger, startle). Cataplexy is one of the classic symptoms of the tetrad of narcolepsy. During cataplexy, respiration, voluntary eye movements, and consciousness are not compromised.

central apnea: Cessation of airflow at the mouth and nose because of a decrease in or absence of respiratory effort.

central hypopnea: Diminution of airflow at the mouth and nose resulting from a decrease in respiratory effort.

Cheyne-Stokes respiration: Breathing pattern characterized by regular "crescendo-decrescendo" fluctuations in respiratory rate and tidal volume.

chronobiology: The study of temporal, primarily rhythmical, processes in biology.

circadian: About a day.

circadian rhythm: Innate daily fluctuation of physiological and behavioral functions generally coupled to the 24-hour light-dark cycle. Periodicity may be measurably different (e.g., 23 hours, 25 hours) when time cues are removed.

circasemidian: About half a day.

circasemidian rhythm: An innate daily fluctuation of physiological and behavioral functions that last about half a day.

conditioned insomnia: Sleeplessness produced by the development of conditioned arousal. This conditioned arousal was developed during an earlier experience of sleeplessness and may be caused by a negative association between the characteristics of the customary sleep environment and sleeping (e.g., perseveration about disturbed sleep).

constant routine: A chronobiological test of the endogenous pacemaker. A 36-hour baseline monitoring period is followed by a 40-hour waking episode of monitoring with the subject on a constant routine of food intake, position, activity, and light exposure.

cycle: Characteristics of an event exhibiting rhythmical fluctuations. One cycle is defined as the activity from one maximum or minimum to the next.

deep sleep: Common term for combined NREM Stage 3 and 4 sleep; slow-wave sleep.

delayed sleep phase: A condition in which the major sleep period is displaced to a time later during the 24-hour continuum. The onset of the major sleep period occurs at a time later within a given 24-hour sleep-wake cycle. Wake time occurs at a similar later time.

delta activity: EEG waveform activity with a frequency of less than 4 Hz. In human sleep stage scoring, the minimum criteria include an amplitude of at least 75 μV and a duration of 0.5 second (2 Hz) or less.

delta sleep stage: Sleep stage in which EEG delta waves are prevalent or predominant (NREM Stages 3 and 4); slow-wave sleep.

diurnal: Pertaining to the daytime.

drowsiness: A state of quiet wakefulness occurring before sleep onset. Diffuse, slowed alpha activity is usually present if the eyes are closed. This rhythm then is replaced by a relatively low-voltage, mixed-frequency EEG background characteristic of Stage 1 sleep.

duration criteria: Criteria established in the International Classification of Sleep Disorders for classifying the duration of a particular disorder as acute, subacute, or chronic.

dyssomnias: Disorders of sleep or wakefulness other than parasomnias (i.e., disorders of initiating or maintaining sleep and disorders of excessive sleepiness).

early morning arousal: Premature morning awakening.

electroencephalogram (EEG): A recording of the electrical activity of the brain by means of electrodes placed on the surface of the head. Data obtained by EEG combined with chin muscle EMG and EOG provide the basis for sleep stage scoring. Electrodes are placed according to the International 10-20 System. A central region electrode (C3 or C4) is referentially recorded as the standard electrode derivation from which state scoring is done.

electromyogram (EMG): A recording of electrical activity from the muscles. The chin EMG, combined with EEG and EOG recordings, provides the basis for sleep stage scoring. Sleep recording in humans typically uses surface electrodes to measure activity from the submental group of muscles. These maximally reflect changes in resting activity of skeletal muscles.

electrooculogram (EOG): A recording of voltage changes resulting from changes in position of the globes of the eyes. Each globe is a functional dipole with an anterior (corneal) positive potential and a posterior (retinal) negative potential. The EOG, combined with the EEG and chin muscle EMG, provides the basis for sleep stage scoring. Sleep recording in humans uses surface electrodes placed near the eyes to record the incidence, direction, and velocity of eye movements.

end-tidal carbon dioxide: Carbon dioxide value of exhaled air, usually determined at the nares by an infrared carbon dioxide gas analyzer. The value reflects the alveolar or pulmonary arterial blood carbon dioxide level.

entrainment: Synchronization of a biological rhythm by forcing stimuli such as environmental time cues. During entrainment the frequencies of the two cycles are the same or are integral multiples of each other.

epoch: A measure of duration of the sleep recording that typically is 20 or 30 seconds in duration, depending on the paper speed of the polysomnograph. At a paper speed of 10 mm per second, one page of recording corresponds to one epoch. In some sleep literature an epoch refers to a cluster of periodic limb movements.

excessive sleepiness: A subjective report of difficulty in maintaining the alert awake state, usually accompanied by a rapid entrance into sleep when the person is sedentary or by the appearance of frequent episodes of microsleep during periods of behavioral wakefulness. The term may also refer to an excessively deep or prolonged major sleep period. Excessive sleepiness can be objectively measured by electrophysiological tests, such as the Multiple Sleep Latency Test. Excessive sleepiness more commonly occurs during the daytime; however, it may be present at night in a person who has the major sleep episode during the daytime.

extrinsic sleep disorder: Disorder that originates, develops, or arises from causes outside the body. The extrinsic sleep disorders are a subgroup of the dyssomnias.

final awakening: The amount of wakefulness that occurs between the final wake-up time and the arise time ("lights on").

final wake-up: The clock time at which an individual awakens for the last time before the arise time.

first night effect: The effect of the laboratory environment and polysomnographic recording apparatus on the quality of the subject's sleep during the first night of recording. Sleep is usually of poorer quality than would be expected in the subject's normal sleeping environment. The subject usually habituates to the laboratory by the second night of recording. For most clinical applications and diagnostic purposes, a single night of recording in the laboratory is sufficient.

fragmentation: The interruption of any stage of sleep because of the appearance of another stage or wakefulness. Fragmentation leads to disrupted NREM-REM sleep cycles. The term is often used to refer to the interruption of REM sleep by movement arousals or Stage 2 activity. Sleep fragmentation connotes repetitive interruptions of sleep by arousals and awakenings.

free-running: Refers to the natural endogenous period of a chronobiological rhythm when time cues are removed. In humans the free-running state is most commonly seen in the tendency to delay some circadian rhythms, such as the sleep-wake cycle, by approximately 1 hour every day when a person has an impaired ability to entrain or is without time cues.

hertz (Hz): A unit of frequency; cycles per second.

hypercapnia: Elevated carbon dioxide tension in the blood.

hypersomnia: Excessively deep or prolonged major sleep period; sleep in excess of the age-related norm during a 24-hour period. Hypersomnia may be associated with difficulty in awakening.

hypnic myoclonia: Sleep starts; hypnic jerks.

hypnogogic: Occurrence of an event during the transition from wakefulness to sleep.

Hypnogogic hallucination: See *Hypnogogic imagery*.

hypnogogic imagery: Vivid sensory images occurring at sleep onset but particularly vivid with sleep-onset REM periods. Hypnogogic imagery is a feature of narcoleptic naps, with the onset occurring with REM sleep. It may occasionally be frightening, as occurs with terrifying hypnogogic hallucinations.

hypnogogic startle: Sleep starts; a sudden body jerk (hypnic jerk) observed normally just at sleep onset and usually resulting, at least momentarily, in an awakening.

hypnopompic (hypnopomic): Occurring during the transition from sleep to wakefulness at the termination of a sleep episode.

hypopnea: An episode of reduced airflow (by at least 50%), as measured at the nose and mouth, lasting for at least 10 seconds. It is often associated with a fall in blood oxygen saturation.

indeterminant sleep: A term used to score sleep in infants when criteria for active or quiet sleep are not met.

insomnia: Difficulty in initiating or maintaining sleep; difficulty in sleeping. This term is used ubiquitously to indicate any and all gradations and types of sleep loss.

intermediary sleep stage: A term sometimes used for NREM Stage 2 sleep. It is often used, especially in the French literature, for stages combining elements of Stage 2 and REM sleep.

into bed time: The clock time at which a person gets into bed. This is the same as bedtime for most people; however, it may be different for individuals who spend time in wakeful activities in bed, such as reading or watching television.

intrinsic sleep disorder: Disorder that either originates or develops from within the body or that arises from causes within the body. The intrinsic sleep disorders are a subgroup of the dyssomnias.

K-alpha: Refers to a microarousal characterized by a K-complex followed by several seconds of alpha rhythm.

K-complex: A sharp negative EEG wave followed by a high-voltage slow wave. The complex duration is at least 0.5 second and may be accompanied by a sleep spindle. K-complexes occur spontaneously during NREM sleep and begin and define Stage 2 sleep. They are thought to be evoked responses to internal stimuli; however, they can also be elicited during sleep by external (particularly auditory) stimuli.

light-dark cycle: The periodic pattern of light (artificial or natural) alternating with darkness.

light sleep: A common term for NREM Stage 1 sleep (sometimes Stage 2 is included when light sleep is differentiated from deep sleep).

maintenance of wakefulness test (MWT): Similar to the Multiple Sleep Latency Test (MSLT) and used to objectively assess degrees of daytime sleepiness or the ability of an individual to remain awake under soporific conditions. A series of measurements of the interval from "lights out" to sleep onset is made. In contrast to the MSLT, in which patients are instructed to "try to sleep," patients are instructed to "try to remain awake." Long latencies are indicative of an ability to remain awake. This test is typically used to assess the effects of medication on the individual's ability to remain awake.

major sleep episode: The longest sleep episode that occurs on a daily basis; the conventional or habitual time for sleeping.

microsleep: An episode, lasting up to 30 seconds, during which external stimuli are not perceived. The polysomnogram suddenly shifts from waking characteristics to sleep. Microsleeps are associated with excessive sleepiness, performance deficits, attention span problems, and automatic behaviors.

mixed apnea: Cessation of airflow measured at the nose and mouth secondary to a combination of decreased respiratory effort *and* intrinsic upper airway obstruction.

montage: The particular arrangement of recording electrodes by which a number of derivations are displayed simultaneously in a polysomnogram.

movement arousal: A body movement associated with an EEG pattern of arousal or full awakening.

movement time: In sleep record scoring, the time when the EEG and EOG tracings are obscured for more than half the scoring epoch by muscle artifact (created by body movement).

Multiple Sleep Latency Test (MSLT): A series of measurements of the interval from "lights out" to sleep onset, used in the objective assessment of excessive sleepiness. Subjects are placed in a darkened room and allowed a fixed number of opportunities (and length of time) to fall asleep during their customary awake period. They are instructed to "try to sleep." Excessive sleepiness is characterized by short latencies. Long latencies are helpful in distinguishing physical tiredness or fatigue from true sleepiness.

muscle tone: Resting muscle potential or resting muscle activity.

myoclonus: Muscle contractions in the form of abrupt jerks or twitches generally lasting less than 100 msec. The term should not be applied to the periodic limb movements of sleep, which characteristically have a duration of 0.5 to 5 seconds.

nap: A short sleep episode that may be intentionally or unintentionally taken during the period of habitual wakefulness.

nightmare: An unpleasant or frightening dream that usually occurs during REM sleep. Occasionally it is called a dream anxiety attack or anxiety dream. It is differentiated from a sleep terror by its timing (late in the sleep period, during REM sleep), its mild associated autonomic discharges, and its storylike quality.

nocturnal confusion: Episodes of delirium and disorientation close to or during nighttime sleep.

nocturnal dyspnea: Respiratory distress that may be minimal during the day but becomes pronounced during sleep.

nocturnal penile tumescence (NPT): The natural periodic cycle of penile erections that occur during sleep, typically associated with REM sleep; sleep-related erections.

nocturnal sleep: The typical nighttime or major sleep episode occurring within the circadian rhythm of sleep and wakefulness; the conventional or habitual time for sleeping.

non–rapid eye movement (NREM or non-REM) sleep: One major part of the sleeping state, apart from REM sleep. It comprises sleep Stages 1 to 4, which constitute levels in the spectrum of NREM sleep "depth" or physiological activity.

NREM-REM sleep cycle: A period during sleep composed of a NREM sleep episode and the subsequent REM sleep episode. Each NREM-REM sleep couplet is equal to one cycle. Any NREM sleep stage suffices as the NREM sleep portion of a cycle. An adult sleep period of about 6½ to 8½ hours generally consists of four to six cycles. The cycle duration increases from infancy to young adulthood.

NREM sleep intrusion: An interposition of NREM sleep, or a component of NREM sleep physiology, into REM sleep; a portion of NREM sleep not appearing in its usual sleep cycle position.

NREM sleep period: The NREM sleep portion of the NREM-REM sleep cycle. Episodes consist primarily of sleep Stages 3 and 4 early in the night and of sleep Stage 2 later in the night.

obesity-hypoventilation syndrome: Hypoventilation during wakefulness in obese individuals. Because the term can apply to several different disorders, its use is discouraged.

obstructive apnea: Cessation of airflow measured at the mouth and nose, lasting longer than 10 seconds and resulting from intrinsic upper airway obstruction. Obstructive apneas are often associated with blood oxygen desaturation and arousal.

paradoxical sleep: REM sleep.

parasomnia: A disorder of arousal, partial arousal, or sleep stage transition. It represents an episodic disorder (e.g., somnambulism, sleep terror, enuresis) occurring during sleep rather than a disorder of sleep or wakefulness per se. Parasomnias may be induced or exacerbated by sleep. A parasomnia is not a dyssomnia.

paroxysmal nocturnal dyspnea: Respiratory distress and shortness of breath caused by pulmonary edema, which appear suddenly in the recumbent position and often result in awakenings.

period: The interval in time between occurrences of a defined phase or moment of a rhythmical or periodic event (e.g., the interval of time between one peak or trough and the next).

periodic leg movement (PLM): A rapid partial flexion of the foot at the ankle, extension of the great toe, and partial flexion of the knee and hip that occur during sleep. The movements occur with a periodicity of 20 to 40 seconds in a stereotyped pattern. Each movement lasts approximately 0.5 to 5 seconds.

periodic movement of sleep (PMS): See *Periodic leg movement.*

phase advance: A shift of the sleep period to an earlier position in the 24-hour continuum (e.g., a shift of the sleep period from 11 PM–7 AM to 8 PM–4 AM represents a 3-hour phase advance).

phase delay: A shift of the sleep period to a later position in the 24-hour continuum. It is the exact opposite of phase advance (e.g., a shift of the sleep period from 8 PM–4 AM to 11 PM–7 AM represents a 3-hour phase delay).

phase transition: One of the two junctures of the major sleep and wake phases in the 24-hour sleep-wake cycle.

phasic event (phasic activity): Brain, muscle, or autonomic events of a brief and episodic nature occurring in sleep. Phasic events are characteristic of REM sleep and involve eye movements, muscle twitches, and other physiological phenomena. The usual duration is from milliseconds to 1 to 2 seconds.

photoperiod: The duration of light in a ligh-dark cycle.

Pickwickian: A term applied to an obese, sleepy individual who snores and has alveolar hypoventilation. The term has been applied to many different disorders, and therefore its use is discouraged.

PLM-arousal index: The number of sleep-related periodic limb movements per hour of sleep that are associated with EEG evidence of arousal.

PLM index: The number of periodic leg movements per hour of total sleep time; sometimes expressed as the number of movements per hour of NREM sleep because the movements are usually inhibited during REM sleep.

PLM percentage: The percentage of total sleep time occupied with recurrent episodes of periodic limb movements.

polysomnogram: The continuous and simultaneous recording of multiple physiological variables during sleep. Typical parameters continuously monitored include the EEG, EOG, EMG, ECG, respiratory airflow (nasal and oral), respiratory efforts (chest and abdomen), oxygen saturation, and leg movements.

polysomnograph: A biodmedical instrument for the measurement of physiological variables of sleep.

polysomnographic: Describes a recording on paper, computer disc, or tape of a polysomnogram.

premature morning awakening: Early termination of the nocturnal sleep episode, with an inability to return to sleep. It reflects interference at the end, rather than at the commencement, of the sleep episode. It is a characteristic sleep disturbance of some individuals suffering from depression.

quiet sleep: NREM sleep in infants (and animals) whose specific NREM sleep Stages 1 to 4 cannot be determined. Early in infancy a tracé alternant EEG pattern characterizes quiet sleep.

rapid eye movement sleep (REM sleep): A stage of sleep with highest brain activity, characterized by enhanced brain metabolism and vivid hallucinatory imagery or dreaming. Spontaneous rapid eye movements occur, resting muscle tone is suppressed, and awakening threshold to nonsignificant stimuli is high. The EEG reveals a relatively low-voltage, mixed-frequency background with notched theta activity ("sawtooth" waves). REM sleep occupies approximately 50% of a newborn's total sleep time. This decreases to approximately 20% to 25% of the total sleep time by 3 to 5 years of age and persists at this level throughout adulthood. REM sleep is also termed paradoxical sleep and active sleep.

record: The end product of the polysomnographic recording process.

recording: The process of obtaining a polysomnographic record. The term is also applied to the end product of the polysomnographic recording process.

REM density (REM intensity): A function that expresses the frequency of eye movements per unit of time during REM sleep.

REM sleep episode: The REM sleep portion of an NREM-REM sleep cycle. Early in the night it may be as short as 0.5 minute, whereas in later cycles it may last longer than an hour.

REM sleep intrusion: A brief interval of REM sleep appearing out of its usual position in the NREM-REM sleep cycle; an interposition of REM sleep in NREM sleep. Sometimes this term is used to refer to the appearance of a single, dissociated component of REM sleep (e.g., eye movements, muscle atonia) rather than the appearance of all REM sleep parameters.

REM sleep latency: The interval from the time of sleep onset to the first appearance of REM sleep.

REM sleep onset: The designation for commencement of a REM sleep episode. Sometimes it is used as a shorthand term for a sleep onset REM period.

The term may also be used to categorize sleep onset during infancy, when sleep is entered through REM sleep rather than NREM sleep. In these cases the REM sleep latency is typically less than 15 minutes.

REM sleep percent: The proportion of total sleep time constituted by the REM stage of sleep.

REM sleep rebound: Lengthening and increase in frequency and density of REM sleep episodes, which result in an increase in REM sleep percentage above baseline levels. REM sleep rebound follows REM sleep deprivation, once the depriving influence is removed.

REM sleep volume: See *REM sleep percent.*

respiratory disturbance index: Synonymous with apnea-hypopnea index; the number of central, obstructive, and mixed apneas *plus* hypopneas per hour of total sleep time.

restlessness: Persistent or recurrent body movements, arousals, and brief awakenings in the course of sleep; refers to the quality of sleep.

rhythm: An event occurring at an approximately constant period length.

sawtooth waves: A form of EEG theta rhythm that occurs during REM sleep and is characterized by a notched appearance in the waveform. The waves generally occur in bursts lasting up to 10 seconds.

severity criteria: Criteria for establishing the severity of a particular sleep disorder according to categories: mild, moderate, or severe.

sleep architecture: The NREM-REM sleep stage infrastructure of sleep understood from the vantage point of the quantitative relationship (and progression) of these components to one another. Architecture is often plotted in the form of a histogram (hypnogram).

sleep cycle: See *NREM-REM sleep cycle.*

sleep efficiency: The proportion of sleep in the episode potentially filled by sleep; the ratio of total sleep time to time in bed.

sleep episode: An interval of sleep that may be voluntary or involuntary. In the sleep laboratory the sleep episode occurs from the time of "lights out" to the time of "lights on." The major sleep episode is usually the longest daily sleep episode.

sleep hygiene: The conditions and practices that promote continuous and effective sleep. These include regularity of bedtime and arise time; conformity of time spent in bed to the time necessary for sustained and individually adequate sleep (i.e., the total sleep time sufficient to avoid sleepiness when awake); restriction of beverages, foods, and compounds (which tend to disrupt sleep) before bedtime; and employment of exercise, nutrition, and environmental factors so that they enhance, not disturb, restful sleep.

sleepiness: Somnolence; difficulty in maintaining alert wakefulness so that the person falls asleep if not actively kept aroused. Sleepiness is not synonymous with a feeling of physical tiredness or listlessness. When sleepiness occurs in inappropriate circumstances, it is considered excessive sleepiness.

sleep interruption: Breaks in sleep resulting in arousal and wakefulness.

sleep latency: The duration of time from "lights out," or bedtime, to the onset of sleep. Onset of sleep is generally defined as the appearance of three consecutive epochs of Stage 1 sleep or one epoch of any other sleep stage.

sleep log (sleep diary): A daily, written record of a person's sleep-wake pattern containing such information as time of retiring and arising, time in bed, estimated total sleep time, number and duration of sleep interruptions, quality of sleep, daytime naps, use of medications, and nature of waking activities.

sleep-maintenance insomnia: A disturbance in maintaining sleep, once sleep has been achieved; persistently interrupted sleep, without difficulty falling asleep. The term is synonymous with sleep continuity disturbance.

sleep mentation: The imagery and thinking experienced during sleep. Sleep mentation usually consists of combinations of images and thoughts during REM sleep. Imagery is vividly expressed in dreams involving all the senses in approximate proportions to their waking representations. Mentation is experienced generally less distinctly in NREM sleep, but it may be quite vivid in Stage 2 sleep, especially toward the end of the sleep episode. Mentation at sleep onset (hypnogogic reverie) can be as vivid as in REM sleep.

sleep onset: The transition from awake to sleep, normally to NREM Stage 1 sleep, but in certain conditions, such as infancy and narcolepsy, into REM sleep. Most polysomnographers accept EEG slowing, reduction, and eventual disappearance of alpha activity, presence of EEG vertex sharp transients, and slow rolling eye movements (the components of Stage 1) as sufficient criteria for sleep onset. Others require appearance of Stage 2 patterns.

sleep-onset REM period (SOREMP): The beginning of sleep by entrance directly into REM sleep. The onset of REM sleep occurs within 10 to 15 minutes of sleep onset.

sleep paralysis: Immobility of the body that occurs in the transition from sleep to wakefulness and is a partial manifestation of REM sleep.

sleep pattern: A person's clock hour schedule of bedtime and arise time, as well as nap behavior; may also include time and duration of sleep interruptions.

sleep spindle: Spindle-shaped waxing and waning bursts of 11.5 to 15 Hz waves lasting 0.5 to 1.5 seconds. Distribution is generally diffuse; however, highest spindle voltages are seen over the central regions of the head. Sleep spindles are an identifying

EEG characteristic of NREM Stage 2 sleep but also are seen during slow-wave sleep. Spindles are generally not seen during REM sleep and do not appear during wakefulness.

sleep stage demarcation: The significant polysomnographic characteristic that distinguishes the boundaries of the sleep stages.

sleep stage episode: A sleep stage interval that represents the stage in an NREM-REM sleep cycle. It is easiest to comprehend in relation to REM sleep, which is a homogeneous stage (i.e., the fourth REM sleep episode is in the fourth sleep cycle unless a prior REM episode was skipped). If one interval of REM sleep is separated from another by more than 20 minutes, they constitute separate REM sleep episodes (and are in separate sleep cycles). A sleep stage episode may be of any duration.

sleep stages: Distinctive stages of sleep, best demonstrated by polysomnographic recordings of the EEG, EOG, and EMG.

sleep structure: Similar to sleep architecture. However, in addition to encompassing sleep stages and sleep cycle relationships, sleep structure assesses the within-stage qualities of the EEG and other physiological attributes.

sleep talking: Somniloquy; talking in sleep that usually occurs in the course of transitory arousals from NREM sleep. Sleep talking can occur during stage REM sleep, at which time it represents a motor breakthrough of dream speech. Full consciousness is not achieved, and no memory of the event remains.

sleep-wake cycle: The clock hour relationships of the major sleep and wake episodes in the 24-hour cycle.

sleep-wake shift (sleep-wake change, sleep-wake reversal): When sleep as a whole or in part is moved to a time of customary waking activity, and the latter is moved to the time of the major sleep episode; common in jet lag and shift work.

sleep-wake transition disorder: A disorder that occurs during the transition from wakefulness to sleep or from one sleep stage to another; a form of parasomnia.

slow-wave sleep: Sleep characterized by EEG waves of a duration slower than 4 Hz; synonymous with sleep Stages 3 and 4 combined.

snoring: A sonorous, rhonchous noise produced primarily with inspiratory effort during sleep because of vibration of the soft palate and the pillars of the oropharyngeal inlet. Snoring represents incomplete obstruction of the upper airway.

somnambulism: Sleep walking; a parasomnia characterized by ambulation during a partial arousal from slow-wave sleep.

somniloquy: Sleep talking.

spindle REM sleep: A condition in which sleep spindles persist atypically in REM sleep. It may be seen in chronic insomnia and occasionally in the first REM period of the night.

Stage 1 sleep: A stage of NREM sleep that occurs at sleep onset or that follows arousal from sleep Stages 2, 3, 4, or REM. It consists of a relatively low-voltage, mixed-frequency EEG, with theta activity and alpha activity of less than 50% of the scoring epoch. EEG vertex sharp transients and slow, rolling eye movements are present. Sleep spindles, K-complexes, and rapid eye movements are absent. Stage 1 sleep normally represents 4% to 5% of the major sleep episode.

Stage 2 sleep: A stage of NREM sleep characterized by a relatively low-voltage, mixed-frequency background EEG activity and the presence of sleep spindles and K-complexes. High-voltage delta waves may constitute up to 20% of Stage 2 epochs. Stage 2 sleep usually accounts for 45% to 55% of the major sleep episode.

Stage 3 sleep: A stage of NREM sleep in which at least 20% and not more than 50% of the epoch consists of EEG waves less than 2 Hz and more than 75 μV in amplitude. With Stage 4 sleep, it constitutes "deep" or slow-wave sleep. Stage 3 is often combined with Stage 4 (Stage 3/4) because of the lack of documented physiological differences between the two stages. Stage 3 usually appears in the first third of the sleep episode and comprises 4% to 6% of the total sleep time.

Stage 4 sleep: Characterized in the same manner as Stage 3 sleep, except slow waves comprise greater than 50% of the recording epoch. Stage 4 sleep usually represents 12% to 15% of total sleep time.

synchronized: A chronobiological term used to indicate that two or more rhythms recur with the same phase relationship. In EEG, it is used to indicate an increased amplitude and usually a decreased frequency of the dominant activities.

theta activity: EEG activity with a frequency of 4 to 8 Hz, generally maximal over the central and temporal cortex.

total recording time: The time from sleep onset to final awakening. In addition to total sleep time, it comprises the time taken up by wake periods and movement time until wake-up.

total sleep episode: The total time available for sleep during an attempt to sleep. It comprises NREM and REM sleep, as well as wakefulness. The term is synonymous with total sleep period.

total sleep time: The amount of actual sleep time in a sleep episode; equal to the total sleep episode less awake time. Total sleep time is the total of all REM and NREM sleep in a sleep episode.

tracé alternant: The usual EEG pattern of quiet sleep in newborns, which is characterized by bursts of slow waves, at times intermixed with sharp waves, and intervening periods of relative quiescence with extreme low-amplitude activity.

twitch: A very small body movement such as a local foot or finger jerk. It is usually not associated with arousal.

vertex sharp transients: Sharp negative potentials, maximal at the vertex, occurring spontaneously during sleep or in response to a sensory stimulus during sleep or wakefulness. Amplitude varies but rarely exceeds 250 μV. These potentials are seen frequently in Stage 1 sleep.

wake time: The total time scored as wakefulness (occurring between sleep onset and final wake-up) in a polysomnogram.

waxing and waning: A crescendo-decrescendo pattern of activity, usually EEG activity.

zeitgeber: An environmental time cue, such as sunlight, noise, meals, social interactions, or an alarm clock that usually helps entrainment to the 24-hour day.

Index

Note: Page numbers in *italics* refer to illustrations; page numbers followed by t refer to tables.

J

K

L

M